DIVING MEDICINE
for Scuba Divers

Published by **J.L. Publications**
P.O. Box 381, Carnegie, Victoria 3163, Australia.
Telephone/Facsimilie: 61-3-569 4803.

© C. Edmonds, B. McKenzie, R. Thomas, 1992.

Cover diving photograph by Max Gleeson.

ISBN 0 9590306 62

DIVING MEDICINE
for Scuba Divers

Dr Carl Edmonds

Dr Bart McKenzie

Dr Robert Thomas

J.L. Publications   Melbourne

FOREWORD

"Diving and Subaquatic Medicine", in its third and highly respected edition, has provided a cornerstone of knowledge for the diving medical professional. Now, "Diving Medicine — for Scuba Divers" is a condensed, simplified and lighter publication for the general diving population. The authors — Drs Edmonds, McKenzie and Thomas, have done an excellent job of providing a comprehensive, useful and up to date resource base for the diver in the field.

The presentation of the material reflects the fact that the authors are experienced divers as well as specialists in diving medicine. Their thinly disguised sense of humour is reflected throughout the text in emphasising important issues and occasionally just lightening the academic loading on the reader. Their treatment of areas of controversy reflects their experience and background in treating diving emergencies. Some readers will find information which may be inconsistent with their teachings. It is strongly suggested that the reader pay attention to the advice that is presented by the authors. Their many years of cumulative experience is reflected in their advice.

This text represents the broadest coverage of diving medical issues that has been focussed upon the general diving public. It does an excellent job of bridging the gap between the "dive rescue" type materials put out by the various agencies, and the other excellent medical texts which focus primarily on physician education. This text should serve the reader well since its intent is clearly designed to stimulate the diving population at large to become better informed on current diving medical issues. Additional resource materials are presented for those who wish more detailed information.

Glen H. Egstrom Ph.D.
Professor Emeritus
Department of Physiological Sciences,
University of California, Los Angeles.

CONTENTS

BACKGROUND

SPECIFIC DIVING (PRESSURE RELATED) DISEASES

AQUATIC DISEASES

GENERAL DIVING MEDICAL PROBLEMS

TREATMENT AND PREVENTION

APPENDICES

A. Diving Medical Library
B. Emergency Contact Numbers
C. DCIEM (Canadian) Sport Decompression Tables
D. US Navy Decompression Tables
E. In-water O_2 Recompression Therapy

Chapter 1

HISTORY of DIVING

Historians are unable to identify the first divers. Probably the techniques they used were similar to those of the native pearl and sponge divers. They may have used a stone weight to ensure rapid descent, but it is unlikely that they could dive deeper than 30 metres, or exceed 2 minutes duration. Later, diving was employed for military purposes (such as destroying ships anchoring cables, boom defences, etc.) and for salvage work. Divers took part in great naval battles between 1800 BC and 400 BC. Alexander the Great was said to have descended in a diving bell (circa 330 BC).

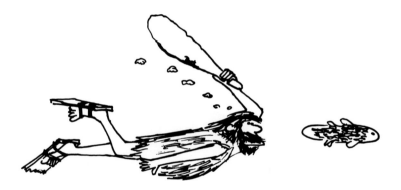

Fig. 1.1

The earliest use of **surface supplied** breathing air by divers was recorded by a Roman historian, Pliny, in AD 77, when a breathing tube connected the diver to the surface. This possibly represents the first "schnorkel". Its use was limited to very shallow dives, since man's respiratory muscles lack sufficient strength to draw air down from the surface. It was also depth limited due to the excessive volume of the breathing tube.

Leonardo da Vinci sketched several designs for diving equipment and submarines. Many diagrams of divers' hoods can be found in other historical texts from 1500 AD onwards, but much of this equipment would not have worked at depths greater than a few feet. They did, however, attest to man's desire to remain below the surface for extended periods. In 1680 Borelli, an Italian, designed a diving set which purported to be a self-contained diving apparatus. Although it was impracticable, the idea was revolutionary at that time. Despite the fact that much diving equipment was primitive and rarely functioned adequately, diving bells were used with success from the 17th century onwards.

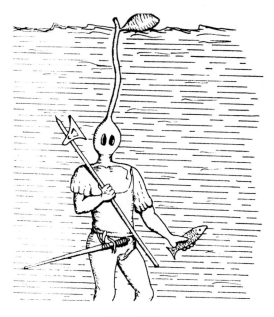

Fig. 1.2
A 1511 concept of surface supply diving.

Diving with a helmet (the equivalent of an upturned bucket which enclosed the diver's head) gradually became an accepted method. It contained air which was pumped down from the surface following the development of efficient air pumps around 1800 AD. Bellows were used to force air down to the divers. This allowed longer and deeper dives and brought to light the many physiological problems caused by the undersea environment.

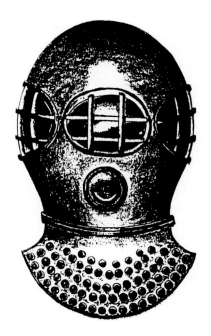

Fig. 1.3
Siebe's first open helmet.

In 1837 Augustus Siebe designed the first effective standard diving dress. This incorporated an air-supply line connecting a pump or compressor on the surface to a diving helmet. The helmet was attached by an airtight seal to a flexible suit which enclosed the diver and was filled with air.

The development of **self-contained** air supplies was impeded by the lack of sufficiently powerful compressors and reservoirs. In 1866 the Frenchmen, Rouquayrol and Denayrouze, invented the first satisfactory demand regulator for self-contained underwater breathing apparatus (SCUBA), but due to lack of suitable compressors and cylinders, its was limited to surface air supply lines.

In 1878 H. A. Fleuss made a workable self-contained (closed circuit) oxygen breathing apparatus utilising caustic potash to remove exhaled carbon dioxide. "Closed" refers to the absence of an outlet for gas (i.e. no bubbles) and means that the exhaled gas is rebreathed. This was the forerunner of modern closed-circuit diving units.

Divers in the late 1800's were capable of reaching depths in excess of 50 metres, but the effects of decompression sickness (or bends) caused much concern and many injuries to divers. It was not until the early 20th century that Dr J S Haldane derived mathematical decompression tables to overcome this physiological problem of deep diving. The first successful tables were based on the assumption that decompression sickness could be avoided by not exceeding a 2:1 pressure reduction between stops. It reflected a mathematical model of inert gas behaviour in a body and was to be the forerunner of current decompression tables. Later observations showed this principle to be incorrect in many cases, but these early tables and the later modified versions, prevented many divers from developing the bends.

Diving research this century has lead to a great improvement in all forms of diving equipment and since 1940 the use of such equipment has increased greatly. The design by Cousteau and Gagnan in 1943, of a proper demand-regulated air supply from compressed air cylinders worn on the back has developed into modern day scuba.

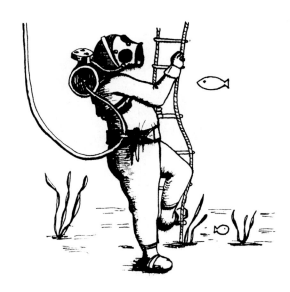

Fig. 1.4
Rouquayrol and Denayrouze's diving suit 1865.

Closed-circuit rebreathing apparatus using oxygen or oxygen/nitrogen mixtures have also been improved considerably since the early units used by Italian Naval divers in their attacks on shipping in Gibraltar in 1941. With the advent of deeper diving, gas economy has become a major problem and for this reason closed-circuit systems have achieved even greater importance.

Diving to depths in excess of 100 metres required not only the development of specialised closed or semi-closed circuit rebreathing apparatus, but also the use of inert gas mixtures with oxygen and other gases. Nitrogen, because of its narcotic effect at depth, has been replaced largely by other gases such as helium and hydrogen. These are not used without complications – as all gases cause specific physiological problems and no ideal mixture yet exists.

The advent of **saturation diving** has completely revolutionised the ability to dive and work at great depth, and for lengthy durations, and this is economically rewarding. The system is based on saturation at any depth of all the diver's tissues by the inert breathing gas. Once this is achieved the body is incapable of absorbing further amounts of gas, no matter what the duration of exposure at this depth. Hence, further exposure does not lengthen decompression times. This practice is now adopted for most diving with extended bottom times at depths in excess of 100 metres.

In an attempt to reduce the risks in deep diving, **one-atmosphere diving suits** (ADS) have been developed out of strong lightweight alloys. These suits are fitted with articulated joints and use mechanical levers or claws for "hands". Some even have mobility and propulsion, but all require backup 'rescue' facilities. They are equipped with self contained rebreathing apparatus and are often used at depths of 200–300 metres. Although somewhat bulky and requiring hoisting gear at the surface, divers can achieve a reasonable degree of movement at depth with the latest models. These suits are also useful for inspection-type work, although much of this is now done by non-manned **Remote Operated Vehicles** (ROV's) with video surveillance.

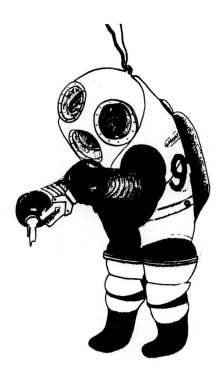

Fig. 1.5
"Jim" one-atmosphere diving suit.

Chapter 2

PHYSICS

To understand the physical and physiological problems which can confront a diver, it is helpful to recall a few basic physical laws of nature. Only a brief and simplified review of the physics of diving is given in this text. For more detailed explanations, refer to the diving manuals.

PRESSURE

Some of the major physical hazards are related to the effects of pressure. Pressure is defined as force per unit area. ie.

$$\text{Pressure} \; = \; \frac{\text{Force}}{\text{Area}}$$

If a force is spread over twice the area, the pressure is halved.

This explains why for example, wide tyres are preferable for driving on beaches. The weight of the vehicle (force) when spread over a large area causes less pressure on the sand. This vehicle is less likely to sink into the sand than one with narrow tyres.

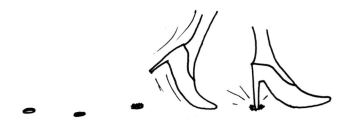

Fig. 2.1

Gases erert pressure because they are made up of lots of fast moving molecules. The greater the number and the faster they move, the greater the pressure.

Pressure on a Submerged Diver

The pressure acting on a submerged diver has two components :

    1. The atmosphere above the water, termed **atmospheric pressure,**
    2. The weight of the water above the diver, termed **hydrostatic pressure.**

ABSOLUTE PRESSURE	GAUGE PRESSURE	DEPTH of SEAWATER
1 ATA	0 ATG	Surface
2 ATA	1 ATG	10 metres (33ft)
3 ATA	2 ATG	20 metres (66ft)
4 ATA	3 ATG	30 metres (99ft)

Table 2.1
Pressure at Depth

Atmospheric Pressure

The atmosphere above the earth is some 150 km high. Although air is very light, this amount of air has significant weight and exerts substantial pressure on the earth's surface.

Atmospheric pressure at sea level is referred to as "one atmosphere" or "one bar". It is the same as 100kPa, 1 kg/cm^2, 760mm Hg and 14.7 psi. At higher altitudes, atmospheric pressure is reduced, a factor which has a significant effect on diving in mountain lakes (see Chapter 6).

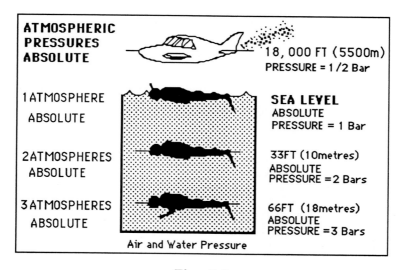

Fig. 2.2

Hydrostatic Pressure

Water is much denser than air and 10 metres (or 33 ft) of sea water exerts the same pressure (weight) as the whole 150 km of atmospheric air. For every additional 10 metres the diver descends, the water will exert a further pressure equivalent to another atmosphere.

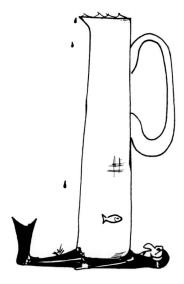

Fig. 2.3

Common units of pressure are (approximately) :

1 ATMOSPHERE	= 10 metres sea water
	= 33 feet sea water
	= 34 feet fresh water
	= 1 kg/cm^2
	= 14.7 lbs/in^2, psi
	= 1 bar
	= 100 kilopascals, kPa
	= 760 millimetres mercury, mm Hg.

Absolute Pressure

The total pressure exerted on a diver at depth will be the pressure due to the atmosphere acting on the surface of the water (atmospheric pressure) plus the pressure due to the depth of the water itself (hydrostatic pressure).

The total pressure acting on the diver is termed the "absolute pressure". It is often expressed in terms of atmospheres and is called "atmospheres absolute" or "ATA".

To calculate the absolute pressure acting on a diver at a given depth in terms of atmospheres, divide the depth in metres by 10 (since every 10 m sea water exerts 1 atmosphere pressure) and add 1 (the pressure of the atmosphere above the water). (The depth in feet, divided by 33 + 1 also calculates absolute pressure).

e.g. the absolute pressure at 40 metres is [40 ÷ 10] + 1 = 5 ATA

Gauge Pressure

Pressure in diving is generally measured by a **pressure gauge**. Such a gauge is normally set to register a pressure of zero at sea level and so it ignores the pressure due to the atmosphere (1ATA).

The pressure registered by a gauge at 10 metres sea-water depth would thus be one atmosphere gauge (1ATG) or equivalent units. Gauge pressure is converted to absolute pressure by adding 1 atmosphere pressure.

Partial Pressure

With a mixture of gases, the proportion of the total pressure contributed by each of the gases is termed its partial pressure (its part of the pressure). The partial pressure contributed by each gas is proportional to its percentage of the mixture. Each gas contributes the same proportion to the total pressure of the mixture, as its proportion in the composition of the mixture.

e.g.   air at 1 ATA contains 21% oxygen, hence the partial pressure of oxygen is 0.21 ATA and air at 1 ATA contains 79% nitrogen, hence the partial pressure of nitrogen is 0.79 ATA.

GAS LAWS

Gases behave in nature and in diving according to several laws. Knowledge of these laws is important to the diver because they influence the duration of the air supply and affect the gas containing spaces in the body such as the ears, sinuses and lungs. They also cause other diving illnesses.

Boyle's Law

This defines the relationship between pressure and volume. It states that the **volume of a given mass of gas varies inversely with the absolute pressure (if the temperature remains constant).**

Stated simply, for a given amount of gas, if the pressure is increased, the volume is proportionally decreased and vice versa. This means that if the pressure is doubled, the volume is halved and vice versa.

Stated mathematically : V varies as $\dfrac{1}{P}$ (where V = volume and P = pressure)

It follows that for a given amount of gas, the volume multiplied by the pressure always has a constant value.

i.e. $P \times V$ is constant.

So if a sample of gas has an original volume of V_1 and an original pressure of P_1, and either the pressure or volume are changed, the new volume V_2 and the new pressure P_2 will multiply out to the same value.

$$\text{i.e. } P_1 \times V_1 \;=\; P_2 \times V_2$$

This law can easily be demonstrated by a piston and cylinder such as a bicycle pump. If the piston is pushed into the cylinder half way, and the escape of gas prevented, the pressure in the cylinder will be found to have doubled. By this process, many litres of air can be crammed into a bicycle tyre but at the cost of an increase in pressure in the tyre (and hard work). Compressors work in this way, squeezing 2000 or more litres of air into a scuba cylinder – but at a high pressure.

Since pressure increases with depth, the consequent reduction in gas volume becomes very important to the diver because his body has numerous air spaces.

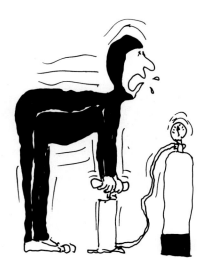

Fig. 2.4

Descent Problems : The air in the diver's middle ear and sinuses will contract in volume as the diver descends. If these volume changes are not compensated for by adding more air (**"equalisation"**), then pressure damage (**barotrauma**) to the tissues will result. For example :

> If a 6 litre bag is filled at the surface (1 ATA) and taken to 20 metres
> depth (3ATA), the volume will be reduced by a factor of 3, to 2 litres.
> $$P_1 \times V_1 \;=\; P_2 \times V_2$$
> $$\therefore \quad 1 \times 6 \;=\; 3 \times V_2$$
> $$\text{i.e. } V_2 \;=\; 2 \text{ litres}$$

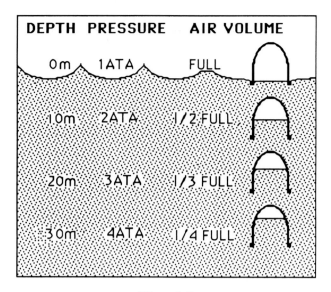

Fig. 2.5

In the same way, if a **breath-hold diver** takes a full breath at the surface and descends to 20 metres (3 ATA), the volume of air in his lungs may be reduced from 6 litres to 2 litres. The chest and lungs cope with compression better than distension. The limit for breath-hold diving is not known, but now has been shown to exceed 100 metres in certain individuals.

Ascent Problems. An average male diver's lungs may contain about 6 litres of gas. If a diver takes a full breath at 20 metres (3 ATA) from his scuba set and returns to the surface (1 ATA) without exhaling, the volume of gas in his lungs will increase from the 6 litre total lung capacity to 18 litres (6×3 litres).

This can be easily calculated this way :

$$
\begin{aligned}
P_1 \times V_1 &= P_2 \times V_2 \\
P_1 &= 3\,ATA, \ V_1 = 6 \text{ litres}, \ P_2 = 1ATA, \\
V_2 &= ? \text{ litres} \\
\\
V_2 &= \frac{P_1 \times V_1}{P_2} \\
&= \frac{3 \times 6}{1} \\
&= 18 \text{ litres}
\end{aligned}
$$

The lungs would have to expand to 18 litres to accommodate this volume – well beyond their rupturing point, causing **burst lung (pulmonary barotrauma)**.

An important practical observation of Boyle's Law is that **the greatest volume changes take place near the surface. This means that the greatest danger from barotrauma is near the surface — and this applies with descent as well as ascent.**

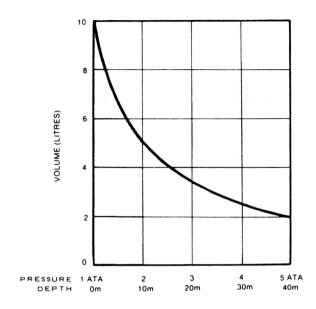

Fig. 2.6

This diagram shows changes in gas volume caused by pressure change
at various depths. Note that maximal volume change is near the surface.

For example, if a diver has 4 litres of air in his lungs at 40 metres depth (5 ATA) and ascends 10 metres without exhaling (to 4 ATA), the volume in the lungs will increase to 5 litres :

$$P_1 \times V_1 \quad = \quad P_2 \times V_2$$
$$5 \times 4 \quad = \quad 4 \times V_2$$
$$\therefore V_2 \quad = \quad 5 \text{ litres}$$

Some people could possibly accommodate this expansion without lung damage.

If the same diver started at 10 metres depth (2ATA), and then ascended 10 metres to the surface, without exhaling, the pressure would change from 2ATA to 1ATA. The air in the lungs would expand from 4 to 8 litres. This would rupture the lungs.

Although the dives involved the same ascent distances, the volume change, and hence the danger, in response to Boyle's Law, is much greater near the surface.

Many divers are not aware of this and have a fallacious belief that if they confine their diving to shallow depths they will minimise the risk of barotrauma.

Buoyancy compensators are similarly affected by depth changes in response to Boyle's Law. **Wet suits** are also affected and lose their buoyancy and insulating properties with depth.

Charles' Law

Most divers will have noticed that bicycle pumps and air compressors become hot during use. As the volume of gas is compressed, and so heat is produced. This is explained by Charles' Law.

This Law states that **if the pressure remains constant, the volume of a given mass of gas varies directly with the absolute temperature** (absolute temperature is obtained by adding 273 to the temperature in degrees Celsius).

In other words, at a fixed pressure, if gas is heated it expands, and if gas is cooled its volume contracts.

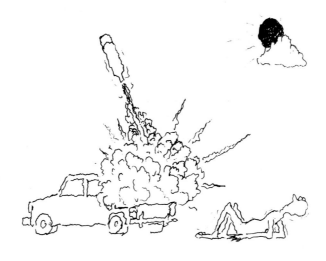

Fig. 2.7

General Gas Law

Charles' and Boyle's laws can be combined into the General Gas Law : $\dfrac{PV}{T}$ is constant

For the non mathematically minded this means that for a given amount of gas, the pressure multiplied by the volume, divided by the temperature, always comes to the same value – so if one of these factors is varied, it has an effect on the other two.

If a gas sample having $\dfrac{P_1V_1}{T_1}$ has one of these factors changed,

the new set of values $\dfrac{P_2V_2}{T_2}$ will multiply out to the same answer

i.e. $\dfrac{P_1V_1}{T_1} = \dfrac{P_2V_2}{T_2}$

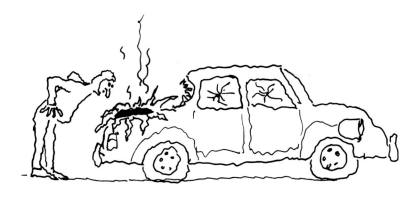

Fig. 2.8

Stated in another way; if a gas is compressed, its volume decreases and it gets hotter. If the gas is heated and the volume is prevented from expanding, the pressure rises.

The consequence of this law has lead to the demolition of several perfectly good automobiles (and divers!) following the storage of full scuba cylinders in the boot, in hot weather. Similarly, inflatable boats used by divers are often pressurised to the maximum and are then left in the sun. As the temperature rises, the pressure of the contained air increases and finally the volume increases until the boat explodes.

If gas is allowed to expand rapidly, it cools. Cooling from the expansion of previously compressed air, as it is breathed from a scuba cylinder, can lead to the regulator freezing up during cold water diving.

Problem : If the temperature of a scuba cylinder is 37°C after being disconnected from the compressor and its pressure gauge reads 199 ATG, what is the pressure after it has cooled to 17° C?

$$\frac{P_1 V_1}{T_1} = \frac{P_2 V_2}{T_2}$$

now because V_1 and V_2 are the same (the cylinder volume is unchanged), the equation can be written :

$$\frac{P_1}{T_1} = \frac{P_2}{T_2}$$

and this can be rearranged to :

$$P_2 = \frac{P_1 T_2}{T_1}$$

Substituting the figures : (note that the cylinder pressure is in ATG and needs to have 1 atmosphere added to get ATA, also that the temperatures have to be converted to degrees absolute by adding 273 degrees)

$$\therefore P2 = \frac{(199+1) \times (273+17)}{(273+37)}$$

$$= 187 \text{ ATA}$$

Dalton's Law

With a mixture of gases, the total pressure exerted by the mixture, is the sum of the pressures that would be exerted by each of the gases if it alone occupied the total volume. That is, the total pressure is the sum of the partial pressures.

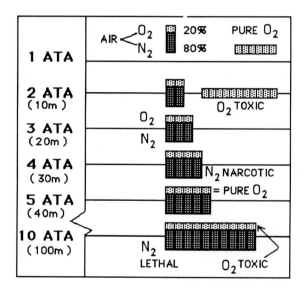

Fig. 2.9

As the overall pressure increases (with descent underwater), so the partial pressure of each constituent gas increases.

e.g. if air contains approximately 21% oxygen (O_2) and 79% nitrogen (N_2), then in a sample of air at a given pressure, O_2 will contribute 21% of the total pressure and N_2 will contribute 79%.

At atmospheric pressure the partial pressure of O_2 in air is $^{21}/_{100}$ of 1 ATA. i.e. 0.21ATA while the partial pressure of N_2 is $^{79}/_{100}$ of 1ATA i.e. 0.79ATA.

To calculate the partial pressure of a gas, multiply the percentage of gas by the absolute pressure.

This law is important when considering the toxic effect of gases at depth or the use of O_2 for treatment purposes.

Problem: Since O_2 can cause convulsions when breathed at greater than 1.8 ATA, would it be safe to breathe a mixture of 50% O_2 and 50% N_2 at 30 metres (4 ATA) ?

The partial pressure of O_2 = 50% × 4ATA = 2ATA

This oxygen / nitrogen mixture would be potentially toxic at this depth.

Henry's Law

This law describes the dissolving of gas in a liquid and states that the **quantity of gas which will dissolve in a liquid at a given temperature is proportional to the partial pressure of gas in contact with the liquid.** This means that if the pressure of gas exposed to a liquid increases, then more gas will dissolve in the liquid.

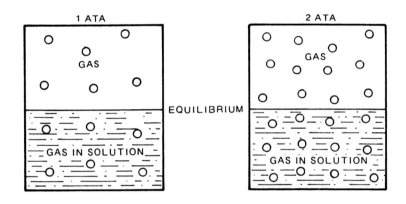

Fig. 2.10
This diagram shows how more gas molecules are dissolved in a liquid as the pressure of gas exposed to the liquid is increased.

An illustration of this law can be seen whenever a soft drink bottle is opened. During the manufacture of these drinks, carbon dioxide is dissolved in the liquid under pressure and the pressure is maintained by the lid on the bottle. When the bottle is opened and the pressure released, the liquid will not allow as much gas to be dissolved and so the excess gas is released from solution in the form of bubbles.

At sea level (1ATA) the human body contains approximately 1 litre of N_2 dissolved in the tissues. Whenever a diver breathes compressed air at depth, more N_2 will dissolve in the body because the partial pressure of N_2 in the air being breathed is increased. This is the cause of **nitrogen narcosis**.

Under certain circumstances, when the diver returns to the surface this N_2 can come out of solution in the form of bubbles. These bubbles cause tissue injury which is the basis of **decompression sickness** ("bends").

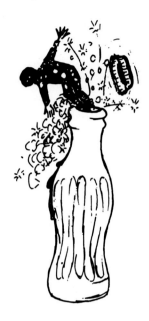

Fig. 2.11

Diffusion of Gases

If a diver were to pass wind in a confined room, all the occupants of the room would soon be aware of the fact but, fortunately, not necessarily the source.

This process of distribution of gas is termed diffusion. It is caused by the rapid random movement of gas molecules to all parts of a contained space. Gas molecules, being only single or small groups of atoms are able to easily diffuse through watertight membranes such as blood capillaries or cell walls. This process allows O_2 and other gases to pass from the lungs to the blood and tissues, and then back.

GASES OF IMPORTANCE TO DIVERS

Air

Air consists of a mixture of $O_2 + N_2 +$ a trace of carbon dioxide (CO_2), and minute amounts of rare gases. Rare gases such as Neon (Ne), Argon (Ar) and Xenon (Xe), and Hydrogen (H_2) exist in trace amounts only.

The exact composition of air is :

Oxygen (O_2)	—	20.94% by volume
Nitrogen (N_2)	—	79.02% by volume
Carbon Dioxide (CO_2)	—	0.04% by volume

Some less reputable suppliers of air fills for scuba tanks provide free additives to the compressed air, such as dust, oil, hydrocarbons, rust, water vapor and carbon monoxide (CO).

Oxygen – O_2

This is a colourless, odourless, tasteless gas which is indistinguishable from air to breathe.

It is essential for metabolism and maintenance of life yet in quantities exceeding those in air it is **toxic** to man. Its proportion in air (21% or more specifically, a partial pressure of 0.21 ATA at sea level) is critical. A little more than this causes O_2 toxicity, a little less will not support human life. For this reason most gas mixtures breathed by deep divers contain an inert gas – usually either N_2 or helium (He), mixed with O_2 to ensure that the O_2 composition is maintained at a partial pressure close to 0.2 ATA (0.16 – 0.40 ATA).

O_2 supports combustion vigorously and can cause normally non-flammable substances (such as the occupants of a recompression chamber) to burn brilliantly if it is present at a sufficiently high partial pressure.

Divers should be aware of the potentially explosive and combustible properties of oxygen, as they may require to use it in first-aid, or be inadvisably enticed into diving with high oxygen mixtures.

Nitrogen – N_2

This gas which is the major constituent of air is also colourless, odourless and tasteless. N_2 dissolves well in body fluids and tissues, causing **narcosis** at depth and **decompression sickness** when it bubbles out of solution, after ascent.

It is termed an **"inert gas"** because it does not take part in human biochemical processes. The Creator appears to have included this gas in air to prevent us from developing O_2 toxicity, and to reduce the fire hazard.

Divers vary this N_2/O_2 ratio (Nitrox, oxygen enriched air or mixed gas diving) in an attempt to improve on nature, extend diving durations, and reduce narcosis.

Carbon Dioxide – CO_2

This gas is also colourless, odourless and is said to be tasteless. However if a diver inhales a mouthful of CO_2 from a buoyancy vest inflated from a CO_2 cartridge it will be found to taste very nasty, due to its formation of carbonic acid in water.

CO_2 is a by-product of cellular metabolism and we exhale approximately 5% of CO_2 in our breath.

If a diver rebreathes some of his exhaled gas by using faulty breathing equipment or an excessively large snorkel the CO_2 will accumulate in the body leading to toxicity. These effects are discussed further in Chapter 22.

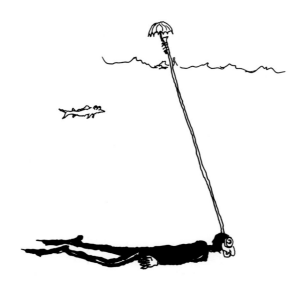

Fig. 2.12

Carbon Monoxide – CO

This gas is colourless, odourless and tasteless. It cannot be detected by a diver and even in trace amounts can cause loss of consciousness or death.

It is usually produced as a product of incomplete combustion of carbon containing compounds and is a constituent of internal combustion engine exhausts and cigarette smoke.

Air contaminated by carbon monoxide, if supplied in scuba cylinders or by surface supply to divers, may have lethal results (see Chapter 23).

Helium – He

This is a colourless, odourless, tasteless gas which is very light and very expensive. It is obtained from underground natural gas sources found in the USA.

It is used to dilute O_2 in gas mixtures breathed at great depths because it has little tendency to produce narcosis (e.g. Heliox = 90% He + 10% O_2).

Due to its very low density it readily escapes through small leaks in pipes and valves making it difficult to retain. It is also a very effective conductor of heat, causing serious problems with **hypothermia**.

The low density of He alters the normal process of speech production causing "Donald Duck" **like speech** when a diver breathes this gas.

Hydrogen – H$_2$

A very light weight gas that can replace N_2 to reduce narcosis at depth. Unfortunately it can combine explosively with O_2 and the resultant water (H_2O) is not sufficient to 'put out the diver'. It is sometimes used with very low O_2 percentages, at great depths, by skilled professional divers. It shares many problems with He.

Inert Gases :

Neon – Ne, Argon – Ar, Radon – Rn, and Xenon – Xe

These are more biologically inert gases which are present only in trace amounts in the atmosphere. They are of little importance to recreational divers.

Oil Gases

Because of lubrication needs in the compressor, oil vapors and hydrocarbons can be produced which may then contaminate the air supply.

BUOYANCY

It is important for divers to understand the factors affecting buoyancy. These are :

Density

Density is defined as **mass per unit volume** (density = mass Π volume).

For our purposes, mass can be considered to be the same as weight, so density is equivalent to weight per unit volume.

A substance is more dense than another if the same volume has more weight. Try lifting a bucket of water and then a bucket of lead for an illustration.

Specific Gravity

Specific gravity (S.G.) is the density of a substance compared to the density of fresh water which is given a value of one.

Lead has a specific gravity of 13.5 so it is 13.5 times as dense as water.
e.g.1000 cc of water will weigh 1 kg., while 1000 cc of lead will weigh 13.5 kg.

The concept of specific gravity is important since the specific gravity of a substance determines whether it will float or sink in water.

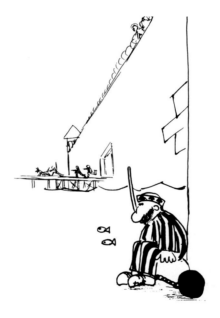

Fig. 2.13

A substance with a specific gravity greater than 1 (i.e. denser than water) will sink. Lead, with a specific gravity of 13.5, does not float well, whereas oil, with a specific gravity of 0.8, floats easily - producing an oil slick.

The human body has a specific gravity of slightly greater than 1, depending on its content (fat has a specific gravity less than 1, and bones are greater than 1) but the air content of the lungs provides enough buoyancy to allow most people to float.

Archimedes Principle

The ancient Greek Archimedes (apparently while reclining in his bath) discovered that when an object is immersed in a fluid, it appears to be lighter, and that the apparent loss of weight (or **buoyancy**) is equal to the weight of water displaced by the object.

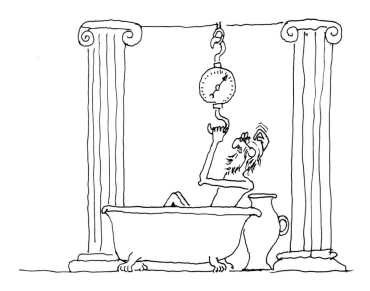

Fig. 2.14

That is – the buoyant effect will be equivalent to the weight of fluid of equal volume to the immersed object.

Depending on whether the weight of fluid displaced is greater than, equal to or less than the weight of the object, an object immersed in the fluid will either float, remain suspended or sink. Even an object which sinks will still appear to be lighter than it would out of the fluid.

Sea water is denser than fresh water because of the salt content, so a greater weight of sea water will be displaced by an object. Hence objects in sea water are more buoyant than in fresh water.

Air (in the lungs, buoyancy compensator and wet suit) provides buoyancy. Unfortunately air in these compartments varies in volume in response to the pressure changes with varying depth, making constant buoyancy adjustments necessary. This is usually accomplished by adding air to, or releasing it from, the diver's buoyancy compensator.

Divers go to considerable lengths to vary their buoyancy to help them submerge, to stay at a given depth , or to ascend or stay afloat in an emergency.

PHYSICAL EFFECTS OF THE ENVIRONMENT

Temperature

Heat is a form of energy, the level of which can be estimated by measuring the body temperature.

Heat energy flows from areas of high temperature to areas of low temperature. The heat transfer which is important to the diver is **thermal conduction** (or transfer of heat by direct contact), and may cause **hypothermia** (low body temperature).

Since normal body temperature is 37∞C and oceanic water temperature is commonly 12–20∞C, the diver is almost always immersed in water at a lower temperature than his body. Usually the water temperature decreases with depth, but there may be layers of water at different temperatures (thermoclines) – especially with still water.

Cold water creates a strong temperature gradient along which heat flows from the body, resulting in a continuous heat loss to the water. This process is assisted by water having a high capacity to conduct and absorb heat.

Since the maintenance of normal body temperature is essential for physiological functioning, the diver needs to take steps to minimise heat loss. This may be achieved by inserting a layer of air (which is a poor conductor of heat) between the diver and the water. It is conveniently contained in minute cells in a wet suit or under a rubber skin in a dry suit.

Light and Colour

Substances which transmit light have have a tendency to slightly alter the path of the light rays which pass through them. This process is termed **refraction**. The degree to which they do this is termed the refractive index. Each time light passes through an interface between substances with different refractive indices, its path is bent.

When a diver views objects underwater, light must pass through the water, the face mask glass, and the air in the mask before it reaches his eyes. The light rays are refracted at each of these interfaces and the distortion makes objects appear larger and closer by a factor of about 25%.

Until the diver adapts to this distortion, it may be difficult to judge size and distances. This creates practical difficulties with simple tasks such as spearfishing.

Light rays are scattered by particles in the water making shadows less pronounced and reducing the ability to see clearly over large distances.

Clear focusing of the eye depends heavily on the refraction of light rays passing between the air in front of the eye and the cornea (the clear surface at the front of the eye). If the eyes are opened underwater without a face mask, the absence of this air–cornea interface results in very blurred vision.

Water absorbs colours to differing degrees. In clean oceanic water, red is absorbed in the first metre, orange in the first five metres, yellow in the first ten, and green and blue at greater depths. This explains why most things, regardless of their colour on the surface, appear to be coloured shades of blue or green at depths beyond about ten metres.

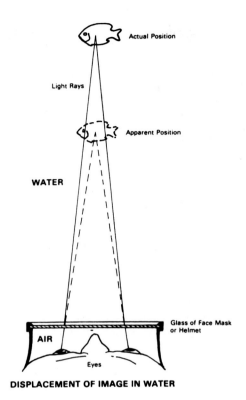

DISPLACEMENT OF IMAGE IN WATER

Fig 2.15

Inshore waters often contain yellowish products of vegetable decay which absorbs most colours except green. As a result, clean oceanic water appears blue, while inshore and estuarine water appears green from the surface.

Because deep water is lit mainly by blue and green light, coloured corals and fish at these depths look less brilliant unless illuminated by a torch or camera flash.

For safety reasons, it is advisable to wear conspicuously coloured diving equipment. However, the absorption of light underwater needs to be considered when choosing these colours. Red, for instance, which is easily visible on the surface, appears black at depth because of the significant absorption of red light by the water.

Fluorescent orange or **yellow** paint or fabric affords better visibility because the fluorescent dye actively emits light of its own colour and also provides a good contrast against natural aquatic backgrounds.

Sound

Sound waves in air usually get reflected at the air–water interface, and therefore shouting instructions to submerged divers is not of much value. Underwater, the sound wave travels much faster than in air, and this makes localisation of the source much more difficult. An example of this is the concern experienced when divers hear outboard engines, but cannot identify the distance or direction of the boat.

Altitude

If the diver is exposed to altitude (less than 1 ATA) a variety of effects may endanger the diver. Some equipment may be affected e.g. pressure gauges, and the diving profile needs to be modified to prevent pulmonary barotrauma and decompression sickness (see Chapter 6).

Chapter 3

PHYSIOLOGY

The functioning of the heart and lungs are of considerable importance to the diver. The cardiovascular and respiratory systems are described here while the physiology of some other organs, such as the ear, are considered in specific chapters.

METABOLISM

The Need for Energy

Energy is a fundamental requirement for all life processes. It is needed for growth, repair, movement and all the active functions of the body. The fuel for this energy comes from **carbon compounds**, which are incorporated in complex molecules in the food we eat. This is biochemically dismantled in the digestive tract into simple chemical compounds which are carried by the bloodstream to the cells. Here they undergo further biochemical processing until ultimately the carbon is combined with oxygen (O_2), forming carbon dioxide (CO_2) and releasing energy.

This is similar to the energy formation which takes place in an automobile engine or a fire, where carbon in fuel or wood is combined with O_2 to produce energy. The body processes will only function under strict conditions of O_2 availability, temperature and acidity.

The body needs a means of transferring food products to the cells, together with delivery of O_2 and removal of CO_2. This is performed by the blood, in the vascular system. It comprises **arteries** which take blood to the tissues, a vast network of microscopic **capillaries** that bring the blood into contact with all the cells of the body, and **veins** which return blood to the heart.

The blood is circulated through the blood vessels by a muscular pump – the heart, and the whole system is called the **cardiovascular** system. It brings O_2 from the lungs to the cells and eliminates CO_2 through the respiratory system.

RESPIRATION

Anatomical Structure

The respiratory tract begins at the mouth and nose and ends in the microscopic air sacs called the **alveoli**, in the lungs.

The **nose**, apart from its decorative function, warms and humidifies the air that we breath. It also filters large particles which might otherwise be inhaled. If the nose is bypassed by breathing through the mouth, a snorkel, or scuba regulator, the lung then has to cope with drier, colder, unfiltered air.

After passing through the mouth or nose, the air then enters the throat where the **larynx** (or voice box) is situated. This is recognised as the "Adams Apple". The larynx produces the sounds of speech as well as helping to protect the lungs from inhalation of foreign material.

When sea-water from a flooded snorkel or scuba regulator enters the larynx, a trap-door like structure called the epiglottis closes over the opening and the vocal cords shut to prevent the foreign material from entering the lungs. If any material passes these structures, the cough reflex, activated by foreign material touching the inside of the air passages, may cause a **coughing** reaction which tends to expel whatever has been inhaled.

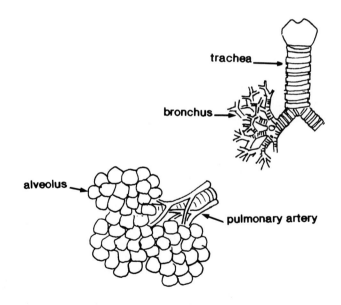

Fig. 3.1
Diagram showing the trachea and bronchial tree, terminating in the alveoli. The relationship between the bronchus, alveoli and branches of the pulmonary artery can be seen.

Below the larynx the air passes through a tube called the **trachea**. This is about as thick as the average snorkel and branches inside the chest into two tubes, the **bronchi**, which lead to the lungs. Those air passages are lined with cells covered with microscopic hairs (cilia) which move a sheet of secreted mucous slowly upwards towards the larynx. Small pieces of foreign material such as dust eventually find their way to the larynx, along with this mucous sheet. It is then either coughed-up or swallowed. The cilia may be damaged by smoking or infection, causing retention of mucous and inhaled material which may eventually obstruct the air passages.

The bronchi divide repeatedly into progressively smaller passages rather like the branches of a tree. These passages have encircling muscles in their walls which, by contraction or relaxation, can vary the diameter of the air passage.

In **asthma** the muscles of the small bronchi become oversensitive and overactive, causing excessive narrowing and obstruction of these air passages. This can occur in response to allergy, cold, infection, anxiety, smoking or other inhalants such as sea water. At the same time, the cells lining these passages produce excessive and thickened mucous. The combination of these factors causes airway narrowing which has serious repercussions for a diver.

The smallest branches of the bronchi end in bunches of microscopic air sacs called **alveoli**. The vast number of alveoli are packed together into the two sponge like organs, the **lungs**. There are about 300 million alveoli in the lungs and the combined area of all the alveoli in the lungs is equal to about half a tennis court. The alveoli are lined by a thin layer of fluid containing a detergent-like substance called **surfactant**. This acts as a wetting agent to prevent the alveoli from collapsing from surface tension.

The surfactant lining of the alveoli can be damaged in disease or by inhalation of water, leading to collapse of the lungs and serious respiratory difficulty.

Each alveolus is surrounded by a network of blood capillaries. These bring the blood into close contact with the air in the alveolus, with only the microscopically thin walls of the alveolus and capillary separating the two.

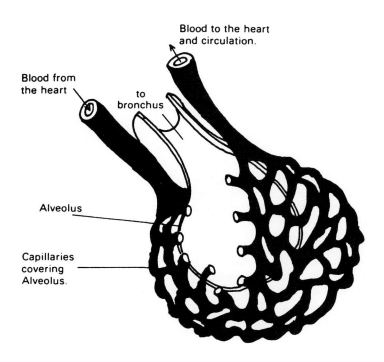

Fig. 3.2
This diagram illustrates an alveolus with its surrounding meshwork of capillaries.

If the wall of an alveolus is ruptured, as it may be in **pulmonary barotrauma** ("burst lung"), then air from the alveolus is able to enter the blood stream where it may cause blockage of distant vessels such as those in the brain. This is called an **air embolism**.

The lungs occupy a cavity about the size of a football on each side of the chest. The lung is covered by a thin membrane called the **pleura** and the inside of the chest wall is lined by a similar membrane. Between the two pleural layers is a narrow space which contains a small amount of lubricating fluid to minimise friction as the lungs expand and contract during breathing. If the outer surface of the lung tears, as it may in pulmonary barotrauma, then air can enter this pleural space causing the lung to collapse. This disorder is called **pneumothorax**.

The chest wall which encloses the lungs is made up of ribs with muscles between them - known as intercostal muscles. At the base of the chest cavity lies a large thin dome shaped muscle called the **diaphragm**. When the diaphragm contracts, it flattens and has a piston like effect, reducing the pressure in the chest cavity and increasing the volume of the lungs. The reduced pressure draws air into the lungs through the air passages.

Contraction of the diaphragm is the main method of **inhalation** in the resting state. It is assisted by contraction of the muscles between the ribs which rotate the rib cage upwards and outwards, enlarging the chest cavity and reducing the pressure in the chest. A group of neck muscles which are attached to the rib cage can also assist respiration when maximal breathing is required.

At the end of inhalation the elasticity of lungs and rib cage causes the lungs and chest wall to contract and **exhalation** takes place. With quiet breathing, this does nor require muscular effort. With heavy breathing, exhalation can be assisted by the abdominal and chest muscles.

Respiratory Function

During quiet respiration in adult males, about 500 ml of air is moved in and out of the respiratory tract with each breath. The volume per breath is termed "**tidal volume**". During extremely heavy exercise, the tidal volume can increase 10 fold, up to about 5 litres.

The total amount of air that can be held in the lungs (**total lung capacity** or **TLC**) in adult males is approximately 6 litres. Only about 10% of the air in the chest is exchanged with each breath during quiet respiration. The **vital capacity** (**VC**) is the maximum volume that can be exhaled in one breath, and the **forced expiratory volume** (**FEV**$_{1.0}$) is the maximum volume that can be exhaled in one second.

The **flow of air** through the respiratory passages varies at different stages of respiration. It reaches a peak about midway through inspiration — and during quiet breathing, this peak flow rate is approximates 30 litres per minute. This value increases during exercise to 600–700 litres per minute.

Any breathing system (such as a snorkel or demand valve) which the diver is using, should be capable of handling these large air flows without significant resistance. If this does not occur, then the diver must exert extra effort during respiration in order to overcome this resistance. This problem is compounded when the diver is breathing compressed air at depth because the increased density of the gas will further increase the resistance to airflow in both the equipment and the lungs.

Gas Uptake and Loss

Air, which contains approximately 21% oxygen (O_2) and 79% nitrogen (N_2), is inhaled into the alveoli where it is brought into contact with the blood in the capillaries. This blood contains a lower partial pressure of O_2 than the air in the alveolus and a higher partial pressure of CO_2, since it has just returned from the body which has been using O_2 and generating CO_2. Consequently, there is a pressure gradient causing O_2 to diffuse from the alveoli to the blood, and CO_2 to diffuse from the blood to the alveoli, where it is then exhaled. There is no net movement of N_2 since the N_2 in the alveoli and in the blood is in equilibrium, except when diving.

If the diver breaths air (79% N_2) or another inert gas such as helium, while descending or remaining underwater, this inert gas will pass from the alveoli to the blood because the partial pressure of the gas in the lungs is increasing as the diver goes deeper.

On ascent, the partial pressure of inert gas in the lungs will reduce, and this allows inert gas to move from the blood (returning from the tissues) to the alveoli, and be exhaled.

Respiratory Control

The partial pressures of CO_2 and O_2 in the blood are kept within very strict limits by a sensitive control system. There are sensors in the brain which detect small changes in the blood CO_2. If this increases, then the sensor causes stimulation of the **respiratory centre** within the brain, leading to faster and deeper respiration to eliminate more CO_2.

When a snorkel diver holds his breath, the CO_2 level in his blood increases. This produces respiratory stimulation which compels the diver to take a breath — hopefully after he has had time to return to the surface.

The sensors for blood O_2 partial pressure are in the carotid arteries which supply the brain. Any reduction in the blood O_2 level also leads to respiratory stimulation, but this effect is not as powerful as that caused by CO_2 changes.

Smoking

The ingenious habit of rolling tobacco into a tube of paper, setting fire to it and inhaling the smoke, sabotages the complex respiratory and circulatory process at several points.

Noxious tars in the smoke precipitate out in the bronchi producing chronic irritation, narrowing of the bronchi and causing a persistent outpouring of mucous. This ultimately results in chronic bronchitis. The tar also poisons the cilia, which conduct the mucous up the airway to the larynx, resulting in retention of old mucous in the lungs (smell the breath!).

Various toxins in the smoke ultimately cause destruction of the alveolar walls producing cavities in the lungs and destruction of the lung architecture, resulting in the disease called **emphysema**. This, combined with obstruction of the air passages, makes the smoking diver more liable to air trapping in the lungs and pulmonary barotrauma (see Chapter 11).

The carbon monoxide content of the smoke reduces the capacity of the blood to carry O_2, thereby reducing oxygenation of the tissues.

Some of the chemical constituents of the smoke are absorbed into the blood stream producing changes in the walls of the blood vessels supplying the heart, brain and limbs. Ultimately these become obstructed. In later life this can cause heart attacks, strokes and peripheral vascular disease (gangrene).

CARDIOVASCULAR SYSTEM

Blood

Arteries take blood from the heart. **Veins** return blood to the heart. Arterial blood (which has passed through the lungs), is then pumped to the periphery by the heart and is brought close to all the cells in the body by the capillary system. Here the O_2 diffuses into the cells and the CO_2 diffuses out of the cells into the blood.

The blood transports O_2 and CO_2. The O_2 is mainly carried by an iron containing compound called **haemoglobin (Hb)** contained in the red cells. 100 ml of blood will transport approximately 20 ml of O_2. If the red blood cells are removed, blood plasma will transport only 0.3 ml of O_2 per 100 ml. A drop of blood contains approximately 300 million red cells.

In arterial blood, the haemoglobin is almost 100% oxygenated when the blood leaves the heart to go to the tissues. It is bright red in colour. If for any reason the arterial blood is not adequately oxygenated, it causes the blue colour of the skin (cyanosis) seen in **hypoxia** (see Chapter 20).

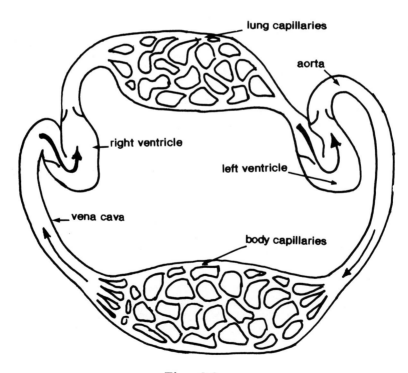

Fig. 3.3
A diagram showing the relationship between the circulations produced by the right and left sides (ventricles) of the heart.

In venous blood, the haemoglobin in red blood cells returns to the heart with 75% of its O_2 load still attached. It is then a blue colour.

The tissues need only 25% of the O_2 carried in arterial blood. This allows a reserve supply of O_2 which can be used during exercise or breath holding.

CO_2 is carried from the tissues by the blood in the veins, back to the lungs . Some of it is dissolved in blood plasma and some bound to the protein of the haemoglobin molecules. Although the CO_2 dissolved in the blood forms carbonic acid, the acidity of the blood is prevented from rising to excessive levels by a system of buffering compounds.

It is possible to increase the O_2 carrying capacity of blood by the use of **hyperbaric oxygen**. In recompression chambers, increased amounts of O_2 can be physically dissolved in the plasma, even though the haemoglobin is fully saturated with O_2.

Heart

The heart is a large muscular pump (about the size of a man's fist) located in the centre of the chest. It is composed of two functionally separate pumps which maintain two distinct circulations. The **right side** of the heart receives venous blood from the body and pumps this blood through the lungs where it picks up O_2 and eliminates CO_2. The **left side** of the heart receives this oxygenated arterial blood from the lungs and pumps it through the body.

Each side of the heart is essentially a two-stage pump which is not unlike a two-stage compressor. The **atrium** is the first or low pressure stage of the pump and it has a thin muscular wall. It receives blood from the veins at low pressure. When it contracts, it propels this blood into the second or high pressure stage – the more thickly walled and stronger ventricle.

The **ventricle** has two valves, one valve preventing blood from flowing back into the atrium, and the other valve preventing blood flowing back into it from the arteries. When it contracts, it pumps blood in only one direction – into the arteries.

Occasionally there may be openings between left and right sides of the heart (patent foramen ovale, septal defects). In divers this allows bubbles to pass from the venous system to the arterial, causing serious manifestations of decompression sickness from dives that should otherwise be safe. People with these heart abnormalities should not undertake Scuba diving.

The heart, being a muscle, requires its own blood supply. This is provided by the **coronary arteries** which originate in the aorta, the main artery of the body. Any obstruction of these coronary arteries will cause damage to the heart muscle – a heart attack.

Partial obstruction of the coronary arteries may produce **angina** (which is pain or discomfort arising from cardiac muscle), because it is receiving insufficient blood supply. Since a heart attack can take some of the fun out of a diving expedition, it is important for divers to have skilled medical examinations to exclude this problem or to help predict which divers will be susceptible to such heart conditions (coronary artery disease).

The resting output of the heart is about 5 litres per minute. The heart has considerable reserve and if the tissues require it, can increase this output several fold by increasing its rate and strength of contraction.

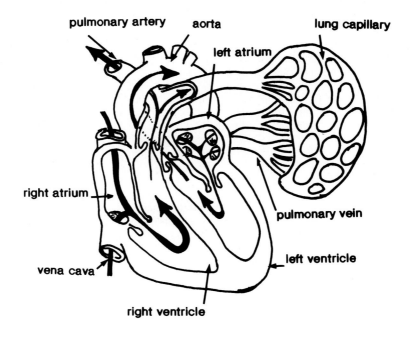

pulmonary artery   aorta   lung capillary

left atrium

right atrium

pulmonary vein

left ventricle

vena cava

right ventricle

Fig. 3.4
This diagram shows a cutaway drawing of the heart to illustrate the flow of blood from the vena cava through the chambers of the heart and the lungs to the aorta.

Circulation

The blood flow from the heart is pulsatile and the **blood pressure** varies depending on the stage of heart contraction. The higher blood pressure during the heart's contraction is called the **systolic blood pressure** and has a normal value of around 100–140mm mercury (mmHg). The pressure when the heart is not contracting is the **diastolic blood pressure** which has a normal value of around 60–90mm Hg. Blood pressure is normally recorded as Systolic / Diastolic – e.g. $^{140}/_{90}$.

Blood vessels can change their internal diameter under the control of the nervous system. This allows for some variation in blood flow to parts of the body depending on specific circumstances. For instance, during exercise the blood vessels dilate allowing more blood flow to the muscles, while under cold conditions the blood vessels to the skin constrict, reducing the blood flow to the skin (appearing pale) and so minimising heat loss.

The constriction or dilatation of the blood vessels also influences blood pressure. Excessively high blood pressure (**hypertension**) can ultimately cause damage to the blood vessels and an excessive strain on the heart. High blood pressure requires treatment, often with drugs which dilate the blood vessels but which may interfere with safe diving.

Blood pressure is constantly maintained by a sophisticated sensing and feedback mechanism. Variations in blood pressure caused by physical activity or standing from a reclining position are quickly compensated for by changes in the diameter of the blood vessel walls.

When a person is in a reclining position, blood pressure is maintained easily and the effect of gravity does not have to be opposed by the contraction of blood vessels. When standing up quickly from this position, blood pressure in the upper part of the body may fall. Occasionally, even in normal people, the heart and blood vessels cannot compensate rapidly enough and fainting or light-headedness can result. This is known as **syncope** or **postural hypotension**.

The cardiovascular system is able to compensate for changes in blood volume, such as those associated with severe bleeding (**haemorrhage**), by constricting the blood vessels and diverting blood from non-essential organs to essential organs such as the brain and heart.

In **pulmonary barotrauma,** air can gain access to the blood as it passes through the lungs. Air bubbles may be carried to vital organs such as the brain and heart, obstructing their blood flow and leading to serious consequences (**air embolism**). In **decompression sickness,** gas bubbles may also be transported by the blood stream.

Chapter 4

DIVING PHYSIOLOGY

BREATH-HOLD DIVING

It is not difficult for a diver to perform a breath-hold dive for a duration of one minute or more. This is possible because there is a reservoir of oxygen (O_2) stored in the lungs (about 1 litre O_2 when the lungs are full), in blood haemoglobin, and in myoglobin in the muscles.

With these reserves the diver is able to hold his breath for some time without the blood level of O_2 becoming dangerously low. Below a threshold blood O_2 partial pressure (about 50mm Hg – half the normal value), the brain ceases to function properly, causing loss of consciousness. At about this stage, the heart also becomes seriously starved of O_2 causing cardiac damage or disturbances of rhythm.

During a breath-hold dive, O_2 is used and carbon dioxide (CO_2) produced, decreasing the blood level of O_2 and elevating that of CO_2. Both effects may stimulate respiration but the CO_2 is the most important. Usually the diver develops an overpowering desire to breath (the **break point**) before the arterial O_2 level falls to a dangerous value. It eventually becomes irresistible and the diver may even take a breath under water, if he is unable to reach the surface in time.

Breath-holding can be extended considerably, with experience and willpower but the break point is eventually reached. This is a safety mechanism to prevent people from losing consciousness from excessively prolonged breath-holding (see Case Histories 33.2 and 33.3).

Hyperventilation

There are some people who find the flaunting of safety mechanisms an overwhelming challenge. The break point can be circumvented by **hyperventilating** (taking a succession of rapid deep breaths) before a dive. This reduces arterial CO_2 so that it takes longer for the blood level to reach the break point during a dive. During this delay, the blood O_2 level may fall below that necessary to maintain consciousness and the diver may become unconscious without any warning. This is called **hyperventilation induced hypoxia**. Using this method some divers have been able to prolong their breath hold dives for extended periods — until their body is found!

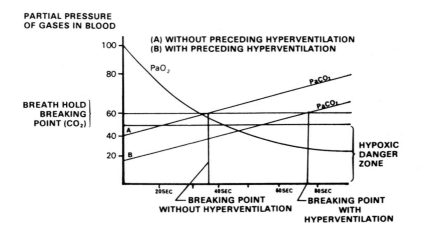

Fig. 4.1

This diagram shows the relationship between the fall of oxygen and carbon dioxide levels in the blood with breathholding. Normally (A) the breaking point is reached before the hypoxic zone is reached. After hyperventilation (B) the breaking point is in the hypoxic zone.

Lung Squeeze

During a breath-hold dive the chest and lungs are compressed by the increasing pressure of water. As the air in the lungs is compressed, the volume is replaced to a limited degree, by expansion and engorgement of the lung's blood vessels. Lung injury from this mechanism is known as lung squeeze, or pulmonary barotrauma of descent (see Boyle's Law, Chapter 2).

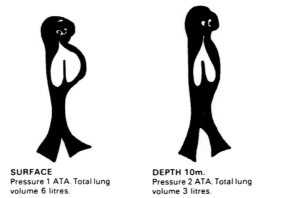

SURFACE
Pressure 1 ATA. Total lung volume 6 litres.

DEPTH 10m.
Pressure 2 ATA. Total lung volume 3 litres.

DEPTH 20m.
Pressure 3 ATA. Total lung volume 2 litres.

Fig. 4.2

Theoretically, the maximum safe depth for most divers should be about 30 metres (4ATA), but it probably varies between individuals, as much deeper breath-hold dives have now been performed – to well in excess of 100 metres.

Hypoxia of Ascent

Most divers will have noticed during a breath-hold dive that the desire to breathe often decreases with depth. This is probably due to the partial pressure of O_2 in the lungs increasing as they are compressed. There is a corresponding rise in the partial pressure of O_2 in the blood which will reduce the hypoxic stimulus to breathing. As the diver ascends however, the lungs will expand and the partial pressure of O_2 in them will correspondingly decrease. This produces an abrupt reduction in the O_2 partial pressure in the blood. It may fall below the threshold and cause unconsciousness during ascent. This phenomenon is termed **hypoxia of ascent**. It is especially common after hyperventilation.

Immersion

A neutrally buoyant diver is exempt from the effects of gravity and this produces physiological changes in the body. The return of blood flow to the heart is increased, allowing for **increased urine production** (which may lead to **dehydration**).

Cold water exposure produces many reflexes, including a desire to urinate. Temperature regulation is more difficult. The pressure variations may influence lung function with head out or vertical positions. Spatial orientation processes are disrupted. Trauma, in the form of physical injury from water movement, marine infections, dangerous marine animals, barotraumas, drowning etc. are dealt with in separate chapters.

Dive Reflex

Aquatic mammals display a reflex known as the "**dive reflex**". This is associated with profound slowing of the heart and redirection of the blood flow away from the muscles and non-essential organs to give a better blood supply to the heart and brain. This reflex is present to a minor degree in humans and can be produced by immersing the face or head in cold water. The heart slowing component of the reflex has been used by physicians to treat certain cardiac disorders associated with a rapid heart rate.

Other similar reflexes can be produced by breath-holding.

Snorkel Diving

All the difficulties associated with breath-hold diving occur with snorkel diving. Snorkel breathing is a convenient way of obtaining air with the head immersed, however it has several physiological and physical limitations (see Chapter 5).

COMPRESSED-AIR DIVING

Scuba allows the diver considerable freedom but has its own limitations. It has all the potential problems of free diving, but includes special problems of its own.

Resistance to Breathing

A major limitation to diving with scuba is resistance to breathing. During maximal exertion, a diver can consume over 70 litres of air per minute at the surface – but the peak flow rate during inspiration is many times this value. Some regulators may have difficulty delivering gas at this rate, adding considerable resistance to breathing.

This problem is magnified at depth because the greater pressure increases the density of the inhaled gas, especially at depths in excess of 30 metres when air is breathed, and 200 metres when helium $/O_2$ (heliox) mixture is breathed. It is likely that resistance to breathing will ultimately limit the depth to which divers can reach.

An idea of the respiratory loads which the diver faces can be gained from the following table :

SCUBA SWIM	SPEED	OXYGEN CONSUMPTION	RESPIRATORY MINUTE VOLUME
Slow scuba swim	0.5 knots	0.8 litres / minute	18 litres / minute
Average scuba swim	0.8 knots	1.5 litres / minute	28 litres / minute
Fast scuba swim	1.0 knots	1.8 litres / minute	40 litres / minute
Maximum scuba swim	1.3 knots	3–4 litres / minute	70–100 litres / minute

Table 4.1

Air Consumption

O_2 consumption is virtually the same for a given amount of exercise whether it is performed at the surface or deep under water. Because compressed air is being breathed at depth, more O_2 will be supplied than is needed by the diver. The actual volume of gas breathed at any depth will be the same as that which would be breathed at the surface. However, since the gas being breathed at depth is at greater pressure, the volume breathed, if converted to atmospheric (surface) pressure, will also be greater.

For example, during maximal effort a diver may consume 70 litres of air per minute at the surface. If he is performing an equivalent amount of effort at 20 metres depth (3ATA), he will still be breathing 70 litres per minute from his scuba regulator at 20 metres, but this will be equivalent to :

$$70 \text{ (litres)} \times 3 \text{ (atmospheres)}$$

$$= 210 \text{ litres per minute at atmospheric pressure.}$$

This type of diving is welcomed by those who make their living selling scuba air fills.

The regulator may not be able to meet the respiratory demands of a diver when certain conditions apply (see Chapter 5). Under these conditions, the diver may be aware of an inadequate air supply and either panic or take other dangerous action, such as a rapid ascent or omission of decompression requirements.

Skip Breathing

It is possible for a scuba diver to minimize his air consumption by deliberately retarding or slowing his breathing rate. This type of breathing pattern obviously limits the reserve of O_2 which will be stored in the divers lungs and haemoglobin, and may lead to retention of CO_2. It reduces the safety margin in the event of air supply failure as well as increasing the likelihood of pulmonary barotrauma, and is recommended only for those with suicidal tendencies.

Other Effects on a Scuba Diver

The physiological effects of scuba diving may parallel those of breathhold diving. Hyperventilation, breathholding, the diving reflexes and the effects of immersion, may all be provoked. The dehydration effect is of importance in aggravating decompression sickness.

Gas Pressures

Because of the increased pressures on the diver, high nitrogen partial pressures cause nitrogen narcosis (or "narks"). Similarly, higher O_2 partial pressures may produce O_2 toxicity in very special circumstances. Gas coming out of solution in the divers body may cause decompression sickness and/or dysbaric osteonecrosis (or "bone rot").

Chapter 5

DIVING EQUIPMENT

This chapter has been included to explain the operating principles and the limitations of some of the equipment currently used in both free and scuba diving.

FREE DIVING EQUIPMENT

Mask

The variety of face masks on the market suggests that the ideal mask has not yet been developed for the multitude of different face shapes.

The mask should cover the eyes and nose but not the mouth. Having the nose included allows the diver to exhale into the mask to compensate for the changes in water pressure, and so prevent **face mask squeeze** (see Chapter 12). The ability to exhale into the mask is also essential to clear a face mask flooded with water. The mask may be shaped so that the diver's fingers can reach and block his nostrils, to make ear equalising easier.

Ideally, the mask should have a small air volume to reduce the effort needed to equalise water pressure during breath-hold diving. The face plate should be close to the eyes, to maximise the field of view. With a basic face mask this is limited by the nose. This problem can be overcome by radical plastic surgery, or reduced by an indented rubber nose piece which allows the glass to be brought closer to the eyes. Clear plastic or glass side panels may also possibly help. Although this arrangement generally improves peripheral vision, it still restricts downward vision – obscuring the harness, weight belt and emergency gear.

Some face masks are fitted with a valve on the undersurface to aid elimination of water. This valve can be an annoying source of water leakage into the mask.

The body of the mask may be made of plastic, rubber, or silicone. The material needs sufficient rigidity to maintain the basic shape of the mask but a soft flanged edge (or skirt) is necessary to allow the mask to adapt to the contours of the face and provide a watertight seal. If the mask is excessively rigid it will not accommodate to water pressure changes, making face mask squeeze more likely. Masks made of silicone rubber are available for use by divers with rubber or plastic allergy.

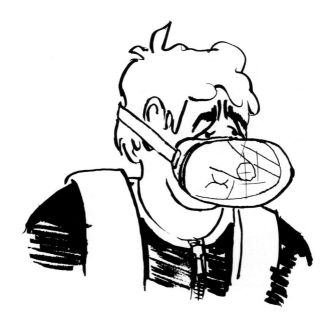

Fig. 5.1

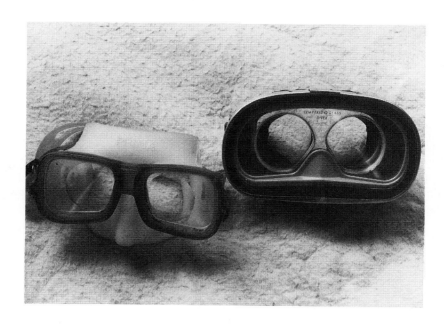

Fig. 5.2
Diving masks with corrective lenses incorporated into or glued onto the faceplate.
The mask on the left is made from silicone rubber, and has replaceable lenses.

The viewing plate of the mask can be made of either glass or plastic. Glass should be "tempered" (safety glass). This will shatter into small cubes rather than sharp splinters if broken, reducing damage to the eyes. Good quality plastic is less likely to break but is prone to scratching.

A mask can be chosen by fitting the mask to the face and gently inhaling through the nose. A mask which seals adequately will then adhere to the face without any air leak. The mask should seal properly without excessive tension by the mask strap. Some mask straps are broadened at the back of the head to distribute the tension over a greater area, as narrow bands are less secure and often cause local tenderness or headaches.

For divers with visual defects, corrective lenses can be ground directly into the face plate or can be made separately and glued onto the face plate with a transparent glue. Lenses of differing refractive index are now available which slot directly into some masks, replacing the "blank" lenses.

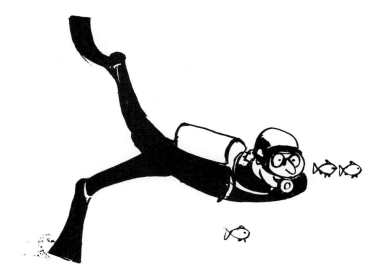

Fig. 5.3

Snorkel

The snorkel allows the diver to breathe while swimming with the face submerged. It can also be used during periods of surface swimming during a scuba dive to conserve compressed air or return to safety without scuba. Because of the limited strength of the respiratory muscles and the effect of water pressure, it is not possible to breath through a snorkel at a depth in excess of about 50 cm (20 inches). The length of the snorkel should be sufficient to allow the diver to swim face down, to look around and to swim through choppy water without the snorkel flooding. It should not be excessively long as this increases breathing resistance and respiratory "dead space". The optimum length is about 30–35 cm.

The snorkel should be of maximum diameter to reduce breathing resistance but not wide enough to create excessive dead space. The optimum internal diameter is approximately 1.5–2 cm. It should have a minimum of angles and curves, and the interior should be smooth. Corrugated tubing or sharp angles increase breathing resistance. Mouthpieces are sometimes made to swivel and rotate in order to minimise drag on the mouth and permit a comfortable hold. This can be assisted by individual 'bite moulding' of the mouthpiece.

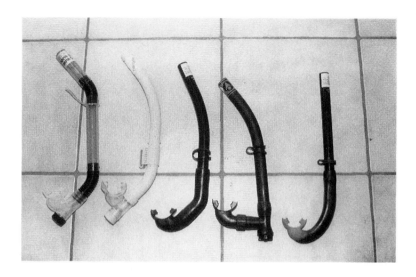

Fig. 5.4
A range of snorkels. Three of these have "purge" valves for eliminating water.

The breathing resistance of a poorly designed snorkel is usually not noticed during quiet breathing, but may prevent the diver from exercising to his maximum capacity when needed. At moderately heavy breathing, as with anxiety-produced hyperventilation or swimming at much greater than 1 knot speed, snorkels restrict the breathing capability of divers engaged in surface swimming.

Several devices have been invented to prevent water entering the snorkel during a dive. These usually employ buoyant objects such as a table-tennis ball or cork which float into, and obstruct the end of the snorkel when it is submerged. This requires an extra U shaped bend in the snorkel which increases resistance and dead space. These devices are unreliable and unnecessary. Divers learn to expel water from the snorkel after returning to the surface.

Some snorkels are now fitted with a small purge valve near the mouth piece which allows most of the water to drain from the snorkel. This reduces the amount of water which needs to be expelled by the diver, and therefore the effort required. It is also a potential source of leaks.

Fins   (Flippers)

The use of fins considerably improves the diver's swimming efficiency. There are several designs available.

Fins have two basic types of foot fitting — one has a shoe integrated with the fin (enclosed heel), and the other has a half shoe fitting and a heel strap (open heels) which allows the diver to wear neoprene boots. These boots can be used for protection when walking over reefs, and offer some thermal insulation to the feet.

The blades of the fins vary in size and rigidity and some types are fitted with vents (venturis). Studies of various fin types have shown that no one type is ideal for all divers. Fins with larger, more rigid blades, allow a more powerful action but require greater strength and are more difficult to manoeuvre. In general, fins of medium size and medium flexibility are suitable for most recreational divers.

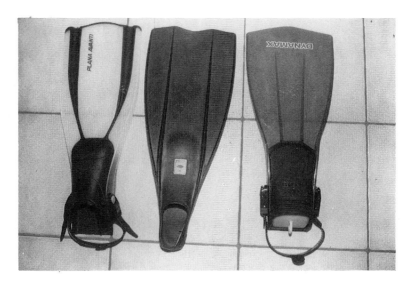

Fig. 5.5
An array of fins. The middle fin has an enclosed heel.

The way fins are used is important. Traditionally, a narrow, straight-leg kicking stroke has been taught. A less graceful wide-kicking stroke using bent knees is more efficient. This comes from directing the thrust of the fin along the direction of movement of the diver.

Fins with integrated shoes can often cause blistering and abrasions ("fin ulcers") around the rim of the shoe fitting. This can be reduced by the use of socks until the diver becomes more accustomed to the particular fins. Correct fitting of the fins is necessary. If too loose, their loss will endanger the diver. An excessively tight fit may cause muscular cramps and fin ulcers.

Wet Suit

The wet suit provides protection, comfort and safety. It is made from rubber or neoprene which incorporates tiny air bubbles, to provide good thermal insulation. It also provides protection from scratching, abrasions and stinging animals.

On the surface and in shallow water, these suits give great buoyancy. To overcome this effect and therefore submerge, accessory weights are usually necessary. At depth however, the air bubbles in the wet suit are compressed, reducing its thickness, buoyancy and insulating properties. The variations in buoyancy may need to be offset by the use of a buoyancy compensator.

A poorly fitting wet suit can cause chafing, especially around the neck and arm-pit. A wet suit with an excessively tight neck can also compress the blood vessels to the brain leading to dizziness and fainting. Tightness around the chest may cause difficulty in breathing. Zippers allow easier access and exit, but contribute to water leakage and reduced reliability.

A wet suit variant containing inflatable gas compartments can partly overcome these problems. These suits can be inflated orally or directly from a scuba tank. Careful venting on ascent is necessary in order to prevent too rapid an ascent with these suits. They are a modern version of the traditional "**dry suit**". Because of the added buoyancy problems, special training is needed to use dry suits.

Weight Belt

A weight belt is used to offset the buoyancy of the body, wet suit and other items of equipment. Ideally the diver should use enough weight to produce neutral buoyancy at the surface (without reliance on a buoyancy vest). The correct amount of weight is found by trial and error and this should be done in shallow water. As the diver descends, compression of the wet suit makes the diver less buoyant. This effect can be offset by the use of a buoyancy compensating vest (B.C.).

A diver without a wet suit will usually require less than 2 kg (5 lbs) weight and many divers will require no weight at all. A diver wearing a wet suit may require 1 kg weight for each 1 mm wet suit thickness. Inexperienced divers tend to use more weights than experienced divers, and are therefore more at risk from buoyancy problems.

The deliberate attachment of up to 10 kg of lead weight, or more, to a neutrally buoyant air-breathing creature in the water has obvious safety consequences. "Lead poisoning" is a common contributor to recreational scuba diver deaths.

Most weights are moulded lead shapes through which the belt is threaded. For comfort these are sometimes curved, and some newer belts incorporate zippered compartments filled with lead shot for better fit to the body. Weights are usually sold as 1, 2, or 3 kg. sizes.

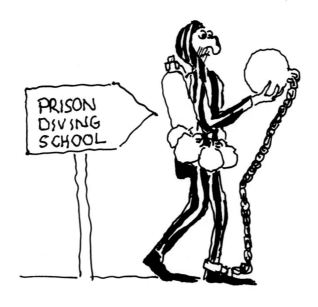

Fig. 5.6

The weight belt should be fitted with a quick release buckle, preferably one which is separate from the scuba harness release. (Exceptions to this requirement are found in saturation diving and in cave diving where a sudden ascent due to inadvertent release of the weight belt could have catastrophic consequences.) The buckle should be easily identified by feel and therefore different from the harness buckle. The strap should not be too long or it will hinder quick release.

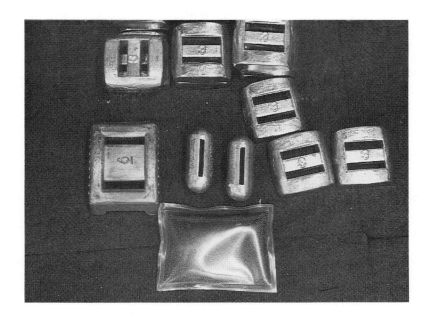

Fig. 5.7
A range of lead weights (and a pouch of lead shot) for use on weight belts.

The weight belt should fit firmly around the waist. If it does not, compression of the wet suit at depth may result in it becoming loose and rotating around the body, and the buckle becoming inaccessible. Some new belts are made from elastic materials which conform irregardless of depth.

In a significant proportion of diving accidents, the diver fails to release the weight belt at the time of the emergency. Training of divers is required to ensure that release of the weight belt is routine in an emergency. When ditching the weight belt, the diver should release the buckle with one hand and hold the weight belt well clear of the body with the other, before dropping it — otherwise entanglement with other equipment is possible. Release of the weight belt will not necessarily cause it to fall.

The attachment of weights to the diver using rope or an ordinary belt buckle which cannot be rapidly released, has sometimes proved more permanent than the diver would have wished.

The weight belt should always be the last item of equipment put on before entering the water, and the first removed before leaving the water. If this advice is followed, then an inadequately equipped diver who does fall into the water, is more likely to float and not drown.

Diving Knife

Contrary to the popular Hollywood image, the diver's knife has limited usefulness in fighting marauding sharks. It is, however, an essential item of safety equipment which can be used to cut the diver free from entanglements such as rope, kelp, fishing lines and nets.

Although stainless steel blades resist rust, inferior quality steels do not hold a cutting edge well. The knife should be of robust construction and of a reasonable size. It should be strapped to the diver at a location where it will not cause snagging (e.g. the inner surface of the calf or arm), and easily accessible. It should not be attached to any item of equipment, such as the weight belt or scuba harness, which may be ditched in an emergency.

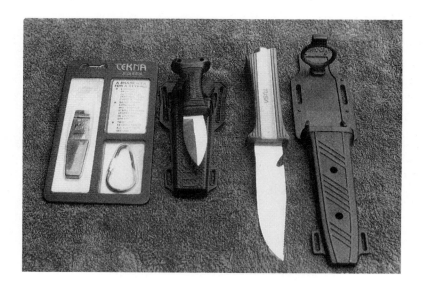

Fig. 5.8
A range of diver's knives.

COMPRESSED - AIR DIVING EQUIPMENT

The use of this equipment has given divers a high degree of freedom underwater and the capacity to go deep and stay there for long periods of time.

Strictly speaking, the term **"scuba"** refers to all **self contained underwater breathing apparatus** but these days it is generally restricted to open-circuit air equipment only (initially called the "Aqualung"). With this equipment the diver breathes compressed air from a cylinder carried on his back, and exhales into the water.

Other equipment used by divers includes **surface supply compressed air breathing apparatus** (Hookah or SSBA) and **rebreathing apparatus** (semi-closed or closed circuit).

Closed circuit and **semi-closed circuit rebreathing apparatus** allows a diver to rebreathe some of his exhaled gas. It includes a chemical "scrubber" or absorber to remove exhaled CO_2. By re-using exhaled gas it make economical use of the gas supply, as well as minimising bubble release into the water. They have obvious advantages for military operations.

Scuba

There are two basic forms of this system — the **twin-hose system** and the **single-hose** type. The twin-hose system is rarely used now and will be discussed only briefly.

The single-hose unit uses compressed air contained within a steel or aluminium cylinder ("**scuba tank**"). It is usually filled to a pressure of 150–200 Bar (2250–3000 psi). Some systems developed in Europe improve endurance by utilising cylinder pressures of approximately 300 Bar (4500 psi). New cylinders manufactured from alloy-mix materials permit greater pressures, and are smaller and lighter. In most countries, laws require that all cylinders are visually and hydrostatically tested every 1–2 years..

A **cylinder valve** fitted with a mechanical tap and connecting yoke is threaded into the neck of the cylinder. Standards require the fitting of a **"burst-disc"** to this valve so that this will burst before the cylinder in the event of overpressure. Attached to this yoke, usually by a universal screw-on or clamp fitting, is a pressure reducing valve (or **first stage regulator**). This regulator reduces the pressure of the gas in the cylinder 150–200 Bar (2000–3000 psi) to an intermediate pressure of just over 7 Bar (100 psi) and supplies air at this pressure to an **air hose** which passes around the diver's shoulder. The first stage regulator is designed to adjust the pressure in the air hose to approximately 7 bar (100 psi) greater than the water pressure at the depth the diver is swimming (the environmental pressure). It automatically maintains this pressure differential as the diver changes depth.

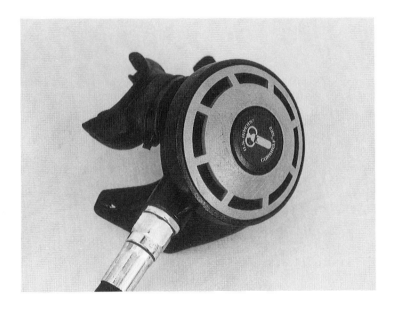

Fig. 5.9
A typical second-stage Scuba regulator.

The **air hose** is a small diameter flexible tube made of pressure resistant material which carries air from the first stage regulator to a **second stage regulator** (or **demand valve**) which in turn supplies air to the diver through the mouthpiece. With inhalation, a diaphragm moves to open a valve in the demand regulator, and air passes from the air hose to the diver, at environmental pressure.

The diver exhales directly into the water through one or more one-way valves which should prevent water from entering the demand valve during inhalation.

It is important that the pressure of the air supply to a diver does not vary as the scuba cylinder empties, otherwise it will become progressively more difficult to breath as the tank pressure falls. Modern first stage regulators are much improved on the 1960–70 models and some have incorporated devices such as "balanced" valves to reduce this problem to some degree.

It is necessary for the diver to create a slight negative pressure in the mouthpiece during each inhalation in order to activate the demand valve mechanism. This negative pressure should be minimal or breathing becomes tiring. A regulator which is easy to breathe from at the surface, may not necessarily be able to deliver the large gas flows required during exertion at depth. When choosing a regulator, divers should refer to independent (e.g. U.S.Navy) testings.

Difficulties are still encountered in obtaining adequate air supply with reasonable respiratory efforts under the following conditions :

   • low cylinder pressures (observable on contents gauges), < 50 Bar
   • cylinder valve not fully opened
   • resistance in the first or second stage regulators (poor design or inadequate maintenance)
   • increased respiration (exertion, hyperventilation, negative buoyancy etc.)
   • at greater depths where the air breathed is more compressed (dense), > 30 metres
   • with other demands on the air supply (inflating buoyancy compensator, octopus reg. etc.)

Some demand valves are bulky and quite heavy, requiring continual tension on the bite and the jaw to retain the mouthpiece. This can lead to painful spasm of the jaw muscles and a dysfunction of the jaw (temporo-mandibular) joint . Malleable plastic mouthpieces are available which attempt to spread the load evenly over the teeth. A soft silastic mouthpiece may be more valuable. Lugs attached to the mouthpiece are designed to keep the mouth open in a comfortable position and to locate and retain the demand valve correctly in the mouth. It should not be necessary to grip the lugs tightly.

Cylinder Valve

The gas outlet from the cylinder to the regulator is controlled by a high pressure valve or tap. A "K" or "J " valve may be incorporated in this assembly. High pressure "burst discs" are fitted by law to all scuba cylinder valves to minimise the risk of explosion if over pressurised.

The **J valve** is a spring loaded valve which restricts the flow of the air from the cylinder when the "contents" pressure reaches 21–35 Bar (300-500 psi). This reminds the diver that he is "low on air". The diver can then open the J valve by pulling a lever on the side of the cylinder, which releases the remaining air in the cylinder for breathing.

This **J valve** has a number of disadvantages. Malfunction of the valve is not uncommon and restriction to breathing may be encountered with a very wide range of pressures (10–70 bar) remaining in the cylinder. If the J valve is accidentally opened during the dive, for example by bumping, the first indication the diver will have of a shortage of air, will be an empty cylinder. The J valve was developed before the availability of economical and accurate "contents gauges" and its use these days is not recommended. These valves were sometimes incorporated in a first stage reducing valve and may sometimes be seen in older equipment.

Most cylinders today are fitted with the simpler **K valve** which has no reserve facility and merely functions as a tap.

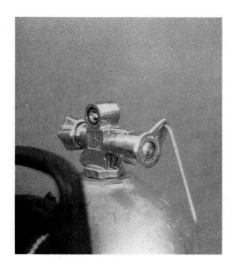 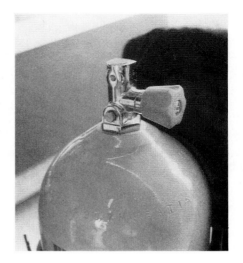

Fig. 5.10
A J and K valve.

Twin Hose Unit

The twin or dual hose unit has both a first and second stage reducing valve combined in a single module attached to the cylinder yoke. Air is delivered by an intake hose to the diver's mouth at a pressure equal to the surrounding water. An outlet hose exhausts the exhaled air to the regulator for release to the water.

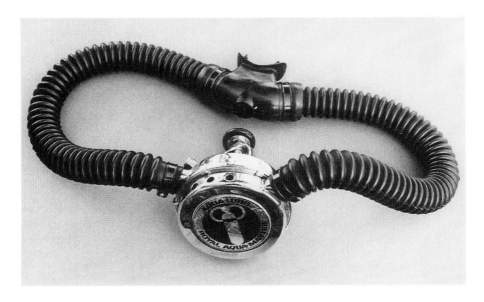

Fig. 5.11
A twin hose regulator.

Since the diver's exhaust gas bubbles are released behind the head from the regulator, they tend not to interfere with vision. The twin hose apparatus has the disadvantage of requiring two bulky corrugated air hoses of around 2.5–4 cm diameter, and it is more difficult to purge the system of water. These units are rarely used today, except by photographers and in sites where regulators may freeze. The twin hoses were very prone to perishing and leakages.

Hookah and SSBA

Air can be supplied to the diver by a hose from the surface, either from a compressor (**hookah unit**) or from a cylinder or bank of cylinders (**surface supply breathing apparatus**).

The air is supplied directly to the demand valve at a pressure which is manually preset according to the depth at which the diver is operating. The first stage reducing valve is located on the cylinder at the surface, and can be adjusted according to the diver's depth. This system can allow almost unlimited diving duration, which poses a risk of decompression sickness if the depth and time of the dive is not monitored.

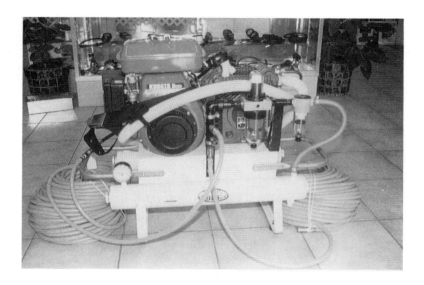

Fig. 5.12
A hookah compressor and motor with capacity for two divers.

If the gas pressure in the hose from the surface fails due to a hose rupture, compressor failure or an empty cylinder, a pressure gradient can rapidly develop between the diver's respiratory tract and the failure site. Unless a non-return valve is incorporated in the gas supply line, near the diver, this pressure gradient can result in parts of the diver returning to the surface through his air hose.

Surface hookah units usually include a small pressurised reservoir as an emergency supply for breathing in case of compressor failure. Many divers carry small compressed air cylinders with them underwater ("pony bottles" or "bail-out bottles") which are connected to the main breathing hose, and can be operated manually in the event of a main supply failure.

Standard Dress or Hard Hat

This traditional piece of equipment uses compressed air delivered by a flexible hose to a rigid brass or copper helmet connected to a heavy duty dry suit. The depth of the dive determines the pressure of the delivered air. A continuous air flow is supplied to the helmet at a rate sufficient to supply the diver's oxygen needs and to flush out exhaled gas. Originally hand powered compressors were used, later superseded by motorised compressors. A bank of compressed air cylinders can also be used as for SSBA.

This system is bulky and requires heavy lead weights (usually boots and chest corsets) to offset the buoyancy of the helmet and the suit. Failure of the gas supply to keep up with the diver's rate of descent, or loss of the air supply (in the absence of a non-return valve), can lead to the diver being compressed into the helmet — causing head or body barotrauma. This is not very comfortable.

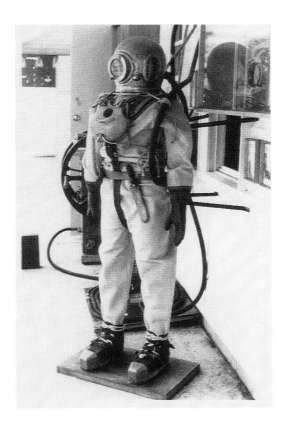

Fig. 5.13
A "hard hat" or
standard dress rig.

A modern variant of this system is used today in deep diving. It utilises a smaller, light-weight fibreglass or aluminium helmet or mask in conjunction with a dry or warmed wet suit, enabling the diver to swim and move more freely. The tethering line may go to a diving bell. The diver usually breathes gas mixtures which include helium, to prevent the development of nitrogen narcosis.

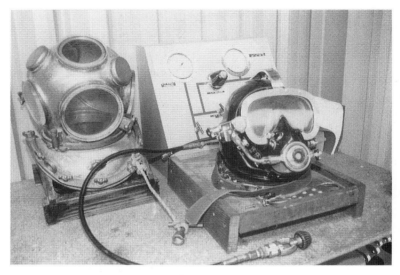

Fig. 5.14
A modern professional diving mask in front
with Standard Dress helmet in the background.

Closed and Semi-closed Circuit
Rebreathing Apparatus

With this equipment some or all of the diver's exhaled gas is passed through a carbon dioxide absorber ("scrubber") and then rebreathed from a breathing bag ("counterlung"). This minimises gas usage, produces fewer bubbles and allows smaller cylinders to be used for an equivalent dive duration.

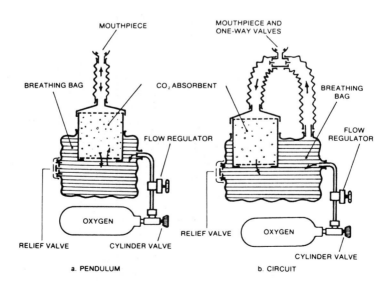

Fig. 5.15
Diagram of two types of closed circuit oxygen rebreathing sets.

A military system, using 100% oxygen in a closed circuit, is employed for clandestine operations (blowing up ships, mine clearance, etc.). Because the diver rebreathes 100% oxygen, there is a risk of oxygen toxicity, so these sets have a practical depth limit of 9 metres.

Closed circuit mixed-gas rebreathing systems are used in deep diving operations to minimise the consumption of costly helium gas. Light weight breathing gas cylinders are more comfortable for the diver to wear and the system is often more economical as regards gas usage.

Some closed circuit mixed-gas rebreathing systems are completely self contained. One early example in the 1960's was the "Electrolung". With this type of apparatus the composition of the gas mixture is monitored by sensors and the gas supply is adjusted electronically by solenoid-operated valves to maintain the gas mixture within preselected parameters.

The safe use of rebreathing systems requires extensive training and they are not suitable for use by recreational divers. Oxygen and carbon dioxide toxicity are common problems (often causing fatalities) while variations in gas mixtures complicate the calculation of decompression. These devices are expensive to purchase, difficult to maintain and those using electronic components are bedevilled by water leakage and unreliability.

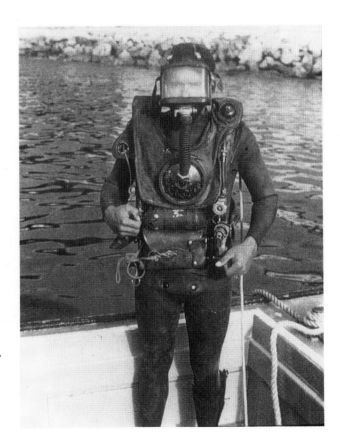

Fig. 5.16.
A military diver wearing
an oxygen rebreathing set.

ANCILLARY DIVING EQUIPMENT

Buoyancy Compensator, Buoyancy Vest, B.C.

This was originally devised as a modified life jacket to provide emergency flotation for the diver at the surface. Its value in compensating for changes of buoyancy due to wet suit compression with depth, was realised and it was modified to allow the gas content to be varied during the dive, depending on the buoyancy needs. It was also variously called a B.C.D. or B.C.V. (buoyancy compensating device or vest) or A.B.L.J. (adjustable buoyancy life-jacket)

Desirable features. When inflated the B.C. should be sufficient to offset the weight of the diver and all his equipment. It should support an unconscious diver so that his face is clear of the water. Ten kilograms (22 lbs) of buoyancy is adequate to achieve this. Most B.C.'s have excess capacity.

The B.C. should have a means of oral inflation, as well as a means of manually inflating with gas from a compressed air cylinder. With modern B.C.s this usually takes the form of an auxiliary "direct low pressure feed" line from the first stage or reducing valve. This direct-scuba-feed allows the B.C. to be inflated using air from the scuba tank. This will often provide unsatisfactory inflation with a low tank pressure at depth, especially if air is also needed for breathing.

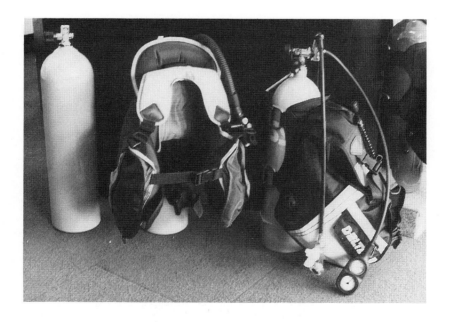

Fig. 5.17
Cylinder, jacket (or vest type) buoyancy compensator attached to cylinder, and full scuba rig with attached regulators and gauges.

Ideally there should be an emergency supply of inflating gas — this may be either a CO_2 cartridge or a small compressed air bottle. If a CO_2 cartridge is used it should have the ability to fully inflate the vest at depth, which usually requires at least 20 gram capacity. The CO_2 cartridge triggering device is especially prone to corrosion and needs to be regularly maintained and inspected before each dive. The toggles which operate these cartridges can snag on passing obstructions, accidentally inflating the vest. This can have disastrous consequences in cave diving, decompression dives and other situations.

Some B.C.s are fitted with a small compressed air bottle for emergency inflation. This is activated by a rotating valve which will not open accidentally. The bottle can also serve as an emergency source for a few breaths of air if a modified demand valve is fitted to the vest. These bottles are usually charged from the main gas cylinder at the surface just prior to fitting the B.C.

The B.C. should have a pressure relief valve to prevent rupture from over-inflation on ascent. There also needs to be an easily accessible air-dumping valve to allow quick release of gas. The direct scuba feed line should also have an easily operated "quick-release" fitting at the B.C. end in case of a jammed inflator valve causing greater inflation than can be released by a dump valve.

The B.C. should be designed so that it will not ride up onto the throat when inflated. This was traditionally accomplished by fitting a crotch strap or attachment to the scuba harness. B.C.s are becoming increasingly more complex and expensive, and may contribute to diver errors and therefore injuries.

Jacket B.C.s incorporating a scuba-tank backpack have become popular in recent years. These are comfortable and convenient to use, do not compress the chest and eliminate many of the straps associated with a conventional scuba-tank harness. With most of these units, however, it is difficult in an emergency to ditch an empty scuba tank on the surface without losing the B.C.

Contents Gauge

It is essential to know the air content of the scuba tank during a dive, to allow a sufficient air reserve for emergency use and for decompression.

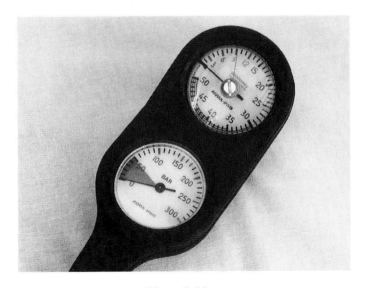

Fig. 5.18.
Depth and contents gauges calibrated in metres of sea water and Bars, respectively.

A "reserve" valve is not an adequate substitute for a contents gauge since it may be inadvertently opened before or during the dive.

To gain maximum advantage from the contents gauge the diver should refer to it frequently, and should be aware of the values in respect to his own diving gas consumption at that depth.

Alternate Air Source

The **octopus regulator** is a second-stage demand valve which can be used by the diver in the event of failure of the main demand valve or which may be used by another diver who has an equipment failure or air exhaustion. This facility eliminates the need for buddy breathing which can be difficult and dangerous to perform in high stress situations or between inexperienced divers.

Obviously, two divers using the same scuba system will halve the endurance of the tank. An alternative is to carry a complete separate emergency **"spare air"** unit with an adequate supply of air to reach the surface. At depth, and with low tank pressure, insufficient air may be available for simultaneous use of the demand valve and the octopus regulator. Other alternative air sources include twin scuba cylinders (and independent regulators) and air breathing from a B.C. supply.

Fig. 5.19
"Spare Air" – an emergency small air cylinder with built-in regulator.

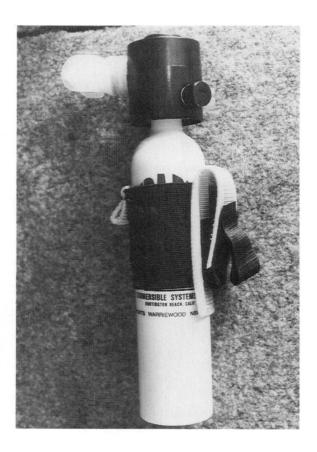

Diving Watch

A reliable, accurate, waterproof watch or dive timer is an essential piece of scuba diving equipment, in order to allow decompression requirements to be calculated.

The device should include some means of measuring elapsed time. A rotating bezel on the face of the watch is a simple and popular way of achieving this. Digital watches with elapsed time counters are also used.

Electronic dive timers, which are automatically triggered after a shallow descent, may not only record the dive duration but also the time between dives (surface interval).

Depth Gauge

It is necessary for the scuba diver to have an accurate knowledge of his depth exposure so that decompression requirements can be determined. A depth gauge should be easily read under all visibility conditions. There are several types of depth gauge currently available. The simplest type uses an air-filled **capillary tube**. As the air in the tube is compressed during descent, water enters the capillary tube and the position of the water interface on a calibrated scale indicates the depth. This type of gauge is very accurate at depths down to about 10 metres but it is inappropriate in excess of 20 metres, due to the small scale deviations available on the gauge at these depths.

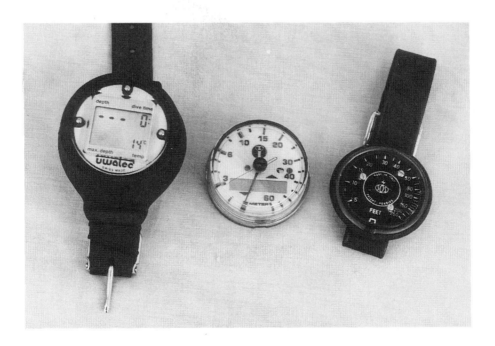

Fig. 5.20
Three types of depth gauge – an electronic (left), Bourdon (centre) and capillary (right).

A **Bourdon tube gauge** incorporates a thin curved copper tube which straightens as increased water pressure compresses the air within the tube. The movement of the tube is magnified by a gearing system which moves a needle across a scale. This type of gauge may become inaccurate due to salt obstructing the water-entry port, repetitive mechanical damage and altitude exposure.

Another type of gauge has a flexible **diaphragm** incorporated into the casing of the **gauge**. The diaphragm moves a needle through a magnifying gear system. This type of gauge has the advantage of relative simplicity and reliability.

Modern micro-processor technology has produced digital depth gauges which measure depth using a **pressure transducer**. This type of gauge is dependant on an adequately charged battery with absolute water-tight integrity for reliable operation.

A device which records the **maximum depth** attained (maximum depth indicator or M.D.I.) is useful as the diver may fail to note the greatest depth attained during a dive. This knowledge is necessary in calculating decompression requirements.

A depth gauge should be regularly recalibrated to ensure its accuracy. Some depth gauges incorporate a capillary depth gauge which will provide a cross check of calibration at shallow depth. Often depth gauges are contained in "consoles" which also contain cylinder contents gauges, timers and compasses.

Decompression Meters (D.C.M.)
(see Chapter 14)

A decompression meter uses a mechanical or electronic model of the gas uptake and elimination by the diver. Unless they follow proven decompression tables, these devices are inherently unreliable. It is impossible to duplicate the very complex gas uptake and loss from a living diver and to allow for individual variation.

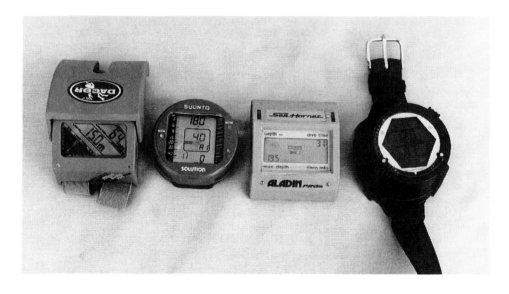

Fig. 5.21
A range of modern decompression meters.

Decompression meters based on decompression theories (or the principles on which the tables were developed), are not yet adequate (1992). They do however, provide a fruitful source of decompression sickness cases for diving physicians. Some meters also incorporate accurate devices for recording times, depths, cylinder contents and even water temperatures.

Some of the better D.C.M.s provide "print-out" capabilities or connections to a computer. These enable accurate graphical representations of a diver's dive profile, and are useful to treating physicians in cases of decompression sickness.

Communication Systems

The safety of the buddy system of diving depends on the two divers being in constant communication. Divers who are not in constant communication are in reality only diving in the same ocean and may or may not be available to assist their buddy in an emergency. Even when they do, third party rescue is often needed.

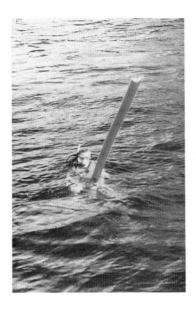

Fig. 5.22
A safety sausage or "divers condom".

A **whistle** may be of value on the surface, in attracting support from the boat crew or other divers. Another system of drawing attention and demonstrating the divers position on the surface, where most accidents either commence or end up, is a depth-resistant **distress signal** (smoke for daytime, flare for night).

A 2 metre orange plastic tube, able to be inflated by scuba or mouth, is of value and is marketed as the **Safety Sausage**. If erect, it is easily seen from aboard boats. Aircraft can identify it more easily when it is laid flat on the water surface. It is also known as the "Diver's Condom".

Underwater a diver can be contacted by a variety of transmitting and homing devices. **Lights** are of real value at night, if the visibility is good.

A **buddy–line** keeps a pair of divers in close contact. It consists of a short length of cord (2–4 metres in length and preferably of floating line) which is attached to each diver's arm by a detachable strap. Any emergency affecting one diver will soon become apparent to the buddy even if he is not watching. Possibly the only instance where the buddy line should be discarded is when snagging is likely, or if a large shark takes a serious interest in one's buddy.

It is a sad fact that most divers bodies are retrieved only after a search — and usually death occurs without the buddy-diver's knowledge. Many deaths could possibly be prevented by the proper use of such simple and cheap systems of communication.

Most divers rely on diving close to each other, with visual communication only. Variations, such as one diver leading the other or diving with a group, results in an antithesis of the buddy system – as there is no clear and complete responsibility of each diver for the other.

Chapter 6

DIVING ENVIRONMENTS

In this chapter, we review some of the problems of diving in various environments and some of the measures taken to reduce the dangers. Inexperienced divers are often oblivious to the potential hazards of special diving environments such as caves, kelp or surf.

We will present only a brief overview. Reference should be made to diving manuals and texts for further details (see Appendix A). Divers are advised to obtain expert tuition from diving organisations specialising in these environments, before they contemplate venturing into these diving areas.

WATER MOVEMENTS

Tidal Currents

Currents of several knots are commonly found in estuaries and ocean sites frequented by divers. These cannot be matched by the relatively puny swimming speeds achievable by a diver. For a short burst, a diver can manage about 1.5 knots, but a sustained speed of about 1.2 knots is the maximum which a fit diver can reach. For a relatively relaxed dive, a current of less than half a knot is acceptable. The problems posed by currents can be lessened by correct dive planning.

Firstly the diver needs to be aware that currents are a factor in the planned diving location. At other times they may be predicted by the tidal charts. This information is best obtained from local divers or maritime authorities. Currents can sometimes be identified by the behaviour of the dive boat at anchor.

The "Half Tank Rule". The best technique is to plan to swim into the current for the first half of the dive and use it to drift back to the boat during the second half. The dive is divided into halves on the basis of the air supply. After subtracting the air pressure to be used as a reserve, allow half the remaining gas for the swim into the current and return using the second half of the supply. In tidal areas, it is necessary to anticipate any change in direction as the tide turns, or both halves of the dive may be into current. The best time to dive in tidal areas is usually during slack water, between tides.

The **anchor line** can be used to advantage. It is much easier to make headway against a current by pulling along a rope or chain, than by swimming. If a rope is attached loosely to the anchor line at the surface and run around the side of the boat, divers can enter the water holding onto this and use it to pull themselves to the anchor line. By using the anchor line, divers can pull themselves down to within 2 metres of the bottom, where the current is often less strong. Avoid swimming onto or dislodging the anchor, which can cast the boat adrift or lift and injure the diver.

Another rope (a **floating** or **Jesus line**) should drift with the current from the back of the boat, for 50 metres or so. This should be supported at regular intervals by buoys or even plastic containers. This line has earned its name by "saving the sinners" who have missed the boat or surfaced down-current.

Another technique used in locations with strong currents is **drift diving**. Because of the fast currents, all equipment should be firmly attached and snagging on environmental hazards and other divers must be avoided. A **float** is towed to mark the diver's position and allow for signals to be sent to the surface craft. A rescue or pickup boat must drift with the divers and the current to another location, where the divers are hopefully recovered. The boat should have a **propeller guard** if it is to be used to rescue the divers. A waterproof **smoke flare** or a **"safety sausage"** (a long fluorescent inflatable plastic float) is a useful backup for a lost diver after an ocean or drift dive. A whistle can be used to attract attention.

Surge

In shallow water affected by waves, a **to-and-fro surge** which is too strong to swim against, may be encountered. This is best dealt with by gripping the bottom (with gloves) during the adverse surge, and moving with the favourable one. A diver contending with a powerful surge can become disoriented from the violent movement, injured from impact with rocks and can exacerbate the danger by panicking.

Surf

A surf entry without proper technique can be hazardous. The fully equipped diver presents a large vulnerable target to waves which can quickly divest him of essential equipment while engulfing him in unbreathable, non-buoyant foam.

The recommended technique of surf entry is to approach the water backwards after donning all equipment including fins before entry. The diver watches oncoming waves over his shoulder while keeping an eye on his buddy. Waves in shallow water should be met side-on to present the smallest surface area. The diver adopts a wide stance and leans into the wave. The fins and mask must be firmly attached as they are easily lost and the regulator is attached to the vest by a clip in a readily accessible position. The diver should descend and swim while breathing through the regulator as soon as possible. Thus he avoids turbulence by diving under oncoming waves.

Floats are towed behind the diver on entry, and pushed in front when returning. Exit is achieved by the opposite process and by using incoming waves to help with progress towards the beach.

ENTRAPMENT

A variety of ropes, cords, fishing lines, nets, kelp and other material can easily snare the diver or his bristling array of equipment. Entrapment of this type can be safely dealt with by a calm appraisal of the situation and a sharp knife. The limited field of view inherent with all face masks complicates these problems and makes the assistance of a buddy invaluable in tracing and untangling or cutting the causes of entrapment.

Kelp

This is a giant seaweed growing in forests from as deep as 30 metres to the surface. It has a long trunk with branching fronds near the surface. It occupies cooler waters and provides a fascinating but potentially dangerous diving environment. A good kelp diver is a slow diver.

A diver can easily become entangled and drowned in kelp, especially near the surface where the fronds are thickest and special diving techniques are necessary for safe kelp diving.

Divers help minimize projections, which cause entanglement, by wearing the knife on the inside of the leg, use flush-fitting buckles and tape over protruding equipment. The water is entered feet first and an attempt is made to push a hole in the kelp fronds, through which the diver passes. Divers should avoid twisting and turning in the kelp. The area near the bottom of the kelp causes the least likelihood of entanglement.

It is important to return to the surface with an ample reserve of air to ensure that the passage through the surface kelp is careful and unhurried. If entangled, be careful when cutting kelp stalks with a diameter similar to the regulator hose – you never know...

Enclosed Environments

Caves, wrecks, under-ice and even diving beneath large over-hangs are potentially hazardous environments which should not be entered without special training and equipment. The following outline is by no means comprehensive. Specialised training and equipment are needed.

❏ Caves.

A diver in a cave usually cannot return directly to the surface in the event of an equipment malfunction or emergency. Even without these problems, it is easy to become lost and be unable to find the surface before the air supply is exhausted. The main problems are – panic, loss of visibility and navigational difficulties. The roof of a cave may collapse after air (expired from scuba) replaces the previously supporting water

Caves are usually dark and lined with fine silt which is easily stirred into an opaque cloud by the use of fins. This is reduced with small fins, slow movements and avoiding the floors and roof. With silt, the natural or artificial illumination sources become valueless, reflecting the light back towards the diver.

All essential equipment and lights are duplicated. A compass is mandatory. Cave divers carry a spare tank and regulator attached to a manifold, with the spare regulator on a long hose so it can be used by another diver following in a narrow passage, if necessary. Totally separate emergency air supplies are recommended.

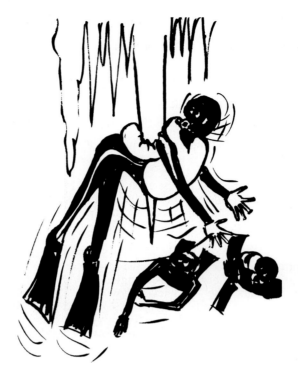

Fig. 6.1

Return to the entrance of the cave is marked by a line which is dispensed from a reel by the dive leader, who goes in first. This allows the way-out to be found by following the rope, away from the leader. Vertical passage to the surface is marked by a heavier shot line which is less likely to entangle the diver ascending in haste.

❑ Wrecks.

Wreck diving shares many of the problems of cave diving as well as presenting some unique problems. In many areas the enduring wrecks are deep, adding the risk of decompression sickness and nitrogen narcosis to the general hazards.

Wrecks frequently contain physically or chemically unstable cargo, toxic chemicals and unfriendly marine animals. Disturbed silt deep in a wreck and sharp jagged metal edges can make navigation through a labyrinth of ladders and passageways difficult. A compass may be of little help as the steel of the wrecks is often magnetised.

❑ Ice diving.

Diving under ice requires special equipment and know-how. It shares many of the hazards and precautions of cave diving but has the added complication of freezing conditions. Being trapped under ice can be an alarming experience for a diver with a frozen regulator. Reliance should not be placed in specialised "ice diving" regulators – in which the water is replaced by oil, alcohol or air. These can also freeze, especially on the surface using octopus regulators, and with overbreathing. Attention has also to be paid to the exit procedure, as holes can "ice-over" rapidly.

ENVIRONMENTAL VARIANTS

Cold Water

This can disrupt the performance of both the diver and his equipment. Diving in cold water requires the insulating qualities of a thick wet suit or dry suit, with gloves, boots and a hood. The wet suit, unfortunately, loses it efficiency when the insulating air layer is compressed with depth.

The cooling effect of compressed air expanding in the regulator, added to the low temperature of the water, makes freezing of the regulator a significant problem. Modified regulators which reduce these occurrences are available but cannot be relied upon.

Night Diving

This is not for everyone. The concept holds real fears for some divers who are perfectly comfortable diving in daylight. Because of the dangers of anxiety reactions and panic, night diving should be avoided by divers who are claustrophobic or feel excessively anxious at the prospect. The lack of visual cues can cause disorientation and imagination runs rife.

Lights well above the waterline, should be displayed on the boat and the shore exit. Torches should not be shone into a diver's face — it blinds him (destroys night vision) — but they may be directed to display one's own hand signals.

The problems centre around impaired visibility. Vision is dependent on artificial light which is very restricted and can easily fail. It is important for the night diver to be able to find and use all items of equipment by touch alone.

Detecting and rescuing divers who develop problems and surface some distance away, may be difficult. An emergency flare, strobe light or chemical light stick (e.g."cyalume") attached to the diver's tank valve is worthwhile carrying for this eventuality, as is a whistle.

Deep Diving

Dives deeper than 30 metres become associated with an increasing number of complications and inappropriate responses to these.

The endurance of the scuba air supply is severely limited at greater depths while the decompression requirements increases almost exponentially, adding a sense of urgency to the dive in the face of a diminishing reserve-air safety margin.

Decompression becomes obligatory for even short dives to depths in excess of 50 metres and requires the provision of extra air for this purpose. Unfortunately, the decompression tables, even if followed exactly, become less reliable as the depth increases, raising the possibility of serious decompression sickness even after a faultlessly executed dive.

Nitrogen narcosis can occur at less than 30 metres (100 ft.) and progressively impairs judgement, attention, perception and an appropriate response to adversity as the depth increases. At depths in excess of 45 metres (150 ft.) mental stability, cognition and judgement are seriously impaired.

Equipment becomes more difficult to manage at these depths. Breathing through the regulator becomes harder. The buoyancy compensator takes much longer to inflate and uses more of the limited air supply. Wet suit compression reduces its insulating properties at the same time as the diver passes into colder deep water. This compression also progressively decreases buoyancy.

The environment beyond 30 metres (100 ft.) is dark, colourless, cold, relatively devoid of marine life, and replete with physiological hazards. In spite of this, some recreational divers feel compelled to experience it, albeit briefly because of the limited air endurance.

The authors recommend that, in view of the increased hazards and the limited diving satisfaction available in deep dives, recreational divers regard 30 metres (100 ft.) as the maximum recommended safe depth. Uneventful dives beyond this depth often impart a false sense of capability – which is then shattered when one or more things go wrong. It is then that the effects of narcosis are demonstrated.

Altitude Diving

Diving in waters located above sea level (e.g. a mountain lake or dam) introduces some potential hazards which are not immediately obvious.

Consider a dive in a mountain lake where the atmospheric pressure is half that at sea level (this would be at an unlikely altitude of about 6000 metres or 18,000 ft. elevation, but makes the calculations easy). The pressure at the surface of the lake is that of the atmosphere, 0.5 ATA. Assume it is a salt water lake (fresh water is slightly less dense and so exerts slightly less pressure at a given depth).

The water in the lake will exert the same pressure at this altitude as it would at any other altitude.

That is, 10 metres of water will still exert a pressure of 1 ATA.

The pressure at 5 metres depth therefore will be 1 ATA, consisting of 0.5 ATA contributed by the atmospheric pressure, and 0.5 ATA contributed by the water.

The pressure at 10 metres will thus be 1.5 ATA.

One might think initially that this would give the diver a safety margin since the pressure at a given depth in a mountain lake is less than that in the ocean. The critical difference, however, is that the diver in the lake is returning to a lower surface pressure.

This can be illustrated by referring to one of Haldane's hypotheses (see Chapter 13). He observed that a diver could spend an unlimited time at 10 metres (2 ATA) and return to the surface (1 ATA) without developing decompression sickness. In other words, a diver could return to a pressure of half the original pressure (i.e. a 2 : 1 ratio) without developing nitrogen bubbles in the tissues.

In the mountain lake, because the surface pressure is only half that at sea level (0.5 ATA), the diver need dive to only 5 metres (1 ATA) and return to the surface to encounter the same 2 : 1 ratio. This makes dive tables designed for sea level unreliable at altitude unless considerable corrections are made.

Decompression at altitude is further complicated by difficulties in estimating depth. A depth gauge calibrated for sea level is likely to be unreliable at altitude. The gauge simply measures pressure and registers this as depth. Since the pressure at the surface of the lake is 0.5 ATA (half that of sea level), the gauge will be straining its mechanism and possibly bending the needle, trying to get its pointer past the zero stop to register what it interprets as negative depth. The gauge may only start to register a depth after it has returned to 1 ATA. This would not happen in the mountain lake until the water pressure and atmospheric pressure added up to 1 ATA – a depth of about 5 metres.

Even a capillary depth gauge, calibrated at sea level, will not really read accurately. At sea level, the air-to-water interface in the capillary will move half way along the capillary at 10 metres, since the pressure there is twice that at the surface. In the mountain lake with a surface pressure of 0.5 ATA, twice the surface pressure will be encountered at about 5 metres depth. So the capillary gauge will reach the "10 metre depth mark" (the half volume mark) at 5 metres.

The lower surface pressure also means that gas volume changes with depth are different. The gas in a diver's lungs will double in volume between 5 metres and the surface in the lake, instead of between 10 metres and the surface as would occur in the ocean. Ascent rates thus need to be reduced if barotrauma is not to increase. The gas expansion in a buoyancy vest will also be greater near the surface in the lake, which can lead to buoyancy changes unexpected by a diver used to ocean diving. If the lake is filled with fresh water, then many other buoyancy problems exist.

Flying after Diving

This creates similar problems to altitude diving. The decompression tables were calculated on the assumption that the diver would be returning to a pressure of 1 ATA. If the diver then goes to altitude either in an aircraft of on a high mountainous road, with nitrogen still in his tissues, bubble formation is more likely, and existing bubbles are liable to enlarge. Special "post diving flying rules" apply.

Diving in Freshwater and Dams

Buoyancy is less in freshwater than saltwater. Depth estimations and calculations are similarly disrupted (10 metres of seawater = 10.3 metres of freshwater). Freshwater is often still, and therefore develops dramatic thermoclines. Trees and other sources of entanglement tend to accumulate and not be destroyed as rapidly as in the sea. Some freshwater currents may cause difficulty. Chemical and sewerage pollution can be a major problem, and some specific freshwater organisms are very dangerous (Naegleria).

Dams have a specific problem with outflow below the surface. A diver may be unaware of the pressure gradient that can develop if part of the body covers an outflow orifice. Such a gradient will tether the diver underwater and may cause grotesque injuries as it forces the diver into and through the opening.

Chapter 7

STRESS DISORDERS, PANIC & FATIGUE

INTRODUCTION

The diving equipment and facilities of the 1950's and 1960's were often spartan and the divers were to some extent influenced by the difficulties produced by the equipment and the environment. Diving was not easy, safe or comfortable and only the dedicated were involved in the sport. The divers who survived were very capable and well adapted to the environment.

The advent of more user-friendly equipment, together with the general popularity of diving, has seen the acceptance of some divers who are less naturally suited to the environment. These divers are more prone to **stress syndromes** when confronted with some of the threatening aspects of the marine world.

Some of the factors influencing the divers ability to cope with the diving equipment and environment will now be considered.

PERSONALITY FACTORS

Some personalities are better suited to scuba diving than others.

Military diving requires exacting physical and psychological standards and this is reflected in the high failure rate, generally about 50%. Many professional diving courses have a similar requirement and failure rate. This prompted researchers to look at the personality characteristics of successful trainees in an attempt to select out those who were not suitable.

In general, successful military divers were psychologically stable, not anxious about the dangers of diving, intelligent, practical, physically fit, self sufficient, good swimmers, capable and confident at water sports.

There is little data available for features which characterise successful and safe recreational divers. While the exacting requirements of a military diver probably are not as necessary, it would seem likely that similar characteristics would be shared by both groups.

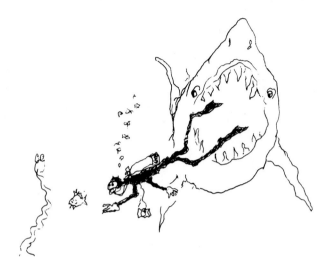

Fig. 7.1

Although there is a high failure rate with military and commercial diving courses, the failure rate in many amateur diving courses is close to zero. The standards set by some diving organisations is a source of grave concern, as it is possible that they may be overly influenced by commercial considerations. Between 5–15% of deaths in recreational divers occur while under training.

STRESS RESPONSES

We all have an inbuilt automatic response to threats in the environment. This involves activation of the nervous system which prepares the body to confront the challenge or flee – the so called **"fight or flight"** response.

With this response, the sympathetic nervous system releases adrenalin into the body, stimulating the heart, increasing blood flow to the muscles, alerting the brain and stimulating respiration. For example, a person suddenly confronted by a mugger is automatically primed to fight or run away. If the mugger is armed, the intellect usually considers the safest option and a decision to quietly hand over money may be taken. This is an intellectual decision appropriate for survival and overrides the autonomic response.

Some divers may respond to certain levels of stress in ways inappropriate to survival. These potentially dangerous stress responses are :

- **Panic** – a psychological stress reaction caused by excessive anxiety
- **Fatigue** – a physical stress response to exertion
- **Sudden Death Syndrome** – a lethal cardiac response to excessive stress (see Chapter 35).

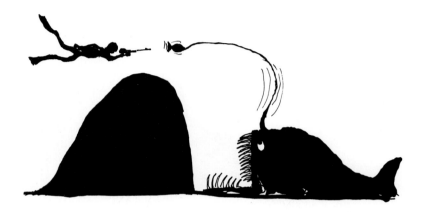

Fig. 7.2

Panic

Panic is probably the most common cause of death in recreational scuba diving. Studies have implicated panic as a contributor to between 40–80% of such diving deaths.

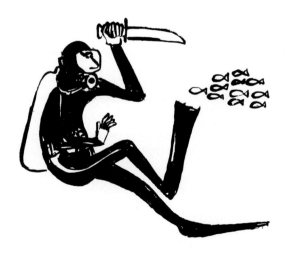

Fig. 7.3

Panic is an extreme and inappropriate response to a real or imagined threat. Behavioural control becomes lost. Some readers will have experienced, or been near to, panic in some real life situations.

In general, the more naturally anxious a diver is, the more likely he is to panic.

As panic develops, the capacity to think rationally and solve the emerging problem deteriorates. The diver becomes more and more narrow minded and eventually may focus on only one goal e.g. reaching the surface – to the exclusion of other vital factors, such as exhaling during ascent.

Factors which upset a diver's emotional equilibrium can contribute to panic. Some of these **contributing factors include** :

Personal Factors	Equipment Problems
❑ Fatigue	❑ Buoyancy
❑ Physical unfitness or disability	❑ Snorkel
❑ Previous medical disorders	❑ Face Mask
❑ Seasickness and/or vomiting	❑ Weight Belt
❑ Alcohol or drugs	❑ Wet Suit
❑ Inexperience	❑ Scuba Cylinder
❑ Inadequate dive plan	❑ Regulator
❑ Dangerous techniques e.g. buddy breathing, free ascents	❑ Low or Out-of-Air Situations
❑ Psychological problems e.g. excessive general anxiety, phobias	❑ Other Equipment
❑ Sensory deprivation – night diving, blue orb syndrome, solo diving	❑ Excessive reliance on equipment e.g. B.C.s
❑ Vertigo and or disorientation	❑ Loss of equipment e.g.face mask or fins
❑ Diving accidents	❑ Misuse of Equipment e.g. B.C. to overcome excess weights
	❑ Entrapment in lines, nets, harness etc.

Environmental Hazards
❑ Tidal currents
❑ Entry or exit problems
❑ White water e.g. surf
❑ Kelp
❑ Caves, wrecks
❑ Ice and cold water
❑ Deep diving – nitrogen narcosis, rapid air consumption, reduced buoyancy
❑ Dangerous marine animals
❑ Poor visibility
❑ Explosives
❑ Boat accidents

Consider the following scene, which has been gleaned from several diving fatalities, to illustrate some of the factors contributing to a panic-related death.

Case history.

Harry was a recently qualified diver who had *borrowed* equipment to undertake an open ocean dive in an *unfamiliar* area. His borrowed wetsuit was a little *tight* around his chest, restricting his breathing.

He decided to use two *extra weights* on his weight belt to help him descend in the ocean conditions, which were somewhat foreign to him. He was *inexperienced* at open ocean diving and the conditions were regarded as marginal so he felt a little *uneasy* about the dive.

His companions were more experienced than him and he was unsure of his ability to make his *air supply* last as long as his buddies. After all, he did not want to be the first to run out of air and force his buddies to shorten their dive.

During the dive he was sure he was using more air than the others but he had no way of checking this as his borrowed scuba set did not have a *contents gauge* .

He became a little more *apprehensive*. They seemed to have swum a long way both from the dive boat and the shore. But he did not want to *inconvenience* his buddy or *embarrass* himself by ascending and checking his distance from shore or inquire about his buddies air supply. He had no idea how much air he had left but he felt that there probably wasn't much.

He became a little more *anxious* and his *breathing rate* increased. He noted some *restriction* to breathing. Was this just *resistance in his regulator* or was he now running out of air?

He activated his reserve valve. Perhaps this would improve the restricted gas flow. It didn't.

There was a tidal current running, which slowed their progress to the planned end of the dive – the safe exit point.

He was hoping that his companions were also running *out of air*, as he appeared to be.

He was becoming more *anxious*. His heart was pounding and his *breathing rate* was increasing. It was becoming harder to get sufficient air from his demand valve.

The difficulty in obtaining enough air settled the matter. He decided to get to the *surface*, fast. In spite of his rapid ascent, he still did not seem to be getting more air from his demand valve. He must be out of gas.

He burst through the surface, gasping for breath. He wrenched off his *face mask* and *demand valve* and gasped air.

The water was choppy and waves washed over his face. He kicked hard with his *fins* to stay on the surface. One of the ill-fitting borrowed fins came off. A wave washed over his face and he *inhaled water* and started coughing. It was a real *struggle* to stay on the surface, he was becoming *exhausted*. He wondered how long he could keep this up. He tried to keep his head well above the waves, but could not.

His buddy noticed he was missing and after a brief search, surfaced. Harry was no where to be seen. An organised search later found his body on the bottom, immediately below where he had surfaced.

His *weight belt* was still fastened, his *buoyancy vest* uninflated. There was ample air in his cylinder and testing of his demand valve revealed normal functioning, but demonstrating the usual resistance with high gas flows.

The autopsy report read **"drowning"**. The **real cause was "death from panic"**.

The story illustrates some of the factors which combined to develop the anxiety which leads to panic and illustrates the irrational responses in a panicked diver. An appropriate response at any one of the steps that lead to the disaster, would have prevented or relieved the situation.

❏ Prevention.

If anxiety is an important precursor to panic, reducing anxiety is an effective counter measure. The most effective way to reduce anxiety is to have confidence in, and familiarity with, the task. This is achieved by **knowledge, training** and repeated **practice** of diving and safety procedures.

A good example is seen in the training of commercial airline pilots. They are required to fly a minimum number of hours per month and to practice and demonstrate emergency procedures at six monthly intervals. They spend many hours practicing emergency drills in a flight simulator. The usually cool and appropriate performance of these professionals in emergencies is a testimony to this approach.

Another important preventive measure is for the diver to know his **limitations** and to stay within them. A diver may be comfortable, confident and competent in one diving situation but not in another. The first allows for safe diving, the second for a panic scenario.

Fatigue

Studies of recreational diver deaths show that **fatigue contributes to about 28% of cases.** This fatigue comes about from a combination of personal, equipment and environmental factors.

❏ Personal.

A high level of physical fitness is an important survival factor in diving. Even the calmest water dive can degenerate into a situation requiring maximal physical exertion due to unforeseen circumstances, such as currents, rescue requirements, etc.

During severe exertion, fatigue and its associated apathy will come sooner to physically unfit divers. Also, fatigue is experienced sooner by anxious or neurotic divers.

As a general rule, scuba divers should be able to swim 200 metres in under 4 minutes, without any equipment. A fit diver will complete this in 3.5 minutes and a very unfit diver may take over 5 minutes.

❏ Equipment.

Much of the diver's equipment, the buoyancy compensator, tank, facemask, and wet-suit either increases resistance to swimming or restricts movement. Excessive weights make swimming more strenuous. Even the best regulators have significant resistance to airflow at high flow rates, significantly restricting breathing. All these factors accelerate fatigue.

❏ Environment.

Fully equipped, a diver cannot swim for long against a current of more than about 1 knot. Rough water and cold exposure will further aggravate this.

Chapter 8

THE FEMALE DIVER

Up to the 1960's, diving was almost exclusively a male domain with a certain associated macho image. Since then, an increasing proportion of female divers have come to enjoy this sport and have proven themselves equal to male divers in every regard.

Despite this, women are not the same as men and there are important consequences of this dissimilarity in diving activities.

History of Women in Diving

Probably the most famous of female diver groups are the **Ama** shell divers of Japan and Korea. These divers were originally men but the work was taken over by women, possibly because of their better tolerance to cold – the men only dived in summer while women were able to dive all year round. Another theory is that the men believed that diving impaired their virility.

The Ama underwent some remarkable physiological adaptations. During the winter months, they increased their metabolic rate by 30%, which allowed them to generate more internal heat. Also, they reduced their skin blood flow by 30%. The fat content beneath their skin was increased, which improved insulation.

There have been numerous famous women diving personalities. In the 1940's, Simone Cousteau dived alongside her husband Jacques Cousteau. In Australia, Valerie Taylor and Eva Cropp became well known because of their diving exploits. In America, Eugenie Clark was known as the 'shark lady' because of her brilliant work in this field. In 1969, Sylvia Earle led the first all woman team of aquanauts in the Tektite II habitat experiment.

Until recent years diving instruction was almost exclusively a male occupation. Many of these instructors basked in a 'superman' role and possessed more experience than knowledge.

In recent years women have become professional diving instructors and have proven to be diligent and highly competent. In general they have been more keen to impress their students by knowledge and skills, rather than strength and bravado.

Women divers must be doing something right. Diving statistics show that while women number about one in three trainees, they account for only one in ten recreational diving deaths.

Scuba Training

Womankind has been described as the "weaker sex." While it is generally true that women are less physically strong than men, there is not a vast difference in their performance in aquatic sports. For example, in the 1988 Olympics there was only a 10–12% difference in times between women and men for swimming events.

In Western society, women are generally regarded as being less mechanically and mathematically adept than men. This prejudice is reflected in attitudes to diver training. In many cases, women are patronised by well-meaning male instructors and companions.

Until recently, culturally acquired lack of assertiveness on the part of many women led them to refrain from asking what appeared to them to be naive questions of their instructors. On the other hand, prejudices by instructors led them to assume women would not be interested in, or understand, the intricacies of equipment functioning or decompression planning. This information tended to be directed towards the males in a training group. Women would often turn to a male friend or buddy rather than the instructor for answers to questions which arose during training. The information that they received was not always accurate.

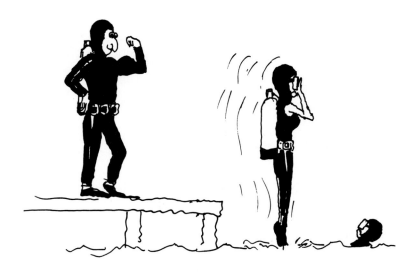

Fig. 8.1

The old stereotype of the woman in a dependent role can lead to problems in diving practice. Thus men and women who are buddied together can become an unsafe combination.

A woman who has her equipment assembled and checked by a male companion, who had the equipment carried to the water and who was assisted into and out of the water, is overall less likely to become a competent and self sufficient diver.

Anatomical Differences

For the same physical size, men have greater physical strength than women. This is because men have a greater muscle mass per unit body weight. This minor difference in strength is not a significant disadvantage in the weightless aquatic environment.

Being physically smaller, the woman has a lower requirement for oxygen at a given level of physical activity and will produce less carbon dioxide. With smaller lungs, women also take smaller breaths. Thus, women can often manage with less air than a male diving companion and so can use a smaller, lighter scuba cylinder. This can offset the apparent disadvantage of diminished size and strength.

Because of differences in body shape, women have different equipment design requirements. There can be difficulty in obtaining appropriate sized wet suits, fins, boots, and gloves.

Particular problems arise with male sized equipment, especially face masks which may not fit well, and large scuba cylinders which are unnecessarily bulky or heavy. Backpacks can be too long and so cover the weight belt, making the release of the belt in an emergency difficult. Standard sized buoyancy compensators may give excessive buoyancy and drag.

Thermal Variations

Women are better insulated than their male counterparts. They have a fat layer beneath the skin some 25% greater then men. They also have a better ability to constrict the blood flow to their limbs, reducing heat loss.

These factors allow women to conserve their heat more effectively in a cold water environment while producing natural buoyancy, which improves their swimming and floating ability.

Menstruation

During menstruation, the average woman is likely to loose 50–150cc blood and cellular debris. There are some physical and physiological consequences of menstruation which will be discussed, but usually there is no reason why women should not dive during menstruation.

For convenience, most women today prefer to wear internal protection such as tampons rather then menstrual pads. In the early days, there was some concern that menstrual blood-loss may act as an attractant to sharks. In fact, females have a much lower incidence of shark attacks than males.

Hormonal changes before and during menstruation tend to cause fluid retention and swelling. There is a theoretical possibility that this might encourage the development of decompression sickness. There is no experimental data to support this conjecture, but it may be wise for women, during this time, to add a safety margin to their decompression requirements.

Some women have significant psychological and physical problems around the time of menstruation, with abdominal pain, muscle cramps, headaches, nausea and vomiting. These may impair their diving ability. Women who suffer from severe problems of this nature, are advised to avoid diving at this time. The psychological disturbances associated with severe pre-menstrual tension and anxiety, may sometimes warrant the avoidance of diving during this time also.

Some female migraine sufferers, have an increased likelihood of migraines around the time of menstruation. The problems associated with migraine are discussed further in Chapter 32 and the recommendations should be followed.

Oral Contraceptives
(the "Pill")

The physiological and psychological consequences of these hormonal tablets may have similar implications to those described above, under "menstruation". In theory, the increased coagulation effects from the pill could initiate or aggravate decompression sickness. In practice this has not been observed. It was considered prudent to cease oral contraceptives in the female team who undertook a long saturation dive during the Tektite No. 2 project. However, the absence of males probably made this decision an uncomplicated one.

Decompression Sickness

Several studies have shown an increased incidence of decompression sickness in women. In the U.S. Air Force, women exposed to altitude chambers had a fourfold incidence of decompression sickness compared with men. A study of women divers showed a 3.3 times increased incidence of decompression sickness compared with men who were exposed to the same dive profile. To place this in perspective, however, the incidence of decompression sickness in this study was only 0.033%. There was no relationship found between the development of decompression sickness and the stage of the menstrual cycle or the taking of oral contraceptive tablets.

The U.S. Navy Diving Training Centre studies have shown no increased incidence of decompression sickness amongst females, but the numbers were small and an increased bubble incidence conflicted with the decreased decompression sickness incidence.

The weight of **evidence** does tend to **suggest** that there might be an **increased** incidence of **decompression sickness among women.** There are several possible explanations for this.

Women are frequently less physically fit than men. Women usually have a higher proportion of body fat for a given weight than men, and the body fat has a high capacity for absorbing nitrogen. Both these factors increase the incidence of decompression sickness .

Navy decompression tables were designed for and tested on physically fit, healthy young male divers. Strictly speaking, the tables should only apply to this population.

Because of this increased risk, it is wise for women divers to apply extra safety factors when using the dive tables : e.g. by reducing the allowable bottom time for any depth or by decompressing for a greater duration.

A modern decompression problem has emerged with **breast implants**. Fortunately, gas filled implants are no longer used, as the barotrauma consequences of diving with these would be horrendous. However, even silicone filled implants do absorb nitrogen during a dive and a 4% expansion in the size of these implants has been recorded after dive profiles commonly used by women sports divers. This is not likely to cause a problem with the implants. However, if these women were involved in saturation diving there is the potential for significant volume changes which could lead to rupture of the implant or tissue damage during or after ascent.

PREGNANCY

There has been considerable controversy over whether pregnant women should dive. This question often arises as most women divers are in the child-bearing age group. The controversy hinges on the conflict between restricting the freedom of an individual and the risks (which have not been fully evaluated) to the unborn child. The potential problems of diving during pregnancy are as follows :

Maternal Effects

❏ Vomiting.

In the second and third months of pregnancy, many women are prone to vomiting – often manifest as "morning sickness". They are more prone to seasickness and to nausea and vomiting underwater during certain conditions. This predisposes to serious diving accidents.

❏ Barotrauma.

From the fourth month onwards, fluid retention and swelling of the lining of the respiratory tract, makes sinus and ear equalisation more difficult and predisposes to barotrauma.

❏ Respiratory function.

There is a progressive decline in respiratory function as pregnancy progresses. There is an increase in resistance to air flow in the lungs. Later, the enlarging baby presses up into the chest, limiting breathing capacity. This combination impairs the pregnant woman's ability to cope with strenuous activity which may be required in an emergency, and may predispose to hypoxia or pulmonary barotrauma.

❏ Decompression sickness.

There are major alterations in blood volume and circulation during pregnancy. This may increase the uptake and distribution of nitrogen and may make the woman more prone to decompression sickness.

❏ Infection.

In the later stages of pregnancy some women develop minor leaks of the amniotic sac, which surrounds the baby with fluid. There is a possibility of infection of this fluid from organisms entering from the water before birth or directly into the womb after birth.

Effects on the Baby

The developing foetus is uniquely at risk from some of the physiological hazards associated with diving.

❏ Development of the foetus.

The foetus begins as a single cell organism and up until after the fourth month it is smaller than a mouse. A small bubble, such as develops during decompression sickness, can then have catastrophic effects.

The **circulation of the foetus** is unique and critical. In an adult diver, venous blood returning from the body passes through the lung capillaries, which filter out the bubbles frequently formed during or after ascent. In the foetus, the blood by-passes the lungs (since the foetus does not need to breathe) and passes directly to the heart without passing first through this filtering network. Even one bubble forming in the veins of a foetus will then be transported directly to the arterial circulation and will embolise to somewhere in its body.

❑ Hypoxia.

The outcome of many non fatal diving incidents is hypoxia, most likely to be caused by salt water aspiration or near drowning. The pregnant diver will not only expose herself to hypoxia in this situation but will also expose the much more susceptible foetus to this.

❑ Hyperbaric oxygen.

Divers are likely to be exposed to hyperbaric oxygen in two situations. By simply breathing compressed air at depth they are inhaling elevated partial pressures of oxygen. In addition, if divers develops decompression sickness or air embolism they will be given hyperbaric oxygen therapy for treatment of the condition.

Some foetal tissues are very sensitive to high partial pressures of oxygen. Great care is taken with newborn premature babies to avoid administration of high concentrations of oxygen because of the danger of retrolental fibroplasia, which causes blindness. The eye of the unborn baby is probably equally sensitive to high partial pressures of oxygen.

The circulation of the foetus contains a channel (the ductus arteriosus) which allows blood to by-pass the lungs. This channel closes after birth under the influence of a raised partial pressure of oxygen in the blood. There is a danger of premature closing of this and other shunts if the foetus is exposed to hyperbaric oxygen because of treatment given to the mother.

❑ Decompression sickness.

As mentioned earlier, women are more susceptible to decompression sickness and there are theoretical reasons to believe that pregnant women are even more susceptible. It is known from doppler studies that showers of bubbles are regularly formed in the veins of divers ascending from many routine non-decompression dives. These bubbles do not usually cause any symptoms.

Some experiments in pregnant animals suggest that the foetus is more resistant to bubble formation than the mother but that bubbles do form after some dives, especially those deeper than 20 metres. Because of the unique circulation of the foetus even a few bubbles in the foetal circulation can have disastrous consequences.

Experiments with pregnant animals have produced conflicting results. One study on pregnant sheep (which have a placenta similar to a human) showed that the foetus developed bubbles in its circulation even after dives of less than 30 metres (100 ft.) within the US Navy no-decompression limits. These results are disturbing when considering the vulnerability of the foetus to any bubble.

Other studies have shown an increased incidence of abortion, birth defects and still-births in pregnant animals after decompression.

Exposure to hyperbaric oxygen has also been shown in some studies to cause birth abnormalities and death.

Human Data

Japanese female divers, the Ama, often dive until late pregnancy, and have a 44% incidence of premature delivery with a high incidence of small babies when compared with non-diving women from the same area.

Margaret Boulton from the University of Florida carried out a survey on 208 women who dived during pregnancy. She found an increased incidence of abortion, still-birth, low birth weight and death of the infant within the first month. Of the 24 women who reported diving to 30 metres (100 ft.) or more, three had children with congenital defects. This contrasts with an incidence of 1 in 50 in the general population. One of the infants had an absent hand, a very rare abnormality.

An Australian case report suggested that the effects of diving may be similar to Thalidomide during pregnancy.

It is difficult to draw firm conclusions from these studies because the numbers are too low for statistical validation. They are however consistent with many of the animal studies.

The Bottom Line ---

There is considerable evidence suggesting that diving during pregnancy is harmful to the foetus. It is generally accepted that unnecessary drugs, alcohol and smoking should be avoided during pregnancy because of the risk to the foetus and we recommend a similar conservative approach to diving. The sacrifice of not diving during pregnancy may be easier to cope with than the guilt, valid or not, of giving birth to a malformed child.

One interesting issue to consider by women who contemplate diving during pregnancy is that the foetus, who will have to live with any birth defect which may result, cannot be consulted when the decision to dive is made.

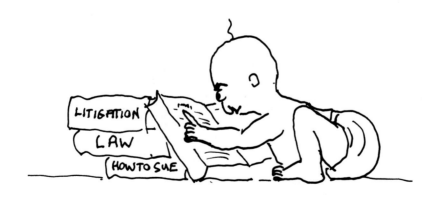

Fig. 8.2

Chapter 9

EAR BAROTRAUMA

ANATOMY OF THE EAR

The ear is divided anatomically into the outer, the middle and the inner ear.

The **Outer Ear** comprises the visible part of the ear (the pinna) and the ear canal. The pinna gathers sound waves and reflects them into the ear canal and onto the ear drum.

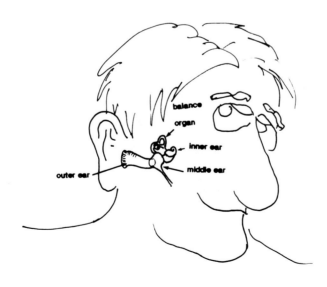

Fig. 9.1

The **Middle Ear** is a pea sized cavity enclosed in a solid bony part of the skull. It is separated from the ear canal by the paper thin **ear drum**. There are several structures opening into the middle ear space.

  • The **Eustachian Tube** joins the middle ear with the throat, allowing air to enter the middle ear cavity.

  • The **Mastoid Sinus** (air pockets in the mastoid bone) also come off the middle ear.

There are two openings on the inner bony surface of the middle ear space called the **Round** and **Oval Windows,** because of their shape. These openings connect the middle to the inner ear. The oval window is a tough membrane attached to the end of one of the three interconnecting middle ear bones (ossicles), while the round window is closed by a thin delicate membrane.

The **Ear Drum (or Tympanic Membrane)** is connected by the three tiny ear bones - the malleus, incus and stapes - to the oval window across the middle ear space. This bony chain, which is barely visible to the naked eye, transmits the sound vibrations from the ear drum to the inner ear.

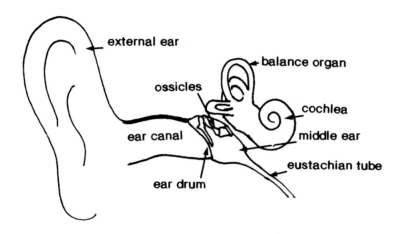

Fig. 9.2

The **Inner Ear** contains the **Hearing** and **Balance** organs. It is entirely encased in bone and filled with fluid. The hearing organ (the **Cochlea**) is a spiral shaped structure containing fluid which surrounds nerve cells sensitive to sound vibrations.

A system of **3 semi–circular canals** is also filled with fluid, and is the balance organ which is sensitive to position and movement. It is also called the **Vestibular System (or Vestibular Apparatus).**

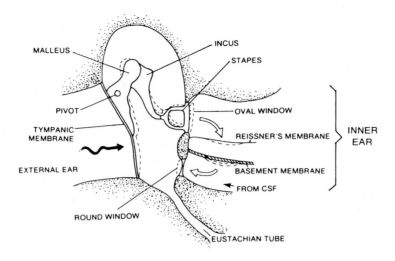

Fig. 9.3
Middle ear communications with External and Inner ear.

THE MECHANISM OF HEARING

The hearing system works in an ingenious way. Sound vibrations, reflected by the outer ear, are directed down the ear canal causing the ear drum, at the end of the ear canal, to vibrate. These vibrations are transmitted and magnified by the bony chain system of levers, to the oval window.

They are then converted to pressure waves in the cochlea fluid. As the fluid is incompressible, so the inward movement of the oval window is compensated by the round window bulging out.

The cochlea is tuned so that vibrations of various frequencies resonate in specific areas, allowing the ear to distinguish between differing frequencies of sound. This stimulates nerve fibres within the cochlea and the impulses are perceived as sound when they reach the brain.

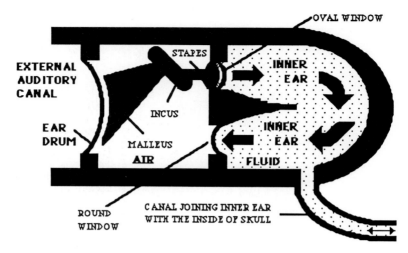

Fig. 9.4
Schematic drawing of Inner Ear with Round and Oval Windows.

MIDDLE EAR BAROTRAUMA OF DESCENT

(MIDDLE EAR SQUEEZE, AEROTITIS MEDIA)

The main risk of barotrauma to the ears is encountered on descent and the commonest site is the middle ear. About one quarter of diving trainees experience this, to a variable degree.

Water pressure around the diver increases as he descends. This pressure is transmitted to the body fluids and tissues surrounding the middle ear space causing compression of the gas space in the middle ear (Boyle's Law). The diver is aware of this and compensates for the reduction in gas volume by **"equalising the ear"** or **"clearing"**. In this manoeuvre air is blown up the Eustachian tube to replace the volume of gas compressed in the middle ear space. The ways of doing this are described later.

If the diver fails to equalise, water pressure will force the ear drum inwards, stretching it and causing a sensation of pressure. At the same time, reduced gas volume in the middle ear is compensated by blood and tissue fluid, swelling the lining of the middle ear space. Ultimately, the blood vessels become over distended and rupture, bleeding into the middle ear space. This tissue damage takes days or weeks to resolve. Sometimes the ear drum itself will tear or rupture.

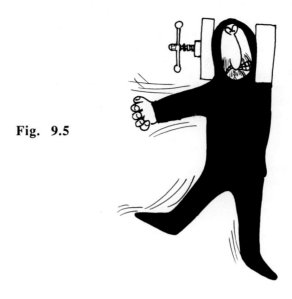

Fig. 9.5

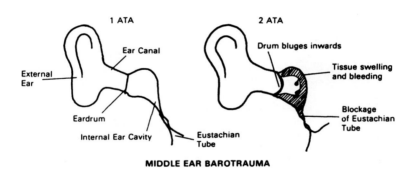

MIDDLE EAR BAROTRAUMA

Fig. 9.6
If equalisation does not occur, the middle ear space
is partly filled with blood and swollen tissues.

The depth at which this damage occurs depends on the size of the middle ear space and the flexibility of the ear drum. It is normally reached at 1–2 metres and if the diver does not equalise by the time he has reached this depth, barotrauma of the ear is likely.

Clinical Features

A sensation of **pressure** is the first symptom of damage or impending damage to the ear. This pressure sensation may develop into **pain**, which is usually severe, sharp and localised to the affected side. It increases as the diver descends, unless he equalises the middle ear spaces.

If the diver continues descending until the **ear drum ruptures**, he will experience relief of the pressure or pain, followed by a **cold feeling** in the ear. This is due to the sea-water which enters the middle ear space, cooling the bone and tissues near the balance organ. Thermal currents may be produced within the balance organ, causing stimulation and dizziness. Cold sea-water may also be noted trickling down the throat, running down the Eustachian tube from the middle ear space after rupture of the drum.

Ear barotrauma, especially when associated with rupture of the ear drum, may be accompanied by **dizziness.** This sensation is termed **vertigo**. It may also be accompanied by **nausea** and **vomiting**. Vomiting underwater is a skill not frequently practised and it can disrupt the air supply and lead to aspiration and drowning.

With lesser degrees of barotrauma, pain or discomfort in the ear may be felt after the dive. There is often a **feeling of fullness** (or "water") in the ear and sounds may appear muffled. Crackling sounds may also be noticed (especially with chewing, swallowing or jaw movements), caused by bubbles of air in blood/body fluid mixtures within the middle ear.

Occasionally blood from the middle ear is forced down the Eustachian tube when the middle ear gas expands on ascent. After surfacing the diver may notice **small amounts of blood** coming from the nose or mouth.

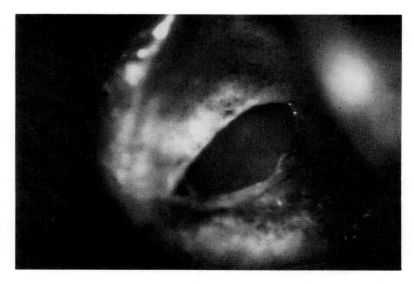

Fig. 9.7
Large perforation of ear drum from a single dive
to 8 metres without adequate equalisation.

Other symptoms due to the ear barotrauma include – a **"squeaking"** sound during equalisation, an **echo** sensation and a mild ache and tenderness over the ear/mastoid area following the dive.

Occasionally a diver has a naturally reduced pain appreciation, so that considerable barotrauma damage can be done despite the absence of much discomfort. These divers are very vulnerable. Others can suffer significant damage after exposure to small pressures, e.g. in a swimming pool – especially if the submersion and pressure exposure is for many minutes duration.

Treatment

A diver who has experienced middle ear barotrauma needs an examination by a diving **physician** to diagnose the condition, and check for complications such as a perforated eardrum or inner ear damage. Assessment of the cause, and advice on prevention of future difficulties is important (see later). **Audiograms** (hearing tests) are essential to test for damage to, and function of, the middle and inner ears.

Occasionally, the doctor may prescribe an oral **decongestant (or nasal spray)** to help open the Eustachian tube, while **antibiotics** may be prescribed if **infection** is present in the nose or throat area, or develops in the blood in the middle ear cavity. This usually presents as a recurrence of pain hours or days after the barotrauma. **Ear drops** do not reach the middle ear and of no value.

Once serious complications have been excluded, active treatment is usually unnecessary. In order to rest the ear and allow healing, diving, flying and middle ear equalisation should be avoided until the barotrauma has resolved. This commonly takes from 1–2 days up to 1–2 weeks.

The length of time away from diving depends on the severity of the barotrauma. The diver should not return to diving or flying until the physician has confirmed resolution of the barotrauma and the ability to equalise the ears. If the ear drum was **perforated**, complete cure may take 1–3 months, even though it may appear to have sealed over within days. Early return to diving predisposes to re-perforation. Occasionally the drum fails to heal and requires surgical "patching" or "grafting" by a specialist. Later, diving may be permitted if repair is complete and easy equalisation of the ear is possible.

It is frequently necessary with the development of symptoms, to perform repeat audiograms to confirm that no inner ear damage has occurred.

INNER EAR BAROTRAUMA

A serious consequence of ear barotrauma is inner ear (hearing and balance organ) damage. The inner ear can be damaged in several ways.

❑ Round window fistula (or "leak").

If the diver fails to equalise the middle ear adequately, water pressure will bulge the eardrum inwards. Since the eardrum is connected to the oval window by the bony chain, this window is forced inwards and the round window bulges outwards. If these movements are excessive, the small end-bone can be pushed through the oval window or, more commonly, the round window may tear. After these injuries, the window may then leak the inner ear fluid (perilymph) into the middle ear.

Round window fistula may also be associated with a **forceful middle ear equalisation manoeuvre**. Increased intravascular pressures in the head associated with this manoeuvre may be transmitted to the cochlea fluid, causing bulging and then rupture of the round window. Alternatively, the sudden displacement of the eardrum after an equalisation manoeuvre may set up a pressure wave in the inner ear fluid which tears the round window.

The fluid which leaks out is crucial to the healthy function of the **cochlea** and its loss leads to damage to the hearing organ. If the fluid loss is not interrupted by healing of the round window or surgical repair, permanent severe **hearing loss** may follow.

The same fluid also bathes the balance organ, and damage to this organ results in **dizziness (vertigo), nausea and vomiting.**

❑ Other pathology.

Permanent hearing loss or balance disturbance, unrelated to round window fistula, can be caused by direct cochlea damage from inner ear barotrauma. The cause may be haemorrhage (or bleeding), inner ear membrane rupture, or air entering the inner ear (from a stretched round window). This hearing loss may be temporary or permanent depending on the degree of damage and its management.

Clinical Features

The cardinal features of inner ear barotrauma are :

- **tinnitus** (ringing or buzzing noises in the ears)
- **hearing loss**
- **vertigo** (a feeling of rotation, rocking or unsteadiness)
- nausea and vomiting
- rarely, **dysacusis** (painful hearing)

One or more of these must be present to make the diagnosis. Fluid may be noted in the middle ear.

Tinnitus is a ringing, buzzing or musical sound in the ear, usually high pitched, due to damage or irritation of the nerve cells of the cochlea.

Hearing loss is due to damage of the cochlea. It may improve, stay the same or deteriorate. Audiograms may differentiate this type of hearing loss from that due to middle ear barotrauma (see Chapter 30).

Vertigo is the spinning sensation due to balance organ damage (see Chapter 31).

Treatment

A diver presenting with any of these symptoms needs **immediate assessment** by a diving physician.

The physician will examine the ear and perform **serial audiograms** to detect any hearing loss, which may not be obvious to the diver. **Tests** of **balance organ function (ENGs)** may be necessary.

Aspirin, nicotinic acid, other vasodilators or anti-coagulants should not be taken.

An expert diving medical opinion concerning **future diving** should be sought if the diver has sustained permanent hearing loss, tinnitus or balance disturbance, as it is probable that further episodes of inner ear barotrauma will cause additional and possibly permanent disastrous effects.

❑ Round window fistula.

This condition can usually be managed conservatively with **absolute bed rest in the sitting position.** Straining, sneezing, nose blowing, loud noise and middle ear equalising should be avoided, to prevent pressure waves in the inner ear.

The round window fistula often heals spontaneously within a week or so with this regimen but if hearing loss progresses or the other features persist, it may be necessary to resort to **surgery** to patch the round window leak.

Once an oval or round window fistula or cochlea injury has healed, the diver's future in this sport is bleak. Flying should be completely avoided for a period of 3 months to allow complete healing of the injury or the surgical repair.

❑ Cochlea damage.

In the absence of a round window fistula, no specific treatment is available for this type of injury. Rest, avoidance of equalisation attempts, and further exposure to barotrauma (flying or diving) is necessary until the condition has stabilised.

PREVENTION OF BAROTRAUMA

Equalisation

Adequate equalisation of pressures in the middle ear space will prevent middle and inner ear barotrauma. This equalisation is necessary whenever increasing depth in the water. It should be performed frequently and before ear discomfort is felt. It is necessary to equalise more frequently near the surface since the volume changes are greatest there (as explained by Boyle's Law). Equalisation should always be gentle to avoid damage. The technique of ear equalisation is a skill which improves with practice. Some divers can equalise without any apparent effort or action.

Upper respiratory tract infections (URTIs) cause congestion of the throat and Eustachian tube openings, making equalisation difficult or impossible. **Hay fever, allergies or cigarette smoking** have a similar effect. Diving with these conditions is risky. A deviated nasal septum may also predispose to aural barotrauma as well as sinus barotrauma (see Chapter 10).

There are several ways of active and voluntary middle ear equalising before and during descent :

❑ Valsalva manoeuvre.

This technique is most frequently used because it is easy and effective. The diver **holds his nose, closes his mouth and blows gently against the closed nose and mouth.** This raises the pressure in the pharynx, forcing air up the Eustachian tubes into the middle ear.

If there is infected material in the throat this can also be blown up the Eustachian tube into the middle ear, leading to **infection.** This is another reason why divers are advised against diving with an upper respiratory tract infection.

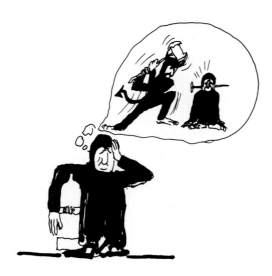

Fig. 9.8

To supplement this manoeuvre, **opening of the Eustachian tubes** can be facilitated by wriggling the jaw from side to side or thrusting the lower jaw forward as the manoeuvre is performed (**Edmonds first technique**).

A drawback of the Valsalva technique is that if it employed too forcefully, it is theoretically possible that damage to the inner ear may result. Another drawback is that the nose must be held closed with the fingers, which is not always easy with some professional diving helmets or full-face masks.

❏ The Toynbee manoeuvre.

This involves **holding the nose and swallowing simultaneously**. This usually causes the Eustachian tubes to open momentarily, allowing air to enter the middle ear.

The Eustachian tubes open only briefly with this manoeuvre and it causes a negative pressure in the pharynx, so only smaller amounts of air are able to pass into the middle ear space. Consequently, this manoeuvre is not as effective as the Valsalva manoeuvre, but it is used successfully by many divers.

❏ Others.

Voluntary Opening of the Eustachian tubes can be performed at will by many experienced divers, by contracting certain muscles in their throat. This technique is difficult to describe but if it can be mastered it is the most convenient and effective of all the techniques because there is little force involved and the manoeuvre can be performed repeatedly.

If difficulty is encountered, the **Lowry technique** ("swallow and then blow at the same time" – a Toynbee + Valsalva combination) or the **Edmonds second technique** ("sniff and blow" – suck the cheeks in with a sniff against the closed nostrils, immediately followed by a Valsalva), may be used.

Diving Technique

Ideally on the day of a proposed dive, the diver should confirm that he is able to equalise easily before setting out on a diving expedition.

All divers should equalise on the surface before descending. This confirms that equalisation is possible and the eardrums balloon slightly outwards, allowing some margin for error if the diver becomes distracted and forgets to equalise during the first metre of descent.

The diver should then **equalise every metre or less as the descent proceeds,** so that no sensation of pressure is felt. This is called **"equalising ahead of the dive"** and is much better than waiting until the pressure (or actual pain) is felt.

If any difficulty is encountered, it is pointless descending further as equalisation will become more difficult due to a **'locking effect' on the Eustachian tube.** This is caused by the pressure difference between the middle ear and the throat. The diver should instead either abort the dive or, if the dive is an important one, ascend a little and repeat the equalisation manoeuvre. The diver should not persist with this "yo-yo" technique. If the ears do not equalise easily, abort the dive.

Descending 'feet first' makes equalisation considerably easier, and is best done on an anchor or shot line. This allows accurate control of the descent rate and depth while allowing the diver to concentrate on equalisation without the distractions of swimming and depth control.

The novice diver and the diver who has difficulty with his ears should use a face mask which allows easy access to the nose to facilitate the various manoeuvres. If one ear causes more problems, then cock this ear to the surface when equalising.

Surgical correction of nasal septal deviations, cessation of smoking and adequate treatment of URTIs and allergies may be needed by those who have these predisposing causes.

Medication

Medication has been used to facilitate equalisation when there is some disorder of the ear, nose or throat. Topical nasal decongestant sprays and drops such as **phenylephrine and oxymetazoline** shrink the lining of the nose and Eustachian tube, reducing congestion and opening the air passages. Some oral medications such as **pseudoephedrine** have a similar effect.

While these drugs can make diving possible when it otherwise would not be, **they permit the diver to dive with conditions which should preclude diving,** such as upper respiratory tract infections. There is an added risk of the drug predisposing to barotrauma during the ascent which is far more dangerous than ear barotrauma of descent.

Because these drugs mask the symptoms of conditions which would otherwise preclude diving, divers are advised that it is **better to avoid diving than to continue while taking these drugs.** They also seem to make other diving disorders more likely e.g. Sudden Death Syndrome.

MIDDLE EAR BAROTRAUMA OF ASCENT

(ALTERNOBARIC VERTIGO, REVERSE SQUEEZE)

This condition is relatively uncommon by itself, but it is often a complication of a middle ear barotrauma of descent. During ascent, air in the middle ear space expands and must escape. The air normally escapes down the Eustachian tube to the throat without any conscious effort by the diver. If very observant, he may actually hear or feel it escape from his ear .

Occasionally the Eustachian tube may obstruct this flow of air, with subsequent air distension and increased pressure in the middle ear cavity during ascent. This causes bulging and possible rupture of the ear drum. There may also be damage to the inner ear, leading to hearing loss (see Chapter 30). The increased pressure in the middle ear may also stimulate the nearby balance organ producing vertigo.

It is usually seen in divers who have recently used decongestants (nasal drops or pseudoephedrine tablets). These may wear off during the dive resulting in congestion of the pharyngeal end of the Eustachian tube more than the middle ear end and permit diving despite minor descent barotrauma.

Clinical Features

Increasing pain is sometimes felt in the affected ear as the diver ascends. Often there may be **vertigo** as well as **nausea** and **vomiting**. After surfacing the diver may feel fullness or dullness in the ear. **Tinnitus** or **hearing loss** may indicate serious damage (inner ear barotrauma).

Vertigo may develop after only a metre or so of ascent (see Chapter 31, Case History 31.2). Many of these symptoms can be hazardous, especially as ascent may be prevented by the symptoms.

First–Aid

If a diver encounters ear pain or vertigo during ascent, he should **descend a little** to minimise the pressure imbalance and attempt to open the Eustachian tube by holding the nose and swallowing (Toynbee manoeuvre). This equalises ears with ascent, since it creates a negative pressure in the throat and relieves the distension in the middle ear.

Occluding the external ear by pressing in the tragus (the small fold of cartilage in front of the ear canal) and pressing the enclosed water inwards may occasionally force open the Eustachian tube. If this fails then try the other techniques of equalisation described above, and attempt a slow ascent.

Treatment

Uncomplicated cases resolve quickly but eardrum rupture or inner ear damage may need **specialised care. All cases need expert diving medical assessment, for diagnosis and advice.**

EXTERNAL EAR BAROTRAUMA

(EXTERNAL EAR SQUEEZE)

If the external ear canal is obstructed, the enclosed gas will be compressed during descent. This will be accommodated by outward bulging of the eardrum and swelling and bruising of the skin lining the ear canal.

Obstruction of the canal can be caused by a tight fitting **hood, wax** in the ears, **bony growths (exostoses)** in the ear or the wearing of **ear plugs**. As this condition can be encountered at depths as little as 2 metres, **ear plugs should not be worn during any type of diving.**

The symptoms include discomfort and pain on descent, bleeding from the external ear and the other pressure effects of barotrauma on the middle ear, including difficult equalisation.

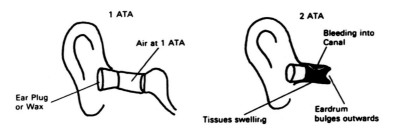

EXTERNAL EAR BAROTRAUMA (EAR SQUEEZE)

Fig. 9.9

Chapter 10

SINUS BAROTRAUMA

ANATOMY OF THE SINUSES

The sinuses are air filled cavities contained within the bones of the base and front of the skull. Apart from causing inconvenience to divers, their exact function is unknown.

There are four main groups of sinuses, with openings into to the nose :

- **Maxillary sinuses** in the cheek bones
- **Frontal sinuses** in the skull above the eyes
- **Ethmoid sinuses** in the thin bone at the base of the nose
- **Sphenoidal sinuses** situated deep inside the central part of the skull.

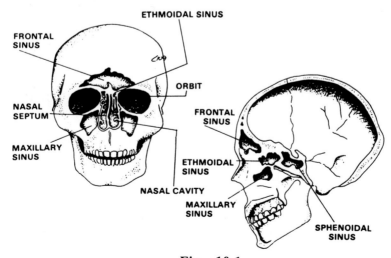

Fig. 10.1

Location of sinuses in the skull. They are connected by canals to the nose.

All the sinuses are lined by a soft mucous-secreting tissue which is richly supplied with blood vessels. Each sinus communicates with the nose by its own narrow opening called the **ostium,** and through these, the sinuses are normally permanently open to the atmosphere.

The **mastoid sinus** or antrum is a similar structure that opens into the middle ear cavity. It more often reflects the pathology of the middle ear and reference should be made to Chapter 9 for this.

THE MECHANISM OF SINUS BAROTRAUMA

As the water pressure changes during a dive, the sinuses normally equalise automatically by free passage of gas into or out of their openings.

Problems are inevitable, however, if these openings become obstructed. Obstruction can be due to **congestion** associated with **allergy, smoking, respiratory tract infection** or the **overuse of topical decongestants**. Other causes of ostia obstruction include chronic sinus inflammation (**sinusitis**), nasal inflammation (**rhinitis**), folds of tissue (**polyps**) and plugs of **mucous**.

When the sinus is blocked during descent, the gas in the sinus is compressed causing sinus barotrauma of descent. The shrinking volume is replaced by swelling of the sinus lining, tissue fluid or bleeding – partly filling the sinus.

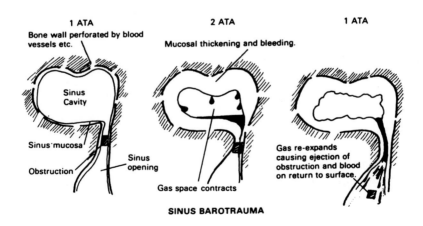

SINUS BAROTRAUMA

Fig. 10.2

If the sinus opening is obstructed, increased pressures cause congestion and swelling of the sinus lining (mucosa) and eventually bleeding. Ascending then causes re-expansion of the original gas within the sinus, often producing expulsion of the obstruction along with any blood contained.

This tissue fluid and blood, which may take days or weeks to absorb, represents a rich nutrient medium for bacterial growth, promoting sinus **infection** (see Chapter 28).

During ascent, blood and tissue fluid from the descent barotrauma may be discharged into the nose by the gas expanding in the sinus, causing an apparent **nose bleed** from the same side as the injured sinus.

If the sinus opening becomes obstructed during ascent, the expansion of gas flattens the sinus lining against its bony wall, causing pain and injury to this delicate tissue. This is called sinus barotrauma of ascent. Rarely, the bony walls of the sinus may rupture, with the expanding gas passing into the eye socket (**orbital emphysema**), the brain cavity (**pneumocephalus**) or tracking elsewhere. Sinus barotrauma of descent is more common than ascent, but they may often coexist.

CLINICAL FEATURES

Sinus Barotrauma of Descent

This condition usually presents during descent with a sensation of **pressure,** developing into a **pain** in the region of the affected sinus. It is usually felt **over the eye** (frontal or ethmoidal), **the cheek bone** (maxillary), or deep in the **skull** (sphenoidal) depending on which sinus is involved.

Maxillary sinus barotrauma can also present as pain in the **upper teeth.**

The pain may settle during the dive and recur as a dull pain or headache afterwards.

A small amount of **blood** issuing from the nose during or after ascent is a frequent accompaniment of sinus barotrauma.

Sinus Barotrauma of Ascent

This presents with pain in the affected sinus during and after the diver's ascent. Bleeding from the sinus frequently drains through the nose or can be spat out.

Severe headache persisting after the dive suggests either infection (sinusitis) or sinus tissue damage.

TREATMENT

Any case of suspected sinus barotrauma accompanied by headache after a dive requires medical assessment, because decompression sickness and many other conditions can also present as headache.

Normally sinus barotrauma resolves without any treatment. Significant bleeding into the sinus may drain more rapidly if topical nasal and oral decongestants are used.

The diagnosis may be confirmed by X–Rays or CT scans (preferred) of the sinuses.

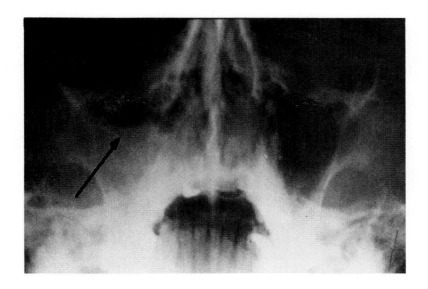

Fig. 10.3
Sinus x-ray showing fluid level (opaque area almost filling cavity below right orbit) in right maxillary sinus after barotrauma of descent. Left sinus cavity appears clear and filled only with air (black).

Increasing pain in the sinus, with fever or malaise developing after the dive suggests **infection** which is treated with decongestants and antibiotics.

Diving and flying should be suspended until the condition has resolved, usually from 2–10 days.

PREVENTION

Active and frequent middle ear equalisation, using positive pressure techniques, fortuitously assists by forcing air into the sinuses during descent and preventing barotrauma.

Diving should be avoided if the diver is suffering from any upper respiratory tract infection, to reduce both the risk of barotraumas and the infection complications. Smoking and allergic nasal congestion (hay fever) increases the risk of sinus barotrauma by obstructing the sinuses. A deviated nasal septum may also contribute to the development of sinus barotrauma, and if so, it can be surgically corrected.

Nasal decongestants used at the time of diving tend to reduce the congestion of the sinus ostia (at least at the nasal end), but may not prevent sinus barotrauma of ascent. For this reason they should be avoided. It is better for the diver to be prevented from descending (sinus barotrauma of descent) than to be prevented from ascending (sinus barotrauma of ascent).

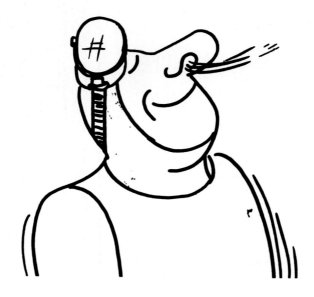

Fig. 10.4

Chapter 11

PULMONARY BAROTRAUMA

(LUNG BAROTRAUMA)

Pulmonary barotrauma is lung injury caused by pressure changes. In divers it can occur on ascent or descent. Barotrauma of ascent is relevant for scuba diving, and barotrauma of descent for free diving (breathhold).

PULMONARY BAROTRAUMA OF ASCENT

("BURST LUNG")

This is second only to drowning as a cause of death in recreational scuba divers.

The lungs of a male diver normally contain about 6 litres of air, contained in the alveoli and air passages. If a diver takes a full breath at 20 metres (66 ft.) and returns to the surface, that 6 litre volume expands to 18 litres since the pressure at 20 metres is 3 ATA and at the surface, 1 ATA.

In this situation, to avoid over distension of his lungs, the diver must exhale 12 litres of air (measured on the surface) before reaching the surface. If he does not exhale this air, the pressure in his lungs increases and once it exceeds about 80mm Hg. above the pressure around the diver, the lungs will rupture. Even if he does exhale correctly, he can still encounter problems if there is some obstruction to the venting of air from some part of the lung.

A pressure differential of 80mm Hg. is equivalent to the pressure change between one metre depth (approx. 4 ft.) and the surface, making pulmonary barotrauma a real possibility even for a scuba diver in a swimming pool.

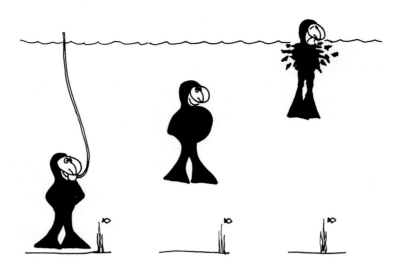

Fig. 11.1

Predisposing Factors

❑ Breath holding.

This may be due to failure to read "Diving Medicine – for Scuba Divers", **panic, ignorance, forgetfulness or spasm of the larynx after inhalation of water.** Breathholding during ascent can lead to excessive distension of the lung, and their rupture.

❑ Air trapping.

Anything preventing air from leaving all or part of the lungs can lead to barotrauma.

Several factors may predispose to air trapping. Obstruction of the bronchi is frequent in; **asthma, acute and chronic bronchitis, respiratory tract infections.** This obstruction may allow air to enter the lungs but restrict exit of air – a ball valve effect. Other conditions which can cause this include **tuberculosis (T.B.), tumours of the lung, calcified glands, cysts in the lung and emphysema. Heavy smoking** may cause **mucous obstructions.**

❑ Disorders of lung compliance.

Lung compliance is a measure of the stretching ability of the lungs. One published study investigated pulmonary barotrauma in Navy divers who had correctly exhaled during ascent and were medically fit. Studies of the lung compliance of these divers showed their lungs to be more "stiff" than normal, and therefore presumably more prone to tearing when slightly over-expanded.

Divers with **scars or fibrosis in the lungs** may have localised reduction in lung compliance which may cause shearing forces and tearing in these areas. Fibrosis of this type may be found after inflammatory lung disease such as **sarcoidosis, tuberculosis, lung abscess** or even some **severe pneumonias.**

Lung tearing has rarely been described in **breathhold divers.** These divers developed pneumothorax and mediastinal emphysema during breath hold dives — the tearing of the lungs being caused by the diver taking very large breaths, with excessive respiratory pressures. On investigation, these divers were found to have relatively small lungs and relatively large chest cavities. Full expansion of the chest cavity in these divers led to over-expansion of the lungs and subsequent tearing.

❏ Rapid ascents

Any partially obstructed airway may restrict airflow. This can be overwhelmed by the massive volume changes which occur during rapid ascents. This risk can be reduced by adhering to the recommended ascent rate of 1 metre per 3 sec (18 metres or 60 ft. per minute), upon which most decompression tables are based, or slower.

A slower ascent rate of 8 metres (or 25 ft.) per minute is strongly recommended by the authors. This rate may also help to reduce the risk of developing serious decompression sickness. The bottom time should be reduced accordingly.

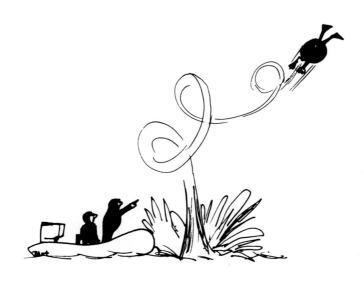

Fig. 11.2

❏ Emergency ascents.

The sudden failure of gas supply, especially at considerable depths, tends to alarm even the most sanguine diver. The subsequent emergency ascent is often undertaken at very high ascent rates. Breathholding due to anxiety, and a rapid gas expansion, together greatly increase the likelihood of barotrauma.

❏ Free ascent training (or "Emergency swimming ascent").

A "free ascent" is a manoeuvre in which the diver breathes from compressed air equipment, takes a breath and then returns to the surface without breathing further from the equipment. Naturally, he must exhale to exhaust the expanding gas – but he may still encounter several problems during ascent. Most divers, aware of the dread consequences of breath holding, tend to exhale excessively and may run out of breath before surfacing.

In the Australian Navy free ascent training, salt water aspiration syndrome and near drowning were not uncommon accompaniments of these exercises. Because of the hazards of this training technique, a **recompression chamber** and a **specialised diving physician** had to be available immediately adjacent to the ascent site.

Unless closely supervised the rate of ascent is usually excessive, especially from greater depths since the diver knows that he only has one lung full of air to sustain him until the surface is reached. In fact he has the equivalent of 3 lung fulls of air when compressed air is breathed at 20 metres depth. The excessive rate of ascent causes rapid gas expansion and damage if airways are partially obstructed.

This outmoded training technique was designed to prepare the divers to cope with an "out-of-air" situation in days before contents gauges, octopus rigs, and emergency air supplies were common.

Unfortunately the death rate of the procedure made it a dubious prophylactic. Also, the tendency of divers to over-inhale before commencing the ascent made the procedure more hazardous and not at all similar to the out-of-air situation, where lack of air is usually detected after exhalation. Thus, the lungs in a real "out-of-air" situation are not fully inflated. As this 'real situation' usually happens without any inspiratory capability it is presumably safer.

❑ Submarine escape.

Escape from a sunken submarine usually involves a rapid, buoyancy-assisted free ascent. This technique is practiced by most navies from depths of 20–30 metres in specially made submarine escape training facilities (SETF). Ascent rates are very fast and pulmonary barotrauma is not uncommon in spite of good training and thorough preliminary medical examinations.

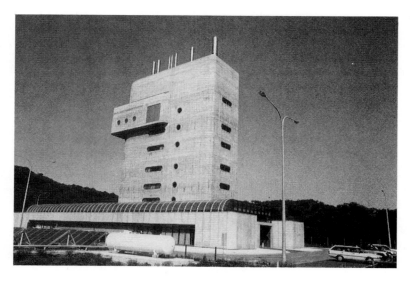

Fig. 11.3
The Royal Australian Navy's S.E.T.F. in Western Australia.

The emphasis on escape procedures demonstrates the optimistic outlook of submariners since the submarines generally operate in water depths which exceed the crush depth of the submarine's hull.

❑ Buddy breathing.

This technique is not easy to perform and unsuccessful attempts at buddy breathing, especially during ascent, are often followed by one diver abandoning the procedure and undertaking a free ascent to the surface. The diver tends to over-inhale prior to handing over the regulator and then breathhold during ascent, while waiting for its return. These conditions are conducive to pulmonary barotrauma.

Mechanisms of Injury in Pulmonary Barotrauma

If the lungs rupture due to excessive gas pressure, any or all of four consequences can follow :

- **Lung tissue damage**
- **Emphysema (gas in the tissues)**
- **Pneumothorax (gas in the chest cavity)**
- **Air embolism (gas bubbles in the blood)**

Lung Tissue Injury

If the lungs are over distended, generalised tearing of the lung tissues with severe diffuse damage to the lung structure is likely. Bleeding, bruising, and generalised destruction to the lungs causes severe breathing difficulties.

❑ Clinical features.

Shortness of breath, pain when breathing, coughing, coughing-up blood, and shock are the principal manifestations. Death may follow rapidly.

❑ Treatment.

The diver should be examined and treated for other manifestations of pulmonary barotrauma. Lung tissue damage alone has no specific treatment apart from basic resuscitation measures (see Chapter 40 and 42). The patient should be given oxygen and taken immediately to hospital.

Surgical Emphysema

Tearing of the alveoli allows gas to escape into the tissues of the lung. Air tracks along the lung tissues to the **mediastinum** in the midline. From here it migrates into the **neck** or, in severe cases, even further, tracking around the heart sac (pericardial sac) or even into the **abdominal cavity.**

If the diver has performed a long or deep dive and still has a nitrogen load in his tissues, nitrogen will continue to diffuse into these air spaces to expand them over the next few hours.

The presence of the air in the tissues causes damage by compressing the blood vessels, nerves, larynx, or oesophagus. In severe cases air can compress the heart causing malfunction.

❑ Clinical features.

It may take some time for symptoms to develop, as the air migrates slowly through the tissues. Air in the mediastinum and around the heart may cause **chest pain** and **shortness of breath.** Air in the throat leads to **voice changes** (the voice developing a "tinny or brassy" note), shortness of breath and/or **swallowing difficulties**. A **"crackling sensation"** may be felt under the skin around the neck – and especially just above the collar-bones (supra-clavicular space). It feels like "rice bubbles beneath the skin" or "cellophane paper", on pressing. The diver may complain of a sensation of **fullness in the throat**.

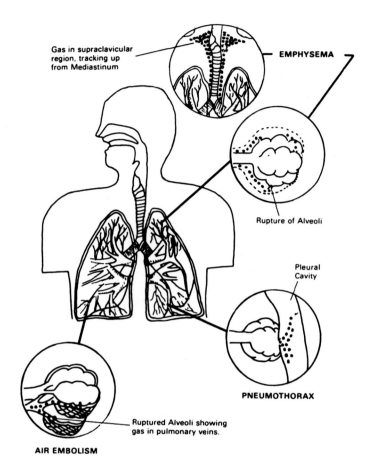

Gas in supraclavicular region, tracking up from Mediastinum

EMPHYSEMA

Rupture of Alveoli

Pleural Cavity

PNEUMOTHORAX

Ruptured Alveoli showing gas in pulmonary veins.

AIR EMBOLISM

PULMONARY BAROTRAUMA OF ASCENT

Fig. 11.4
The various manifestations of a ruptured lung on ascent.

❏ Treatment.

The diver should be examined and treated for the other manifestations of pulmonary barotrauma. Mild surgical emphysema alone responds to **100% oxygen.** (see Chapter 40). This causes a diffusion gradient for nitrogen (between the air space and the nitrogen-free blood) which eliminates the air bubbles. If not treated, the condition will slowly resolve, but it may last many days.

Severe surgical emphysema, especially if causing compression of the airway or blood vessels, will respond to **recompression** in a recompression chamber. Again, breathing oxygen produces a diffusion gradient of nitrogen out of the air spaces. If air is breathed, more nitrogen may diffuse into the tissues, making the surgical emphysema even worse when the diver is decompressed.

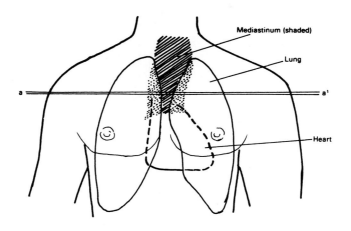

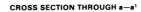

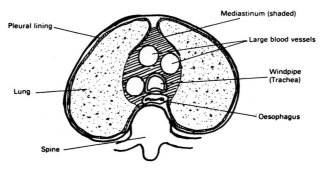

Fig. 11.5

The location of the mediastinum can be seen from this frontal view and cross section. It is located deep in the chest between the lungs and above the heart, and its connection with the neck tissues can be noted.

Pneumothorax

If the lung ruptures near its surface, air gains access to the pleural space, between the lung and the chest wall (pneumothorax). The elasticity of the lung causes it to collapse like a burst balloon and the lung space is replaced by an air pocket.

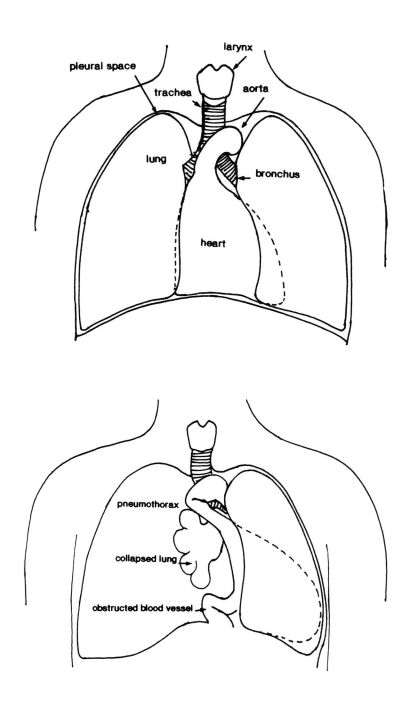

Fig. 11.6

These schematic diagrams show a normal chest (as seen on x-ray) at the top, and a pneumothorax below, with collapse of the right lung. As air in the right side expands with further ascent, it pushes the heart and midline structures towards the left side of the chest, causing a "tension" pneumothorax on the right.

Occasionally a valve effect allows air to pass from the air passages into the pneumothorax but prevents its return. As more and more air collects in the pneumothorax, the pressure in the thoracic cavity rises and forces the contents of the chest (including the heart and lungs) to the opposite side. This is called a **tension pneumothorax** and its effect on cardiac function is catastrophic and rapidly fatal if not treated.

Bleeding may take place into the pneumothorax, leading to a **haemo-pneumothorax.**

❏ Clinical features.

A pneumothorax is usually heralded by **chest pain**, often made worse by breathing, and causes **shortness of breath**. Respiration becomes rapid and the heart rate increases.

With a **tension pneumothorax,** as the mediastinum is pushed to the other side, the trachea can be felt to be displaced to that side. The patient becomes increasingly short of breath and may become cyanotic (blue) and shocked. The pulse is difficult to feel as the blood pressure falls.

With severe cases of burst lung, a pneumothorax will be evident very soon after the diver reaches the surface, but in milder cases, the symptoms of pneumothorax may be delayed for many hours. Symptoms may be brought on by coughing or altitude exposure (e.g. mountain range, travel in aircraft).

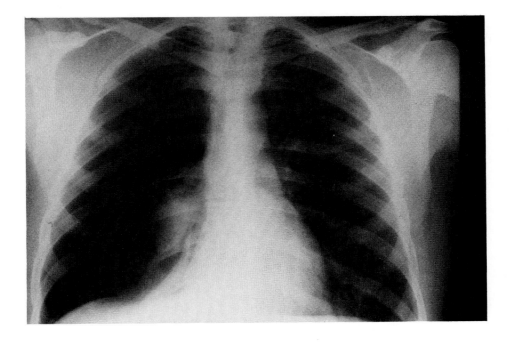

Fig. 11.7
X-ray of diver's chest after suffering pulmonary barotrauma of ascent with a right sided pneumothorax. The right chest cavity appears "black" due to its being filled with air and the collapsed lung (white) can be seen near the midline.

❑ Treatment.

A pneumothorax requires **urgent medical attention**. The extent of lung collapse is assessed clinically and confirmed by a chest x-ray. A large pneumothorax is treated by placing a **tube into the pleural air space** and connecting it to a one-way valve such as a Heimlich valve or an underwater drain. This allows air out of the pneumothorax but prevents its return. The placement of tubes in the chest is beyond the capability of untrained personnel as there are important structures, like the heart, which can be injured in the process. After a period of hours or days the tear in the lung usually heals and the lung re-inflates.

A minor pneumothorax (less than 25% lung collapse) may be treated by the diver **breathing 100% oxygen** (see Chapter 40).

A **tension pneumothorax** is a medical **emergency**. The pressure in the pneumothorax must be relieved by the placement of a needle or tube into the pneumothorax.

If the diver is aware of the possibility of a pneumothorax, he may be able to alert a physician to the possible diagnosis if any of these clinical features present.

Air Embolism

When the lungs rupture, tears in the alveoli walls (and contained blood capillaries) can allow air to enter the blood circulation. This air is conducted to the left side of the heart, from whence it is pumped through the arterial circulation.

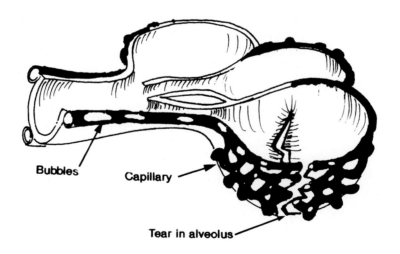

Bubbles   **Capillary** ──

Tear in alveolus ──

Fig. 11.8
Diagram of a ruptured alveolus and capillary vessel from pulmonary barotrauma of ascent. Air bubbles (emboli) are entering the veins carrying blood back to the left atrium of the heart.

The air bubbles obstruct or damage blood vessels in vital organs such as the heart and brain, leading to impairment of function, serious disability or death.

❏ Clinical features.

Symptoms present abruptly, usually immediately or within 10 minutes of the diver reaching the surface. Air bubbles lodging in the brain may cause **loss of consciousness, fits** or **confusion**, a pattern of symptoms similar to a "cerebral stroke".

There is often **loss of function** of parts of the brain causing :

- **disturbances of sensation** such as **numbness** or **tingling**
- **disturbances of movement** including **paralysis** or **weakness**
- **disturbances of vision**
- **disturbances of speech**
- **disturbances of balance** or **co-ordination**
- **disturbances of intellectual function**

Air bubbles lodging in the coronary arteries which supply the heart with blood may lead to symptoms resembling a **heart attack** including **chest pain, shortness of breath** and **palpitations**. Air bubbles lodging in the circulation of the skin cause white or purplish patches (**marbling**).

If a diver surfaces after a deep dive and develops disturbances of brain function it is also possible that he might have **cerebral decompression sickness.** It may not be possible immediately to distinguish between air embolism and cerebral decompression sickness, now both called **acute decompression illness.** Fortunately the initial treatment is similar for both (see Case History 33.5).

❏ Treatment.

Air embolism causes hypoxic damage by obstructing important blood vessels with air bubbles. **Recompression therapy** in a chamber reduces the size of the bubbles and allows them to flow on, into smaller less-important blood vessels. The bubbles ultimately pass into the venous system, may be trapped in the lungs, and are eliminated as nitrogen diffuses out of them.

Divers who develop air embolism after free ascent or in submarine escape training, where a recompression chamber is available nearby, are immediately recompressed to 50 metres – reducing the air bubbles to a $1/6$th. of their original size. Otherwise, **transport** must be arranged urgently.

There is some controversy about the best way to **position** the patient. Divers used to be taught to place the patient in the 30 degrees head down position, to keep the rising bubbles away from to the brain. This caused difficulty with resuscitation and transport however, and the increased venous pressure in the head worsened the cerebral oedema (brain swelling) which accompanies injury.

A more reasonable approach is to place the patient **horizontally, on their side** (the left side is theoretically preferable but this is probably not critical) without a pillow. This will place the head slightly lower than the heart. The patient is likely to be unconscious or drowsy and this position is also good for patency of the airway. This is often called the **coma position**.

The patient should **not be allowed to sit up or stand up** once this position is adopted as there are some case reports of divers rapidly deteriorating after sitting up, even some time after the barotrauma event.

The patient should be given **100% oxygen** to breathe. If the patient is unconscious the principles of airway management, breathing and circulation management (**A–B–C**) take precedence and must also be followed (see Chapter 42).

The **other complications** of burst lung, such as pneumothorax or emphysema, must also be looked for and treated if present.

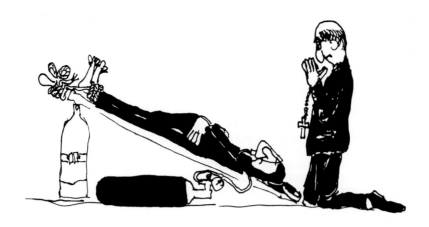

Fig. 11.9
An outmoded form of positioning for acute decompression illness.

The definitive treatment is **recompression therapy** in a well equipped chamber. Urgent transport is necessary in order to minimize brain or other essential organ injury. Unfortunately, even in the best facilities, full recovery is not always possible.

Prevention of Pulmonary Barotrauma
of Ascent

❑ Medical fitness.

Divers should be carefully screened to ensure there are no respiratory problems that predispose to pulmonary barotrauma (asthma, fibrosis, cysts, pneumothorax, infections, etc). Divers who do develop this disease are much more likely to have recurrences, which are then more severe – often with fatal consequences. Thus an episode of pulmonary barotrauma usually precludes further diving.

❑ Diving techniques.

Divers are advised to avoid situations which could lead to them having to perform an emergency free ascent. Such situations include greater **depths, reduced air supply, overweighting** and/or **excessive buoyancy.**

The use of well maintained **good quality equipment** (e.g. regulator), a **contents gauge**, an **octopus rig** or better still, and an **emergency air source** (to avoid the need for buddy breathing) are common sense measures which can be employed.

It is important for scuba divers to remember to **keep breathing normally** at all times, as a relatively small ascent in shallow water while the diver is holding his breath can lead to over-pressure of the lungs and pulmonary barotrauma. **"Skip"** (controlled or reduced) **breathing** is dangerous.

Pulmonary barotrauma is a not uncommon accompaniment of **"free ascent training"** (also called **"emergency swimming ascent training"**). Included in this category is **"ditch and recovery"** drill, where the diver performs a free ascent as he returns to the surface after ditching his gear on the bottom. The greatest volume changes due to Boyle's Law take place near the surface, so that free ascents from even shallow depths are not safe.

The concept of training novice divers in "free ascent" technique is controversial. Obviously it is desirable for all divers to be familiar with safe "free ascent" principles in case of equipment failure. However, if a diver develops a serious air embolism after a free ascent, a fatal outcome is likely unless a recompression chamber with an experienced diving physician is available at the site of the dive. This facility is rarely available in sport diver training. Even a few minutes delay in instituting recompression has a significant negative influence on the outcome of treatment.

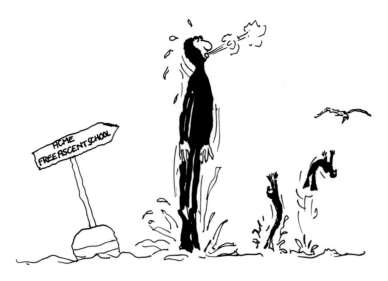

Fig. 11.10

Studies conducted on submarine escape trainees in Sweden showed an almost 4% incidence of EEG (electroencephalogram or "brain wave") changes in these divers indicating sub-clinical brain damage, presumably due to minor air embolism. Studies of free ascents by trainees in the U.S. Navy showed an incidence of pulmonary barotrauma of 1 in 3000.

PULMONARY BAROTRAUMA OF DESCENT

(LUNG SQUEEZE)

There is a theoretical risk of pulmonary barotrauma during descent as well as ascent, although from a different mechanism.

A diver descending during a breathhold dive will have the air in his chest and lungs progressively compressed in accordance with Boyle's Law. Eventually a lung volume is reached when the compression of gas can no longer be accommodated by a further reduction in lung volume, and is instead compensated by the engorgement of blood vessels in the lungs. The lung blood vessels have only a limited distensibility, and can be expected to rupture once this limit is reached, causing pulmonary haemorrhage.

A rapid descent when standard dress equipment is used, or failure of a surface-supply gas pressure in the absence of an effective non-return valve, are also possible causes of pulmonary barotrauma of descent. It is theoretically possible whenever a surface-supply of air is used e.g. standard dress, surface supply from a compressor or compressed air tanks, or pumping the air supply from the surface in commercial devices such as the "Diveman".

Case reports of this condition are infrequent and poorly documented. The theoretical basis of the condition was severely tested when a world record descent to beyond 100 metres was made by a breathhold diver several years ago.

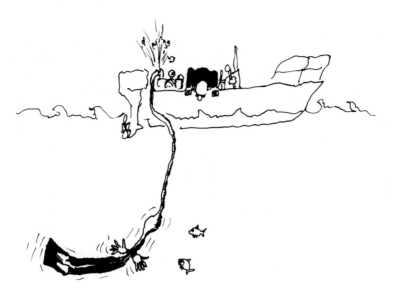

Fig.   11.11

Chapter 12

OTHER BAROTRAUMAS

Barotrauma can develop wherever there is an enclosed gas space adjoining tissues. With descent, the space contracts, pulling tissue and blood into the space (implosions). With ascent, the space expands and disrupts tissue (explosions).

The spaces may be within the body or between the body and the equipment. They include :

- Facial (mask) squeeze
- Skin (suit) squeeze
- Body squeeze and "blow up"
- Gastro-intestinal barotrauma
- Dental barotrauma.

Barotraumas dealt with earlier include lung, ear and sinus barotraumas.

FACIAL BAROTRAUMA OF DESCENT

(MASK SQUEEZE)

During descent the airspace inside a face mask is compressed and the contraction in volume of the gas space is accommodated by flattening of the mask against the face, and later by congestion of the facial skin and eyes.

It can lead to bleeding into the soft tissues under the skin and produce a characteristic **bruised** facial appearance under the mask area. The whites of the eyes may be grossly haemorrhagic ("**red eye**"). It may take 1–3 weeks to clear up.

This condition is easily prevented by exhaling into the face mask during descent, to equalise the mask with the water pressure. More cases have developed since rigid plastic face masks replaced the soft rubber ones. Expanding gas automatically vents around the edge of the face mask during ascent.

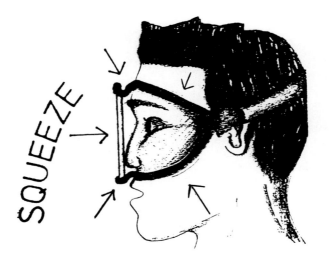

Fig. 12.1

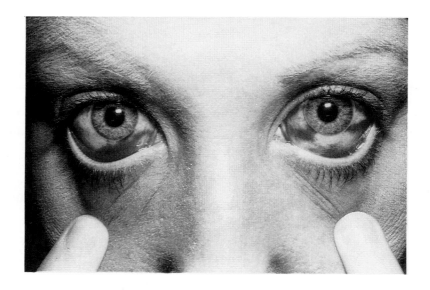

Fig. 12.2
Facial barotrauma from diving with goggles – note the bleeding into the sclera (white parts) of both eyes. Face masks can cause similar eye bleeds, but then the surrounding facial tissues are also bruised.

Divers using goggles run the risk of a similar form of barotrauma on a smaller scale involving the tissues around the eye. In the past, if goggles were used to dive, a method of equalising the space around the eye, such as that shown in the accompanying diagram, was employed.

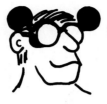

Fig. 12.3

SKIN BAROTRAUMA OF DESCENT

(SUIT SQUEEZE)

Divers using a **dry suit** or a **loose wet suit** may experience this problem. During descent, pockets of gas can be trapped in folds under the suit. Where the suit has folds, the contraction of the gas space is accommodated by the skin being sucked into the space leading to strips or welts of bruising.

It may cause discomfort at the time. After surfacing the diver may notice bruising over the skin, corresponding to the folds.

BODY BAROTRAUMA OF DESCENT

(BODY SQUEEZE)

With the solid metal helmet used in standard diving there is a possibility of the diver descending and the pressure in the air hose not keeping up with the environmental pressure. If this occurs, the diver's body may be forced up into the helmet, and crushed.

This can also happen at a constant depth, when a non-return valve is not used (or is not functional) and the air supply fails. The only treatment for this bizarre injury is to wash out the helmet with a good antiseptic.

Even the modern plastic helmets, used in deep and helium diving, can cause minor variants of this condition.

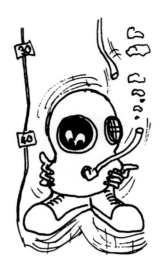

Fig. 12.4

SUIT BAROTRAUMA OF ASCENT

("BLOW UP")

With either dry suit or standard dress, the gas in the suit can expand with ascent, causing increasing buoyancy, more rapid ascent, etc. and a vicious circle develops where the diver may hurtle to the surface and be imprisoned in a balloon-like inflated suit. Special training and emergency procedures are needed for recreational divers who wear this equipment. As well as the physical injury that may result, other barotraumas and decompression sickness are likely.

GASTROINTESTINAL BAROTRAUMA

Gas is normally present in the gastro-intestinal tract. This finds its way into the atmosphere from time to time, as those who consume prunes, baked beans or cabbages will attest.

During a dive, gas may be swallowed when the diver equalises his ears, especially in the inverted (head-down) position. It may accumulate in the stomach and gastrointestinal tract without initially causing any discomfort to the diver. During ascent however, this accumulated gas increases in volume, and can result in cramping colicky abdominal pain, belching and vomiting. Rare cases of stomach rupture have even occurred.

Divers are advised not to equalise their ears in the "head down" position.

Several cases of severe gastric discomfort have been reported during chamber dives when the divers drank carbonated beverages while under pressure. One amusing account relates the opening of a new hyperbaric chamber which was toasted by champagne at 20 metres depth. The occupants were disappointed that the champagne appeared to be flat, but they drank with relish anyway because it tasted good. Their discomfort was exceeded only by their embarrassment during ascent as the gas in the champagne came out of solution and expanded in their stomachs.

DENTAL BAROTRAUMA

This uncommon form of barotrauma has on occasions been given sensational publicity, causing some divers to believe that they carry potential bombs set into their jaws.

Decayed teeth can occasionally contain a small air space which may lead to the tooth crushing inwards (imploding) during descent or fragmenting painfully (exploding) during ascent. The latter happens when there is an opening sufficient to allow air to enter during descent, but insufficient to allow it to escape during a fast ascent. The explosive potential of this occurrence has been overrated.

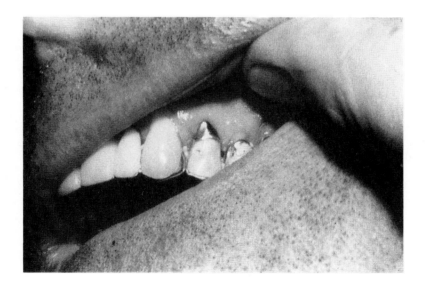

Fig. 12.5
Note the upper tooth fourth from front – the malleable gold filling (once convex) at the base has been pulled inwards and therefore the front and rear facets are flattened due to the effects of increasing pressure reducing the volume of the contained air spaces during descent.

Diving within several days of a tooth extraction may occasionally allow air to enter the tissues through the tooth socket from the positive air pressure generated by breathing through a regulator. This results in air tracking into tissues around the face (**tissue emphysema**). This is rarely serious and is treated by the diver breathing 100% oxygen for several hours to eliminate the air.

Diving after any tooth extractions should be avoided until the tooth socket has healed — usually this takes about a week to ten days.

Chapter 13

DECOMPRESSION THEORY and PHYSIOLOGY

Decompression Sickness (DCS) is an illness caused by the effects of gas coming out of solution to form bubbles in the body after diving. It is due to the effect of Henry's Law (see Chapter 2) following diving exposures. Understanding decompression theories is difficult if not impossible, so the average diver may well bypass most of this chapter, if he is not mathematically inclined.

In sport divers the main gas formed in bubbles is nitrogen (N_2) because these divers almost invariably breath air. However, the same principles apply to other inert gases, such as helium (He), which may be breathed by deep commercial divers.

GAS UPTAKE

When a diver breaths air from scuba equipment at depth, N_2 is breathed at an increased partial pressure. Because gas diffuses from areas of high concentration (high partial pressure) to areas of lower concentration, N_2 is taken up from the lungs by the blood and transported around the body and into the tissues. The greater the depth, the greater the partial pressure of N_2, and therefore the amount of N_2 absorbed. Haldane applied this concept to decompression.

The speed of N_2 distributing to the tissues depends on the their blood flow. Tissues with high metabolic needs such as the brain, heart, kidneys and liver receive most of the blood pumped from the heart. They will also receive most of the N_2 carried in the blood and will have a **rapid N_2 uptake.** Such tissues are termed **"fast tissues"** because of their fast N_2 uptake .

Because blood passing through the lungs immediately equilibrates with any change in inspired N_2, partial pressure, blood is the fastest tissue of all.

Other tissues such as ligaments, tendons and fat with a relatively small blood flow have a relatively slow N_2 uptake. These tissues are termed **"slow tissues"**. Between the two, are tissues of intermediate blood flow such as muscle. Some organs, such as the spinal cord, have both fast and slow tissue components. The rate of uptake of N_2 in a tissue is **exponential** i.e. it varies depending on the amount of gas already taken up by the tissue. As the tissue takes on gas, the uptake slows because the partial pressure gradient decreases.

The filling of a scuba cylinder is an example of an exponential process. When an empty cylinder is connected to a high pressure source, the cylinder initially fills quickly, but the flow slows as the pressure in the cylinder increases and approaches that of the gas source .

The uptake of gas in any tissue is initially rapid but slows with time. Accordingly, it may take a long time for a tissue to become saturated with gas, but fast tissues become saturated sooner than slow tissues.

Since the exponential uptake takes a long time to reach completion, even if it starts rapidly, the concept of **tissue "half times"** is used to compare tissues. The half time is the time taken for a tissue to reach half its saturation level. A fast tissue may have a half time as little as a few minutes, while a slow tissue may have a half time of an hour or more.

GAS ELIMINATION

N_2 is eliminated in a reverse of the uptake process. As the diver ascends there is a reduction in the partial pressure of N_2 in the air he breathes, allowing blood to release N_2 into the lungs. The decrease in the blood level of N_2 causes N_2 to diffuse into the blood from the tissues. Fast tissues naturally unload N_2 quicker than slow tissues.

Theoretically, tissues should lose N_2 exponentially, and most decompression tables are calculated on this assumption. While large amounts of N_2 are lost initially, the process slows with time and it may take 24 hours or longer for all the N_2 taken up during a dive to be released. Diving again during the time of N_2 elimination will mean that the diver will start his second dive with a **N_2 retention** in some tissues. Adjustments are provided in the decompression schedule to allow for this and are incorporated as the **repetitive dive tables.**

In practice, even during routine conservative dives, bubbles of N_2 frequently form in the blood and tissues, interfering with N_2 elimination. It has been estimated that as much as 5% of N_2 taken up by the body after some dives is transformed into bubbles on decompression. These are often termed **"silent bubbles"** since they usually do not produce any symptoms. They do however have a profound and unpredictable influence on the decompression requirements for repetitive diving, because it takes much longer to eliminate gas bubbles in tissues than it does gas in solution.

SATURATION

When tissues are subjected to an increased partial pressure of inert gas during a dive, they dissolve the gas in accordance with Henry's Law. However, there is a limit to the amount of gas which can be dissolved by a tissue exposed to any given partial pressure of gas (i.e. depth of dive). When this limit is reached the tissue is said to be **saturated**.

Our bodies are normally saturated with N_2 at atmospheric pressure and contain about one litre of dissolved N_2. If a diver were to descend to 20 metres (3 ATA) and remain there for a day or more, his body would take up the maximum amount of N_2 possible at that pressure and would then be saturated at that depth. His body would now have about 3 litres of N_2 dissolved in it.

Once the body is saturated with inert gas at a given depth, it will not take up more of that gas, no matter how long the diver spends at that depth. Consequently, once the diver is saturated the decompression requirement does not increase with time. This economy of time is exploited in **saturation diving**, when the diver is kept at depth for very long periods of time (days, weeks, months) but then needs only one lengthy decompression.

BUBBLE FORMATION

The process of bubble formation can be demonstrated easily by opening a bottle of beer (or champagne, depending on taste and income). In a carbonated beverage CO_2 is dissolved in the liquid at a high pressure which is maintained by the lid. When the lid is opened, the pressure of the liquid becomes atmospheric and the partial pressure of CO_2 in solution exceeds the critical limit for bubble formation, causing bubbles to form.

During ascent, the pressure surrounding the diver (the environmental pressure) is reduced. Eventually, the pressure of N_2 dissolved in the tissues may become greater than the environmental pressure. The tissue is then said to be **super saturated**.

The tissues are able to tolerate a certain degree of supersaturation. Nevertheless, Haldane explained that if the pressure of N_2 in the tissues exceeds the environmental pressure by a critical amount, then bubble formation is likely. The pressure differential needed to cause this varies between tissues but with most scuba diving it equals or exceeds 2 : 1 (i.e. the partial pressure of inert gas in the tissues should not be more than twice the environmental pressure). This explains why DCS under recreational diving conditions is unlikely after an isolated dive to less than 10 metres — the pressure at 10 metres is 2 ATA, while the pressure at the surface is 1ATA.

Gas bubbles in the tissue and blood are the cause of DCS. The exact mechanism of bubble formation is complex. It is likely that microscopic gas spaces (**bubble nuclei**) exist in all body fluids and that these form a nucleus for bubble formation during decompression.

Bubbles can form in any tissue in the body including blood. The pressure in each bubble will be the same as the environmental pressure (if it was not, the bubble would expand or contract until it was) and the bubble size is governed by Boyle's Law if the pressure changes.

At the onset of DCS, the pressure of N_2 in the tissues is supersaturated (greater than the environmental pressure) so there is an immediate diffusion (pressure) gradient of N_2 into any bubbles present, causing them to expand.

A bubble of DCS contains mainly N_2 if the diver has been breathing air, but the other gases present in the tissues, such as carbon dioxide (CO_2), oxygen (O_2) and water vapour, also diffuse into it.

Once a bubble has formed its behaviour depends on several factors. Any increase in pressure such as diving or recompression will reduce its size while any decrease in pressure such as ascent in the water, over mountains or in aircraft will expand it. The bubble will continue to grow in any tissue until the N_2

excess in that tissue has been eliminated. Once this has occurred (which may take hours or days) the bubble will begin to decrease in size but it may take hours, days or weeks to disappear. In the meantime the bubble can damage the tissues which host it.

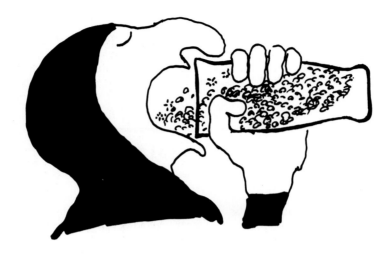

Fig. 13.1

There is good evidence that bubbles frequently form in tissues and blood of recreational divers after routine non-decompression dives, even when the tables have been faithfully followed. These bubbles do not usually cause symptoms but certainly cause doubt about the reliability of the tables.

Tissue damage by a bubble results from several factors. Bubbles in the blood obstruct blood vessels in vital organs such as the brain, while bubbles forming in the tissues may press on blood vessels and capillaries obstructing their blood flow. Bubbles in the blood can also stimulate the clotting process causing the blood to clot in the blood vessels, obstructing blood flow to vital organs, and reducing the ability of the remainder of the blood to clot adequately. In the brain, spinal cord and other tissues, bubble pressure in or on nerves may interfere with nervous system function.

DIVE PROFILES

The type of dive has a significant bearing on where and when bubble formation takes place. **Short deep** dives (i.e. deeper than 30 metres) **tend to cause bubbles in the fast tissues** (blood, brain and spinal cord) while **long shallow dives tend to produce bubbles in the slow tissues** (like the joints). Long deep dives cause bubbles everywhere.

This distribution occurs because :

- in short dives, only the fast tissues take up enough N_2 to form bubbles on ascent and
- in shallow dives, fast tissues eliminate their relatively modest N_2 excess before a critical pressure differential develops.

It can thus be seen why it is important to ascend slowly. The slower the ascent, the longer the time for fast tissues to eliminate N_2 through the lungs, before a critical N_2 pressure-differential develops.

Diving folklore contains a myth that a diver using a single 2000 litres (72 cu.ft.) tank cannot develop DCS. The air supply available was said to limit the diver to safe dive profiles. This is only true at very shallow depths and even then only partly so, e.g. for a dive to 20 metres, the average endurance may be about 30 minutes, which is within the no decompression time given by most tables. Remember though, as mentioned previously, that any dive in excess of 10 metres can produce DCS.

The myth may become more apparent for deeper dives. For example, a single 2000 litre tank will give around 10 minutes duration for a 50 metre dive. According to most decompression tables, a 10 minute dive to 50 metres will require 10 minutes of decompression — but there will be no air remaining to complete these stops. Even if there was sufficient air, dives to this depth have a significant risk of DCS despite the tables being followed correctly.

FACTORS INFLUENCING DCS

DCS is unpredictable. In general, anything that increases blood flow to an organ will increase the rate of N_2 loading. Anything that interferes with blood flow from an organ will reduce the capacity to off-load N_2. Both factors therefore predispose to bubble formation.

❏ Depth.

Any dive deeper than 10 metres can produce DCS although in general, the deeper the dive, the greater the risk.

❏ Individuals.

Some people appear to be more susceptible to DCS than others. Even an individual may vary in susceptibility at different times, and DCS can develop after a dive profile which has been safely followed on many previous occasions.

❏ Adaptation.

Repeated dives to similar depths over a period of time reduce the incidence of DCS. This may be due to the elimination of bubble nuclei. A diver returning to these dives after a break loses the benefits of this adaptation or acclimatisation.

❏ Age.

Older divers tend to be more predisposed to DCS (an old diver being defined as anyone older than the senior author of this text).

❏ Obesity.

This appears to be a predisposing factor probably due to increased N_2 solubility (4 : 1) in fat compared to water (obesity is defined as anyone heavier than the biggest author).

❏ Debilitation.

Factors causing the diver to be unwell such as **dehydration, hang-over** or **exhaustion** tend to predispose to DCS.

❏ Injury.

DCS, particularly involving the musculo-skeletal system and joints, is more likely with recent bruises, strains or chronic injuries.

❏ Cold.

Diving in cold conditions makes DCS more likely, especially when the diver is inadequately insulated. More precisely, coldness during the dive inhibits inert gas uptake (because of restricted circulation) but allows more N_2 to dissolve in body fluids — whilst coldness during decompression inhibits inert gas release. Theoretically, it would be better to be cold during the dive and warm on decompression, unless bubble formation occurs. Warming will then reduce gas solubility and increase bubble growth and DCS.

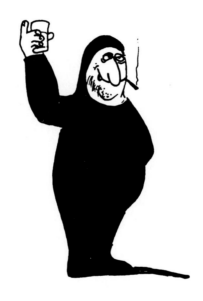

Fig. 13.2

❏ Exercise.

Strenuous exercise during a dive is likely to increase the N_2 uptake by increasing blood flow to muscles, favouring DCS development. Gentle exercise during decompression, by promoting circulation to the tissues probably aids in N_2 elimination. Strenuous exercise after the diver has returned to the surface makes the development of DCS, particularly in the musculo-skeletal system, more likely by promoting bubble formation. Strenuously exercising (shaking) a beer can, before opening it, aptly illustrates this phenomenon. During the first hour after a dive, particularly when there has been a large N_2 uptake, it is best to rest quietly as this is the period of maximal N_2 elimination.

❏ Gender.

There is some evidence that women have a higher incidence of DCS for a given dive profile. There are subtle differences in physiology and body composition which could explain this. The decompression tables in current use only evolved after extensive testing on men alone (see Chapter 8).

❏ Dive profile.

Deep dives (greater than 18 metres), **long dives, decompression dives** and any dives exceeding the **limiting line** (in RN based tables) all have a higher incidence of DCS.

❏ Rapid ascents.

These allow insufficient time for N_2 elimination from fast tissues, thus encouraging bubble formation.

❏ Multiple ascents.

Multiple ascents during a dive mean multiple decompressions and often involve rapid ascents. Bubbles in the blood (fast tissue bubbles) are likely to form during these ascents. The bubbles may not be adequately filtered by the lungs, passing along into the tissues, or may be reduced in size during the second or subsequent descent, allowing them to escape through the pulmonary filter into the tissues. DCS is then more likely.

❏ Repetitive dives.

Each repetitive dive begins with a N_2 load of some degree from the previous dive. Since bubble formation even after routine dives is common, a repetitive dive will often start with the diver carrying N_2 bubbles from the previous dive. These bubbles will be expanded by N_2 taken up during subsequent dives, and make DCS more likely.

❏ Flying after diving.

The jet age often finds divers flying home after a dive holiday within hours of their last (sometimes literally) dive. Jet airliners are pressurised to an altitude of about 2000 metres (6500ft.) above sea level. This means a pressure reduction on the diver of about 25% with a corresponding increase in the degree of N_2 supersaturation as well as a corresponding increase in the size of any bubbles he may be carrying. The increase in size of critical bubbles may be sufficient to provoke symptoms.

❏ Decompression meters (see Chapter 14).

Using computers that are based on largely invalidated **theories,** as opposed to practical diving and decompression table experience, may result in a diver getting much more time underwater while diving — and in the recompression chamber during treatment. Both can be included in his log book if he survives.

> **Note :** The senior (elder) author believes that the only explanation for most cases of DCS lies in the random application of Chaos Theory, which he also does not understand.

Chapter 14

DECOMPRESSION TABLES

Since the work of J.S.Haldane (a British physiologist) early this century, decompression tables have been based on mathematical models of gas uptake and elimination in the body.

The acclaimed **U.S. Navy Tables** are based on Haldane's theories. These include exponential uptake and elimination of inert gases and supersaturation gradients – as described in Chapters 1 and 13 – but have been modified by experimental trials and during extensive international use. When the tables were pushed to the limits (decompression diving, deep diving and approaching non-decompression limits), there was an unacceptable 1–5% incidence of decompression sickness (DCS). Even in divers who appeared unaffected, Doppler (ultrasound) studies often showed bubbles in the major veins during decompression.

In both recreational and navy diving there is only a 1/5,000 to 1/10,000 incidence of decompression illness, due to the fact that most dives do not approach decompression or depth limits, and divers include safety or "fudge" factors. Any table that offers longer duration, or more dives, will result in a greater incidence of decompression illness.

It would seem that it is not possible to make a satisfactory mathematical model of the human body during decompression. Even under normal conditions, the blood flow to some capillary beds shuts off from time to time, while flow to other areas increases. During decompression, Nitrogen (N_2) elimination will virtually cease from an area of shut-down capillaries. As decompression proceeds, this area will have a much higher N_2 concentration than predicted. No mathematical model can predict biological phenomena such as this.

Some of the better known **decompression tables** which have evolved from recent attempts to decompress divers include the following :

- RNPL – BSAC
- Bassett
- DCIEM
- NAUI Dive
- Huggins
- PADI
- Buhlmann
- "New"
- Multilevel Diving .

RNPL/BS-AC AND BS-AC '88 DECOMPRESSION TABLES

These tables were based on the theoretical work of **Hempleman** conducted at the Royal Naval Physiological Laboratory (United Kingdom) in the early 1950's. The principles differed from Haldane's in that it was assumed that the rate of elimination of N_2 was slower than the uptake because of the formation of subclinical bubbles. Rather than the tissues being able to tolerate a certain supersaturation as Haldane supposed, Hempleman assumed that bubbles formed routinely, and that tissues could withstand a certain amount of these bubbles before symptoms developed. The ascent rate was a more conservative 15 metres (50 ft.) per minute so as to reduce the speed of decompression.

These tables resulted in longer decompression and deeper first stops. They compared favourably with the USN tables, at least at recreational diving depths of less than 30 metres. Unfortunately, neurological DCS was more likely if these tables were used at greater depths.

In 1968 new schedules known as the "1968 Air Diving Tables" were devised based on modifications of the decompression theory. These new tables were considered too conservative, and the Royal Navy modified them, metricated them and presented them as the **RNPL 1972 Tables**.

The British Sub-Aqua Club (BS-AC) adapted the RNPL 1972 Tables, creating the **RNPL/BS-AC Tables**. For the RNPL/BS-AC Tables, the initial no-stop limits with deeper dives are sometimes considered dangerously long. Some surface intervals were too short.

In 1988, Hennessy modified the BS-AC procedures, including repetitive dive calculations, and deleted the longer exposures. These **BS-AC '88 Tables** allegedly have more conservative no-stops limits and a safe no-decompression depth of 6 metres, although there are serious doubts as to whether they really are always safer than the earlier or other comparative tables, especially for decompression stop dives. They presume subclinical bubbles during repetitive dives, and assume that decompression after these dives will eliminate nitrogen more slowly. Progressively longer decompression is required for each repetitive dive.

These tables are comparable with the current Buhlmann and DCIEM Tables for non-decompression diving (see below). For dives requiring decompression stops, they are sometimes, but not always, more conservative than the USN tables and usually less conservative than the Buhlmann or DCIEM tables.

BASSETT TABLES

Dr.Bruce Bassett (a USAF physiologist) concluded that the current US Navy Tables resulted in an excessive incidence of about 6% DCS when pushed to the limit.

Bassett reduced the no-decompression limits of the USN tables. He recommended an ascent rate of 10 metres (30 ft.) per minute, with a 3–5 minute safety stop at 3–5 metres for all dives greater than 9 metres. The total time underwater, rather than the bottom time was used to calculate the repetitive group after a dive. Bassett's tables are safer than the US Navy tables for sports divers.

Knight and **Lippmann (Australia)** modified the Bassett Tables for repetitive dive use.

DCIEM TABLES

The **Defence and Civil Institute of Environmental Medicine of Canada** uses a different model for decompression based on tissue compartments arranged in series, rather than in parallel as with the US Navy (originally Haldane) model.

It is a very well researched table. Although based on a decompression theory, it has been modified by extensive human testing in cold water and hard working conditions, with Doppler (ultrasound) monitoring. The single no-decompression times, and most repetitive dives, are more conservative than the US Navy tables and are recommended for recreational diving.

NAUI DIVE TABLES

These tables are based on the US Navy tables with **"fudge factors"** included. The no-decompression levels are reduced and a "safety" decompression stop at 5 metres for 3 minutes is recommended. The actual dive time is defined as the duration between commencing descent and reaching either the safety stop or the surface.

HUGGINS TABLES

These tables are also based on the US Navy tables, but made more conservative by recalculating them based on lower "M" value (maximum supersaturation gradients) and recalculation of repetitive diving groups to consider all the tissues (not just the 120 minute tissue as in the US Navy tables). This may make the table more applicable for multi-level diving.

PADI TABLES

The initial PADI Tables were, like the Bassett Tables, based on the US Navy Tables.

The PADI Recreational Dive Planner, and later the "Wheel", however is often less conservative than the US Navy tables, allowing longer repetitive dives after shorter surface intervals. Selective practical testing of the tables was performed using Doppler (ultrasound) monitoring.

BUHLMANN TABLES

The Swiss decompression expert, Professor Buhlmann, has conducted many theoretical and practical investigations on the Swiss model, which includes 16 theoretical tissue compartments with widely ranging half times. The testing of these tables at altitude has been more extensive than for most other tables.

The permitted duration of deep dives exceeds the US Navy tables, but the ascent rate is reduced to 10 metres per minute. All no-decompression dives require a stop of one minute at three metres.

It is believed that shorter initial dives will minimise bubble formation on the first dive and so improve the nitrogen off-loading during ascent. This allows longer times for the repetitive dives.

"NEW" TABLES

The imminent release of "new" tables is a permanent rumour. The difficulty in producing mathematical models which truly reflect human decompression physiology upon which to base the tables, as well as the difficulty and expense of testing them, makes the frequent development of tables based on truly new models unlikely. However, tables based on recycled mathematical models do frequently arise.

MULTI–LEVEL DIVING

Recreational divers often have a need to dive at different depths during the dive (usually depending on the bottom terrain). To allow for this, a number of ingenious modifications were made to the conventional tables, to give an indication of the decompression requirements. Sometimes the repetitive group residual N_2 concepts of the US Navy tables are used to assess each of the various depths.

Some tables have specifically included multi-level diving in their decompression requirements. These include the Huggins, DCIEM and BSAC – 88 tables. Many of the computers, especially those based on decompression theory, allow for multi-level diving (and this is probably a major reason why they are less safe).

Multi-level diving is almost totally based on theory. There have been no adequate and comprehensive trials performed to show their reliability. One obvious error was that they often allowed divers to dive from a shallow plateau to a deeper one, with little penalty. Most proponents now realise the danger of this and recommend the opposite sequence — a triumph of empirical practice and commonsense over mathematical theory.

DECOMPRESSION METERS (COMPUTERS)

These meters are based on three different principles :

❏ Mechanical models of gas transfer.

These meters rely on the movement of gas through small orifices to simulate uptake and elimination of nitrogen by compartments of the body. They are obviously a gross oversimplification but one, the **SOS meter**, is moderately safe for single shallow non-decompression dives to less than 24 metres.

❏ Electronic models of existing tables.

These devices record the depth and time of a dive and relate this to one of the existing decompression tables which is stored in its memory. One has even been incorporated into a wrist watch. They save the diver the trouble of recording his depth and time, and reading the tables.

These meters have not been very popular, since they do not offer any greater endurance than that offered by the conventional tables and represent quite a great expense merely to save the diver the trouble of reading a decompression table.

❏ Electronic models based on decompression theory.

These meters are programmed with one of the mathematical models on which the conventional tables have been based (usually the model for the US Navy or Buhlmann tables) and this is integrated with a multi-level diving calculation.

In general, for multi-level and repetitive dives they allow greater underwater exposure for less decompression, a concept initially attractive to a keen diver. What they omit are the inevitable "fudge factors" which go with conventional tables, such as rounding up to the next deepest depth and longest time increments. With the meter, if the dive is to 19 metres for 36 minutes, that data (not 21 metres for 40 minutes) is precisely what is used to calculate the decompression. To overcome this, shorter no-decompression times were often included and slower ascent rates have been advised. Nevertheless, the dive **profiles** and repetitive dives which they permit are **often dangerous** and this has been reflected in the number of DCS cases which they have produced.

With time, the manufacturers have included progressively more safety factors such as maximum depth restrictions, more conservative repetitive dives and safety stops. Many did not even admit that there was a risk of DCS with use of the meter when they were originally marketed.

❏ Disadvantages of decompression meters.

The main attraction of these meters is convenience coupled with maximum diving for minimum decompression. This is important to divers who have a limited amount of free time available for their sport. The price paid for longer duration and less decompression is an increased risk of DCS.

When each of the conventional decompression tables was first formulated from a mathematical model, it had to be extensively modified after human testing. Essentially, the meters are offering the tables as they were, before they were modified for safety.

Most of the new (1987–92) meters are (like the old SOS meters) conservative for short single, shallow dives. The dangers increase with longer, repetitive or deeper diving, and are then even less safe when applied to a multi-level profile — especially if deeper diving follows shallow diving.

The other problem is reliability. Most have a high rate of mechanical failure – despite the exorbitant cost of the equipment. Electronics, batteries and salt water are not very compatible. A prudent diver will ensure that backup recordings are made and kept.

Nevertheless, decompression meters will continue to be popular. They are perceived as an alternative to personal responsibility and are easy solutions to a difficult problem (decompression calculation). To question the value of the computers is tantamount to questioning the integrity of their owners and brings a deluge of unsolicited testimonials reminiscent of "snake oil therapies".

❏ Safety suggestions (the DCM Ten Commandments).

If you must rely on decompression meters, the following recommendations are made :

1. Do not dive within the 24 hours before using the DCM.
2. The DCM should be used on **all** dives, if it is used on **any**.
3. Ensure a back-up documentation of the dive profile and details.
4. In multi-level dives, the depths should be progressively shallower.
5. Repetitive dives (on the same day) should be progressively shallower.
6. Repetitive dives should have surface intervals of at least 2 hours.
7. With multiple days diving, every fourth day should be non-diving.
8. Add an extra decompression safety stop for 5 minutes at 5 metres,
   on each dive in excess of 15 metres depth, if practicable.
9. Do not do dives that require decompression or go into the decompression mode.
   Stay as far away from those dives as possible.
10. Do not presume that the DCM is accurate for diving at altitude or for altitude exposure
   (flying).

Chapter 15

DECOMPRESSION SICKNESS CLINICAL FEATURES

CLASSIFICATION OF SYMPTOMS

It is probably simplest to classify the clinical features of decompression sickness (DCS) according to the organ or system involved. In the past it was traditional to describe them as Type 1 (minor – musculo-skeletal or joint) or Type 2 (serious – cardio-pulmonary and neurological) DCS.

ONSET OF SYMPTOMS

The clinical features of DCS are seen during or after ascent. In the majority of cases, symptoms will be evident within six hours, and 50% within the first hour of the dive. Less commonly, a delay in onset of 24 hours or greater has been described. The time of onset of symptoms depends to some degree on the type of dive. Deep dives (greater than 30 metres), especially those which require decompression or are close to the no-decompression limits or in which decompression has been omitted, are likely to present early. In extreme cases, symptoms may present during ascent or the decompression stops. In general, the earlier the symptoms, the more potentially serious the DCS.

Symptoms may be initiated or aggravated by exposure to altitude (driving over mountains, air travel), exercise or breathing certain gases. Divers should be advised of the serious complications of flying after diving.

JOINT PAIN (MUSCULO-SKELETAL DCS, BENDS)

Pain in or near one of the muscles or tendons around the joints is the **most common presenting feature of DCS from shallow diving.** The shoulder is most often affected while the elbows, wrists, hand, hips, knees, ankles are less frequent. It is not unusual for two joints to be affected, commonly adjacent ones e.g. the shoulder and elbow on the same side. It is rare for multiple joints to be affected in a symmetrical pattern.

Symptoms may begin with discomfort or an abnormal feeling in or near the joint. Over the next hour or two, pain and other symptoms may develop. The pain is generally of a constant aching quality (like a toothache), but occasionally may be throbbing. The diver may hold the joint in a bent position to reduce the pain — the stooping posture which was adopted by Caisson (tunnel) workers affected by DCS near the hip, led to the term "bends".

The joint is usually not tender to touch but movement may aggravate the pain. Pressure, as from a blood pressure cuff (sphygmomanometer), may relieve the pain.

If not treated, pain usually continues for several uncomfortable days before slowly subsiding. In mild cases, minor and fleeting discomfort lasting only a few hours ("**niggles**") may be the only manifestation.

Symptoms are often found around a joint which has been subjected to unusual exertion or strain during or after the dive or which has suffered a recent or chronic injury.

There may occasionally be difficulty distinguishing between DCS and other causes of a painful joint such as strain, injury or arthritis. In the latter conditions, the joint is usually tender to touch and may be red and swollen. It is often bilateral and symmetrical and involves smaller joints. Movement usually makes the pain much worse, and local pressure application produces no relief. These signs are uncommon in DCS.

> **In general, any pain in or near a joint after compressed air dives in excess of 10 metres (or shallower with repetitive or prolonged dives) must be assumed to be DCS until proven otherwise.**

NEUROLOGICAL DCS

DCS can affect the **brain and/or the spinal cord.** The clinical features are due to disturbance of activity in the nervous system, interfering with one or more of its five principal functions :

- **sensation**
- **movement** (including balance and co-ordination)
- **consciousness** and intellectual functions
- **autonomic** functions
- **reflexes** (e.g. knee jerk, cough reflex).

Of these, the first four are easier for the layman to assess.

❏ The Senses.

These include sight, hearing, smell, taste, pain and touch. Numbness and tingling are frequent symptoms. Other abnormal signs include loss of sensation.

❏ Movement.

This includes the ability to move any muscle, the strength of the movement and the ability to co-ordinate it.

❏ Higher function of the brain.

The important intellectual functions are consciousness, orientation (awareness of time, person and place), thinking, speech and memory. Epileptic fits (convulsions) and confusion are possible.

❏ Autonomic functions.

Interference with the control of breathing and heart function may cause shock and collapse. Bladder and bowel malfunction usually causes progressive abdominal discomfort and tenderness until the bladder or bowels are opened.

In **Cerebral (Brain) DCS,** the bubbles of DCS may be located in or near the blood vessels supplying the brain, causing obstruction of blood flow and direct pressure on the neurological tissues. The brain swells like any other tissue when injured, but because it is confined within the solid bone of the skull, the pressure in the skull rises, further impairing blood supply to other parts of the brain. Swelling of the brain (cerebral oedema), as well as expansion of the nitrogen bubbles themselves, often leads to a steady worsening of this condition.

> The onset of cerebral DCS is often heralded by **headache** — probably due to brain swelling. **Numbness** or **tingling** (paraesthesiae), **weakness** or **paralysis** affecting a limb or one side of the body, difficulty with **speech**, **visual** disturbances, **confusion**, loss of **consciousness** or **convulsions** are all possible presenting symptoms of this serious disorder.

The part of the brain responsible for co-ordination (the cerebellum) may also be affected causing inco-ordination known as **"staggers".** The position sense and the balance organs can also be affected.

Spinal DCS has a frequent association with DCS bubbles in the blood and lungs, commonly known as **"chokes".** It also may be preceded by **"girdle pains"** — or pain around the chest or abdomen. Disturbances in movement such as **weakness or paralysis** or disturbances in sensation such as **numbness or tingling** are also common. Interference with nerve supply to the bladder and intestines, may lead to **difficulty in passing urine, or opening the bowel. Paraplegia** or **quadriplegia** may develop.

INNER EAR DCS

The cochlea (hearing) or vestibular (balance) organs may be involved. This type of DCS is more commonly associated with **deep diving, breathing a helium-oxygen mixture. Hearing loss, ringing noises** in the ears (tinnitus), and/or **vertigo, nausea** and **vomiting** are the usual presenting features. This condition must be distinguished from the other major cause of these symptoms in divers – inner ear barotrauma (see Chapter 9).

LUNGS or PULMONARY DCS

Nitrogen bubbles are frequently found in the veins of divers ascending after deep dives, without necessarily the development of overt clinical DCS. When large numbers of these bubbles form, they may become trapped in the small vessels of the lungs, obstructing the blood flow. If excessive bubbles occur, this leads to a disturbance of lung function and a feeling of **breathlessness**, known as the **"chokes"**.

Clinical features also include **a tight feeling in the chest, chest pain** and **rapid breathing**.

HEART or CARDIAC DCS

The nitrogen bubbles which commonly form in the veins of divers after deep dives are usually filtered by the lung vessels.

There is a condition affecting the heart (**patent foramen ovale – PFO**) which is sometimes claimed to be present in about 30% of the population, and in which there is a potential communication between the right and left sides of the heart – between the right and left atria. It is a flap valve, normally kept closed by the naturally higher pressure on the left side (left atrium) of the heart. When large amounts of nitrogen bubbles obstruct the lungs, the back pressure in the right atrium can exceed the pressure in the left atrium. This flap may then open allowing gas bubbles to pass from the right to the left side of the heart, and then be pumped and distributed to any part of the body (similar to arterial gas embolism resulting from a burst lung – see Chapter 11).

Bubbles can occasionally pass down the coronary arteries, which supply the heart, restricting the blood supply to the heart itself. In severe instances this can lead to a fatal destruction of heart muscle (myocardial infarction) just as for a "heart attack" in a non-diving person. Even in less severe cases, life threatening disturbances in cardiac pumping and rhythm may result.

Cardiac symptoms include chest pain, palpitations and shortness of breath.

Bubbles passing through a patent foramen ovale (PFO), or any other cardiac defects, tend to rise because of buoyancy. They can be easily carried into the blood vessels supplying the brain because it has a large blood supply and is located above the heart. This is one cause of cerebral DCS after apparently so called "safe" dives. It may be called cerebral arterial gas embolism or **CAGE,** but is due to DCS, and not pulmonary barotrauma. The term **acute decompression illness** covers both causes.

GASTROINTESTINAL DCS

Obstruction of blood flow to the intestines by nitrogen bubbles can cause dysfunction of the gut. Clinical features include **vomiting** or **diarrhoea, cramping abdominal pain** and **haemorrhage** into the gut. Severe cases can show clinical shock, and can bleed to death.

SKIN MANIFESTATIONS of DCS

These are not common in scuba divers who wear wet suits.

Itching of the arms and legs, sometimes with a rash, is not uncommon after deep recompression chamber dives and with dry suits. This condition is probably due to gas passing from the high pressure atmosphere into the skin. The condition is not serious and requires no treatment.

In more severe DCS, nitrogen bubbles in the blood can obstruct blood supply to the skin, causing patchy white, blue and pink areas – **"marbling"**. Obstruction of the lymphatic system (drainage of tissues) may produce **localised swelling of skin**.

GENERAL SYMPTOMS of DCS

Apathy, tiredness, malaise, and a **generalised weakened state** is a common observation in most cases of DCS. In very severe cases there may be **generalised internal haemorrhages, shock,** and/or **death**.

DELAYED SYMPTOMS of DCS

Prolonged symptoms may be due to damaged nerve, body tissues or bone (see Chapter 17). In these cases there can be a persistence or recurrence of symptoms. Various psychological problems can also supervene on DCS. Even the stressful treatments and peer recriminations can exact an emotional toll on divers.

EVOLUTION OF SYMPTOMS

In assessing DCS, the time of onset of symptoms should be related to the time of ascent. The clinical manifestations and their evolution should be described, together with any aggravating factors.

The manifestations may be progressive (getting worse), static or improving. They may also relapse. Aggravating factors include not only those that predispose to DCS, but also those that precipitate it (see Chapter 13).

A major observation, supporting the diagnosis of DCS, is the favourable response of DCS to raised environmental pressure (re-immersion in the water, treatment in a recompression chamber) and, to a lesser degree, administration of 100% O2.

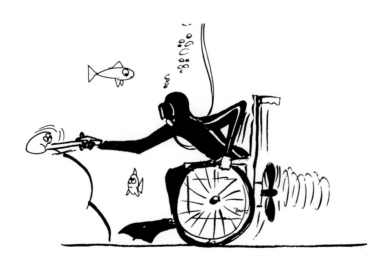

Fig. 15.1

Chapter 16

DECOMPRESSION SICKNESS TREATMENT

FIRST AID

The principles of first aid management of decompression sickness (DCS) are :

- **the basic first aid, A–B–C** — Airway, Breathing, Circulation
- **100% oxygen (O$_2$)**   (see Chapter 42).
- **positioning and rest**
- **fluid replacement.**

❑ **Oxygen therapy** (see Chapter 40).

If the diver breathes 100% oxygen (O$_2$), nitrogen (N$_2$) is removed from the lungs. The breathing apparatus must supply to the lungs as close to 100% O$_2$ as possible. This means an **anaesthetic type mask** – and not the simple oxygen masks that do not produce an air tight seal. 100% O$_2$ in the lungs results in a high diffusion (pressure gradient) of N$_2$ from the blood to the lungs, causing the increased elimination of nitrogen from the blood and tissues – and also from any bubbles there.

Unfortunately 100% O$_2$ can be toxic to the lungs if given for 18–24 hours on the surface. This may complicate the hyperbaric O$_2$ which is given to the diver in a recompression chamber (RCC). Ideally O$_2$ therapy should given under the supervision of a diving physician, however, if expert advice is unavailable, then **all suspected case of DCS should be given 100% O$_2$** from the outset, before and during movement of the patient and transport to the recompression chamber.

Unconscious divers, if not breathing of their own accord, may require assisted ventilation (intermittent positive pressure respiration or I.P.P.R.). Conscious patients can be treated with continuous flow or demand type masks. In such cases, treating personnel must always check the breathing mask on themselves first in order to ensure the oxygen system is working, and that resistance to breathing is not excessive.

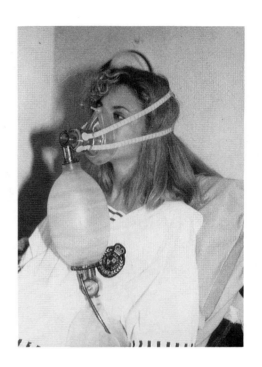

Fig. 16.1
Photograph of diver with DCS breathing near 100% O$_2$ from a Laerdal system (see Chapter 42).

Note reservoir bag (lowermost) and high flow (14 litres per minute) oxygen delivery tube.

❑ Position and rest.

An unconscious diver should be placed on his side in the coma position, to protect the airway at all times (see Chapter 42). If there is any likelihood of air embolism, the diver is best placed horizontal, preferably, on the left side, but not essentially.

Some clinicians recommend that cases of cerebral DCS should be managed with the patient on the side without a pillow, to prevent buoyant gas bubbles reaching the brain through the circulation. Unfortunately, having the head lowered raises the pressure in the brain – and this can aggravate the brain injury thus the Trendelenburg (30º head down) position is no longer recommended.

Due to the buoyancy of bubbles, sitting or standing may be dangerous in patients with air embolism or cerebral decompression sickness where the bubbles are in the blood stream. As a general rule, 100% O$_2$ should be given for at least an hour before allowing the patient to sit or stand. Otherwise, the diver can be allowed to adopt any comfortable position but should be kept relatively still. A diver with "chokes" will be more comfortable sitting up.

❑ Fluid replacement.

Severe DCS results in loss of blood fluids into the tissues. There may be a need to replace this fluid orally or intravenously.

Some authorities have recommended large volumes of oral fluids while the diver is being transported to a RCC in an attempt to replace this deficit. One problem with this (as any party goer will attest), is that the fluid load will promote a vigorous urine flow, so the diver arrives at the recompression facility with a stomach and bladder full of fluid. A patient with spinal DCS may be unable to empty the bladder and will therefore be in considerable pain. If orange juice is used, as advocated by some writers, the glucose content will further delay the emptying of the stomach. Nausea and vomiting may also be induced by such 'acidic' drinks.

On arrival at the RCC facility, the patient will usually be treated on a hyperbaric O_2 (HBO) treatment table. There is a very real risk of nausea, vomiting and convulsions as complications of this treatment. A full stomach can then possibly result in regurgitation of the stomach contents and aspiration into the lungs – further complicating treatment..

If there is no bladder involvement (i.e. the patient can urinate), a litre of clear fluid every 2-4 hours should suffice. This fluid intake should be modified by the patient's thirst. It should be water or a weak electrolyte solution (eg."Gastrolyte") rather than orange juice etc. (unless the diver is also suffering from scurvy).

If the brain or spinal cord is involved and the patient has difficulty in voiding urine, an **in-dwelling urinary catheter** should be inserted whenever possible by a trained physician or nurse. If this is not feasible, care must be taken not to overload the patient with fluids.

Anyone who is trained to institute and monitor an intravenous infusion can be expected to be able to assess the state of hydration and determine the desirability and quantity of intravenous fluids.

❏ Drugs.

Aspirin as a first aid measure has not been demonstrated to be of value in DCS. It may interfere with blood clotting and cause haemorrhage (bleeding) – especially in the stomach. Haemorrhage is already a major complication in spinal cord and inner ear DCS.

The authors have seen one patient with severe DCS bleed to death from an internal haemorrhage just before he was to be given an "experimental last-ditch" anti-clotting agent. We are therefore reluctant to advocate the routine use of aspirin either for pain relief or to inhibit clotting in any DCS case.

Joint pains of DCS can be significantly eased without the risk of serious side effects by the administration of **paracetamol (acetaminophen)** – 1000 mg (or two tablets) 4 hourly.

Other drugs such as steroids, diuretics and special intravenous fluids such as "Rheomacrodex" have been advocated but have not been proven to be beneficial. Anti-epileptics and other drugs such as diazepam ("Valium") may be needed to control fitting (convulsions), and for confusional states.

❏ Expert advice.

Expert advice from a diving physician should be sought as soon as possible. **Appendix B** contains a list of sources for such expert advice.

TRANSPORT OF PATIENT WITH DCS

The diver should be transported with **minimum agitation** and as close as possible to sea level or at **1 ATA**. Mountainous roads should be avoided whenever an evacuation route by land is planned. **100% Oxygen** should be breathed before and during transport (see Chapter 40).

Transportation in aircraft presents problems. Apart from movement which aggravates DCS. environmental pressure decreases with altitude, causing DCS bubbles to expand (Boyle's Law) and more gas to pass from the tissues into any bubbles.

If the patient is evacuated by air, unpressurised aircraft should endeavour to fly at the lowest safe altitude. Even an altitude of 300 metres (1000 ft.) can make the symptoms of DCS worse. However, maintaining such an altitude can be alarming when flying over 297 metre (990 ft.) terrain.

It should be remembered that most commercial "**pressurised**" aircraft normally maintain a cabin pressure of around 2000 metres (6000 ft.), which will seriously aggravate DCS .

Whenever possible the cabin altitude should be maintained at 1ATA. This is attainable by many modern commercial jet aircraft, executive aircraft such as the King Air and Lear Jet, and some military transport aircraft (Hercules C–130). This requirement is not popular with the commercial airlines since it necessitates the aircraft flying at lower than its most efficient altitude, resulting in excessive fuel consumption. This requirement may also limit the range of certain aircraft.

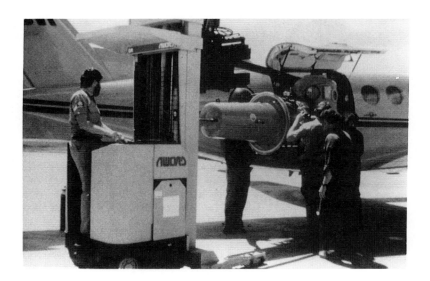

Fig. 16.2

Portable RCC (two-man "Duocom") being loaded into a King Air aircraft. Patient and attendant are contained within RCC which is pressurised. Patient breathes 100% O_2.

DEFINITIVE TREATMENT OF DCS

❑ Therapeutic recompression.

This is the most effective treatment for DCS. Delay increases the likelihood of a poor final result. The diver is placed in a **recompression chamber (RCC)** and the pressure is increased according to a specified recompression treatment table.

The increase in pressure reduces the bubble size (Boyle's Law) and usually relieves the clinical features. It also increases the surface area to volume ratio of the bubble, which may collapse the bubble. The increased pressure in the bubble also enhances the diffusion gradient, encouraging nitrogen to leave the bubble.

The therapeutic recompression schedule determines the depth and duration of the treatment profile. The table selected may depend on factors such as the time elapsed since the onset of symptoms, the depth of the original dive and the type and severity of symptoms, as well as the capability of the treatment facility and the various breathing gases available. The treatment may be amended depending on the patient's response.

In recent years the **Oxygen Treatment Tables** are preferred because of their much increased effectiveness. The injured diver is usually compressed to an equivalent depth of 18 metres (60 ft.) and is decompressed over 2–5 hours. He breathes oxygen from a mask while the rest of the chamber is filled with air. If the whole chamber is filled with oxygen, the **fire risk** increases dramatically.

Because the attendant breathes chamber air, great care must be taken to monitor his dive profile to avoid the embarrassing predicament of an attendant emerging from the RCC with DCS.

The diver breaths oxygen for the duration of the treatment except for 5 minute periods of air – or sometimes heliox (He-O$_2$) breathing – every 25 minutes, to minimise oxygen toxicity to the **lungs**. The regimen is not without hazard as there is a significant risk of **cerebral oxygen toxicity** causing convulsions in such persons.

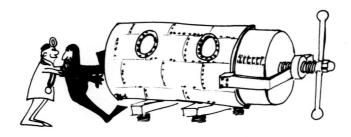

Fig. 16.3

Other tables are available which involve compressing the diver to a depth equivalent of 30–50 metres sea-water (100–165 ft.) in **air, heliox** and **nitrox** mixtures and then decompressing over periods ranging from several hours to several days depending on the severity of the symptoms.

Many other investigations and treatment modalities will be employed by experienced physicians in the RCC, including fluid balance, medications, etc, which need not concern the average diver.

A further emergency procedure, **Underwater Oxygen Treatment,** has been devised for use under expert supervision in remote localities. The diver is **recompressed in the water** to a maximum of 9 metres while breathing 100% oxygen. Details of this procedure are outlined in Appendix E.

Treatment in water with the diver **breathing air** has been used in many parts of the world and water treatment tables are contained in some Navy diving manuals. While success has often been reported and delay in treatment can be avoided, this form of treatment has serious theoretical and practical difficulties which can result in worsening of the diver's condition.

The deep water requirements (30 metres initially, and decompression for 2–4 hours)) renders the patient and accompanying divers prone to cold (hypothermia), gas exhaustion, tide and other current changes. Attending divers may well develop DCS from extra exposures. This form of treatment is not generally recommended, unless other options (RCC, underwater oxygen treatment etc.) are unavailable.

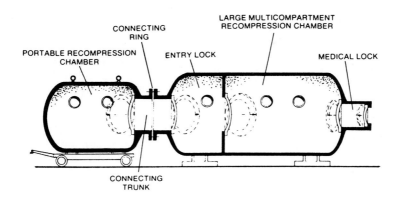

Fig. 16.4

Schematic outline of large static RCC treatment facility showing linking of small portable chamber to the larger fixed unit. Both chambers are pressurised to identical pressures for a "transfer-under-pressure" (TUP).

❑ Hazards of therapeutic recompression.

While therapeutic recompression generally produces dramatic relief of symptoms, it has several life threatening hazards. These include **oxygen toxicity** in the patient, the risk of **fire** and the risk of producing **DCS in the attendant.** It should only be used under the close supervision of a medical officer experienced in its use.

> **Some decompression tables and instructions for their use are published at the end of this book. It is stressed that they are included only as a reference for diving paramedics – not for use by divers.**

PREVENTION OF DECOMPRESSION SICKNESS

There are a number of factors which predispose to DCS. These are described in Chapter 13. Obviously these should be avoided wherever possible. Apart from falsifying a birth certificate, unfortunately, there is little an individual can do about the predisposing factor of age.

Because of the incomplete reliability of the currently available dive tables and the unpredictability of the development of DCS, it is possible for even the most careful, well trained diver to develop this condition. The following suggestions will help reduce the risks.

> **It is important that the diver never exceeds the no-decompression tables and ascent rates. In spite of this, all the dive tables, and especially the dive computers, so far devised have a significant failure rate.**

❑ "Fudge factors".

The rate of development of DCS varies from less than 1% to as much as 15% depending on the table, the depth and the duration of the dive, and if tables are pushed to their limits. The apparent safety of the tables is probably improved by intelligent divers incorporating "fudge factors" of their own. This is especially required for older, fatter and less fit divers.

❑ Accurate depth & time.

It is essential that the diver knows accurately the depths and durations of his diving. A depth gauge which indicates the maximum depth attained is useful, because it is common for divers to descend deeper than they realise. An underwater **watch** or, better, a **bottom timer** is essential.

❑ No-decompression diving.

Although the tables are not totally reliable, they are less reliable for deep diving (greater than 30 metres). It is advisable to avoid pushing the tables to the limits when a no-decompression schedule is followed and to avoid dives requiring decompression.

❑ Slow ascent rates.

A slow ascent is prudent and the diver should certainly not ascend faster than the rate recommended by the tables. Preferably a slower ascent rate should be employed (8–10 metres or 25–33 ft. per minute is a relatively safe rate) and the extra time taken be deleted from the bottom time. i.e. ascend earlier than permitted by the tables.

❑ Routine decompression stops.

Most authorities recommend a routine minimum safety ("decompression") stop at **5 metres for 5 minutes**, after a no-decompression dive to allow partial nitrogen elimination and trapping of venous emboli in the lung vessels.

❑ Dive planning.

When repeated dives are planned, the **deeper dives** should always be **performed first. With multi-day diving,** a rest day is included after each 3 continuous diving days. With deep diving, gradual build up (**acclimatisation**) is achieved by progressively deeper exposures.

❑ Post-dive flying restrictions.

It is advisable to **rest** for an hour or more after a deep or long dive to ensure elimination of nitrogen from the fast tissues. Flying and altitude exposures within 12–24 hours of diving is not recommended.

In addition to the above precautions, the diver is also advised to buy a good quality waterproof rabbit's foot. A healthy scepticism towards reliance on any mechanical equipment, especially if promoted by a glossy brochure or a dive computer salesman, also has good survival value.

❑ Dive computers (See Chapter 14).

Chapter 17

DYSBARIC OSTEONECROSIS

(DIVERS BONE DISEASE, AVASCULAR NECROSIS OF BONE, ASEPTIC BONE NECROSIS, BONE NECROSIS, BONE ROT, CAISSON DISEASE OF BONE)

This was first noticed in caisson (tunnel) workers in the 19th century, and was described as being an area of localised bone death, predominantly occurring in the long bones of the arms and thigh.

If this area of dead bone is located beneath the joint surface of the bones in the hip or shoulder joints, pain and symptoms of arthritis, along with a reduction in mobility of the joint is a common consequence – often occurring in mid or later life.

The exact cause of the disorder is probably a delayed effect of damage caused by gas bubbles produced during a dive (see Chapter 13). In this sense it is a delayed form of decompression sickness.

Cause

Bone is a living organ containing bone cells which constantly absorb and lay down new bone. It has a cleverly designed structure which resembles reinforced concrete or fibreglass and contains fibres of a sinew-like substance called collagen, embedded in a concrete-like calcium material. This is traversed by numerous vessels which supply the blood to the bone cells embedded in the bone. The bone cells permit the repair of fractures and allow the bone to change its structure to accommodate stresses which may vary during the person's life.

If the blood vessels supplying the bone cells are blocked by gas bubbles or any other cause, the bone cells die and the self-repairing ability of the bone stops. It becomes unable to fix the repeated minor trauma which is common around joints and eventually the bone structure collapses causing permanent damage to the major load bearing joints, such as the hips or shoulders.

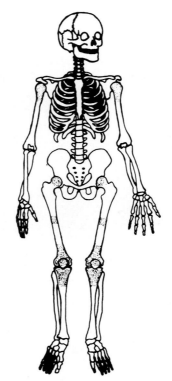

Fig. 17.1

SITES OF DYSBARIC OSTEONECROSIS

The reported incidence of this condition varies from less than 1% in some Navy series, to 80% in Chinese commercial divers. This variance is probably due to factors such as different diagnostic criteria and differing dive patterns and frequency.

Predisposing factors which are commonly associated with osteonecrosis include :

- **age greater than 30 years**
- **inadequate decompressions**
- **experimental dives**
- **deep dives**
- **decompression sickness**
- **long duration dives**

X-Ray changes have been seen as soon as 3 months after a dive and it has been reported following a single deep dive. When joint involvement does occur, the onset of symptoms is usually delayed for many years, reflecting the time required for joint destruction. Fortunately, in most cases the disease does not cause any serious damage to the joints and so produces no symptoms.

Classification of Bone Necrosis

The lesions are classified into two groups :

- **Type A lesions** – which are near the joint surface (juxta-articular).
- **Type B lesions** – which are remote from the joint surface (head, neck and shaft).

❏ Type A lesions.

With these, the joints may become involved as the overlying bone is destroyed and the joint surface collapses. This may produce symptoms which are potentially crippling. Hips and shoulders are more frequently affected.

❏ Type B lesions.

These rarely cause symptoms and are generally of little clinical importance, except to suggest more conservative diving procedures. The most common areas affected are the long bones of the thigh, leg and upper arm. Occasional cases of bone cancer have developed in these lesions.

Clinical Features

When Type A lesions injure the joint, common symptoms are pain, which is usually aggravated by movement, in the affected joint and accompanied by a restriction of joint movement. As the condition progresses, severe osteoarthritis develops and the joint may eventually become frozen and incapacitating, due to pain.

Investigations

X–Rays have been the traditional investigative method but these will only reveal lesions once bone changes have developed. This may take months or years.

Early lesions can now be identified with newer techniques. Injected radioactive Technetium ("bone scans") will bind to an osteonecrotic area and can be detected with a scanner within 2 weeks of the injury. The lesions can also be identified in excellent detail, using MRI (Magnetic Resonance Imaging) scanning. This is unfortunately expensive but has no associated risks of irradiation.

Treatment

The pain associated with movement can be reduced with an anti-inflammatory drug such as NSAIDS. Severe cases may require the fusion of a joint or its replacement with a synthetic joint made of either metal or plastic. While this procedure relieves the pain and increases mobility, a synthetic joint is never as robust as the "natural model" and its endurance is limited.

As the disease is regarded as an occupational hazard of diving, workers compensation claims may help off-set expensive medical costs.

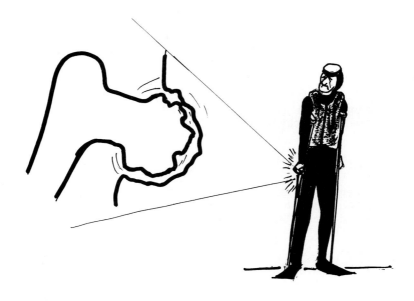

Fig. 17.2

Prevention

Avoidance of the known predisposing factors is obviously desirable. Most sensible recreational divers run little risk of this condition. Generally they should; avoid dives deeper than 30 metres, avoid dives requiring decompression, not approach the no-decompression limits, and ascend slowly.

Occupational divers and other divers who are at increased risk because of their diving practices should have regular routine screening X–ray assessments. Since these investigations can involve worrisome exposure to radiation, their frequency must be weighed against the risk of osteonecrosis development. Divers who are likely to be at risk are required to have a baseline investigation performed before they are employed. For some susceptible occupational divers, follow-up assessments at 5 year intervals are recommended.

In divers who develop decompression sickness, a follow-up bone scan after 2–4 weeks should detect areas of bone damage. MRI imaging can often be better used to determine the extent of the lesion.

Divers with high risk factors who develop unexplained joint pain should be assessed to exclude this condition.

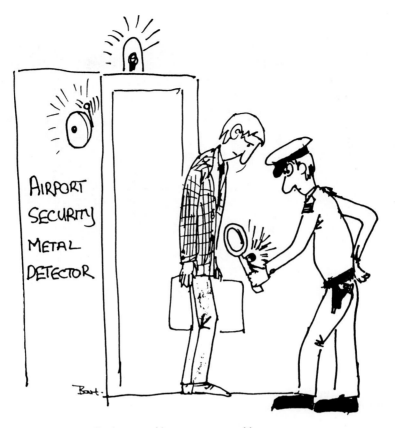

Replacement hips may cause problems.

Fig. 17.3

Chapter 18

NITROGEN NARCOSIS

(COMPRESSED AIR INTOXICATION,
RAPTURE OF THE DEEP,
INERT GAS NARCOSIS, NARCS)

Intoxication in divers is not confined exclusively to beach barbeques and hotel bars. When breathed under pressure, nitrogen (which makes up 79% of air) has an intoxicating effect which, like alcohol, is variable and may lead to pleasure or disaster.

This phenomenon was regarded as an annoyance to the helmet diver who could be pulled to the surface by his attendant if he behaved irrationally, but the consequences to the scuba diver, who's safety is dependent on a buddy exposed to the same effect, can be more serious.

It will be present in all divers breathing air at a depth in excess of 30 metres, although some will notice it earlier. Others may not be aware of the effect, as judgement and perception are affected. The severity of symptoms and the exact depth of their onset varies between individuals. Because of narcosis, diving on air beyond 30 metres (100 feet) is not prudent, and 40 metres is considered unsafe for most recreational divers. 50 metres depth is considered the maximum safe depth for professional divers breathing air.

CAUSES OF NITROGEN NARCOSIS

The exact cause of this narcotic effect is uncertain. Nitrogen is classified as an inert gas because it does not participate in any chemical reactions within the human body. The influence of nitrogen on narcosis must therefore be due to some physical reaction.

When other inert gases such as neon, xenon and argon were investigated, it was found that their narcotic effect at depth correlated approximately with the relative weights of their individual molecules (i.e. their molecular weights). An increased molecular weight caused a greater narcotic effect. It was further shown that the inert gases which were more soluble in fat than water, tended to have a greater narcotic effect. There were unfortunately several inconsistencies in the behaviour of these gases, including hydrogen, which cast some doubt on these generalisations.

Other theories have been proposed implicating oxygen or carbon dioxide toxicity, lipid solubility and enzyme changes in the brain.

CLINICAL FEATURES

The narcotic effect usually becomes effective within a few minutes of reaching a particular depth and does not worsen as exposure continues at this depth. Rapid descents may increase the effect while with ascent it is ameliorated.

The higher brain functions such as reasoning, judgement, memory, perception, concentration and attention tend to be the first affected by narcosis. This often leads to a feeling of well-being and stimulation in a diver secure in his surroundings. In a novice or an apprehensive diver, a panic reaction may follow. Some degree of tolerance develops at a given depth or with repetitive exposures.

The influence of narcosis may not be evident if the dive is uneventful, thus giving a false impression that the diver is in control of the situation. Memory and perception deficits may only be evidenced by a failure to follow instructions or the dive plan, or being inattentive to buoyancy, air supply or buddy signals. When a problem develops, the diver may be unaware of this – attention and perception being focussed elsewhere (perceptual narrowing or "tunnel vision"). Thus emergency signals will go unheeded, emergency air supplies will not be offered, weight belts will not be released, rescue attempts will be crude and amateurish. Survival instincts and responses may be dampened. The safety of both the diver and his buddy are compromised.

Death may supervene due to errors provoked by impaired judgement or perception, and by over confidence. Loss of consciousness may happen without warning and be unnoticed by the diver's buddy. At great depths the diver may lose consciousness from the narcosis itself or the interaction between it and other factors such as carbon dioxide or oxygen toxicity and sensory deprivation.

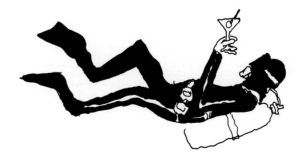

Fig. 18.1

Factors which are known to **increase** the effects of nitrogen narcosis include :

- **low intelligence**
- **fatigue or heavy work**
- **anxiety, inexperience or apprehension**
- **cold (hypothermia)**
- **recent alcohol intake or use of sedative drugs (includes seasickness medications), marijuana etc.**
- **poor visibility**

Factors which tend to **reduce** the effects of narcosis include :

- **strong motivation to perform a given task**
- **acclimatisation following prolonged or repeated exposures**
- **tolerance to heavy alcohol intake**

A diver who can "hold his liquor" is said to have a greater tolerance to nitrogen-narcosis. A plea of "acclimatising to narcosis" is generally not accepted by the courts however, as defence for an alcoholic intoxication charge.

The effect of nitrogen narcosis has been likened by some to that of drinking one martini on an empty stomach for every 10 metres depth (**Martini's Law**). The "olive" appears to be optional.

Martini's Law Table

20 – 30 metres	Mild impairment of performance on unpractised tasks, mild euphoria.

30 – 50 metres	Laughter and loquacity which can be overcome by self control.
	Overconfidence and inadequate responses to danger.
	Perceptual narrowing, fixation on a particular function or exercise.
	Judgement impairment affecting air supply, buoyancy control, navigational errors, decompression obligations, ascent rates, etc. Anxiety.

50 metres	Sleepiness and loss of judgement. Hallucinations may occur.

50 – 70 metres	In a chamber, convivial atmosphere - most talkative, but some terrified.
	Occasional dizziness or uncontrolled laughter verging on hysteria.

70 metres	Poor reasoning ability. Very poor response to signals or instructions.

70 – 90 metres	Poor concentration and mental confusion, stupefaction, loss of memory.

90 metres +	Hallucinations and unconsciousness

Table 18.1

Case History Examples :

1. A group of divers descended into a deep clear freshwater cave in order to savour the pleasant intoxication of narcosis. Their bodies were found some weeks later in a deep confine of the cave. They were victims of over-confidence and impaired judgement induced by nitrogen narcosis.

2. Another diver became so elated during his dive that he removed his regulator and offered it to the other marine inhabitants.

3. A diver developed problems with his air supply but, possibly because of the 40 metre depth and narcosis, he did not attempt to ditch his weight belt. He triggered the dump valve of his BC instead of the inflation valve, and drowned with minimal struggling.

PREVENTION

Avoidance of compressed air diving to depths known to cause narcosis is a good policy. This implies a depth limit of 30 – 45 metres (100 – 150 feet) depending on the diver's experience, his tolerance to narcosis and the task performed. Safe diving beyond 30 metres requires an awareness of the ever increasing risk of this condition and its effects on human performance and judgement. Some experienced professional divers may be able to perform certain practised tasks at depths up to 60 metres with competency, but dives greater than 30 metres should be a source of concern for recreational divers and greater than 50 metres should be regarded as excessive even for professionals.

TREATMENT

A diver incapacitated by narcosis should be protected from injury and inappropriate behaviour, and bought to a shallow depth with a controlled ascent, bearing in mind decompression requirements. Symptoms clear rapidly as the nitrogen pressure is reduced. Any other symptoms present on surfacing (eg. salt water aspiration and near drowning, decompression sickness etc.) are due to complications of experiencing narcosis at depth and not narcosis *per se*.

Chapter 19

HIGH PRESSURE NEUROLOGICAL SYNDROME

(HIGH PRESSURE NERVOUS SYNDROME, HPNS, HELIUM TREMORS)

This condition is a problem for deep commercial diving operations where helium/oxygen (Heliox) mixtures are breathed at depths in excess of 130 metres (430 feet). It causes a serious limitation to very deep diving and gets worse as the depth increases.

It is unlikely to bother the sports diver unless a grave miscalculation of depth or buoyancy has been made.

CLINICAL FEATURES

The first sign is usually a mild uncontrollable tremor, with muscle twitching and difficulty in coordinating movements. If the diver then continues with the descent, confusion, drowsiness, disorientation and unconsciousness may follow. Respiration may also be affected by the incoordination. The tremor particularly affects the hands and arms and resembles the shivering due to cold (which helium breathing may also produce).

The condition is aggravated by rapid descent and thus a slow descent rate is a requirement in all deep diving operations using this gas mixture.

The cause of HPNS is not fully understood. It is probably due to an excitation of a part of the brain by the direct mechanical effect of pressure. Evidence for this is that drug induced anaesthesia in animals can be reversed by simply compressing the animal to depths which provoke HPNS.

TREATMENT AND PREVENTION

Since the effects of HPNS resembled an excitation of the brain, early researchers reasoned that an agent which caused sedation might reverse the condition. Nitrogen narcosis is a common cause of sedation during diving, and so divers affected by HPNS were given a small concentrations of nitrogen to breathe, producing effective reduction of some of the symptoms of HPNS. This helium-nitrogen-oxygen mixture (Tri-mix) is now used in most deep diving. Small percentages of nitrogen have been included to reduce the HPNS – but not enough to cause significant nitrogen narcosis. The added nitrogen also permits better speech comprehension, because helium distorts sound production in the human larynx.

Chapter 20

HYPOXIA

(ANOXIA)

Hypoxia refers to an inadequate level of oxygen (O_2) within the cells. **Anoxia** occurs when there is no O_2 left at all in the cells, and is uncommon. Without O_2 most cells, especially those of the brain, die within a few minutes. This is the final out-come of many diving accidents and is often the ultimate cause of death.

Hypoxia is caused by an interruption in the chain of physiological processes (see Chapters 3 & 4) which bring O_2 from the outside air (or breathing gas) to the body's cells. There are **four links** in this chain where interruption can cause hypoxia, supplying a logical classification.

CLASSIFICATION OF HYPOXIA

Inadequate Oxygen content in Arterial Blood (HYPOXIC HYPOXIA)

In diving, the most common form of hypoxia is **hypoxic hypoxia**. Either there is inadequate O_2 getting to the lungs because the diver has, for a variety of reasons, only water to breathe, or the lungs are unable to convey inhaled O_2 to the blood from alveolar damage due to near drowning. The most common causes are thus an inadequate air supply and/or salt water aspiration or drowning.

The commonest cause is an inadequate air supply. This can also arise from an inadequate concentration of O_2 in the breathing gas (e.g. a gas mixture in which O_2 has been inadvertently omitted or an internally rusty scuba cylinder which extracts O_2). It may develop from equipment failure or obstruction somewhere in the respiratory tract between the nose or mouth and the alveoli, due to :

- upper airway obstruction due to unconsciousness
- tracheal obstruction from inhalation of vomit and
- alveolar damage from salt water inhalation (see Chapters 25 and 26).

O_2 is Taken Up by the Blood but Fails to Reach the Tissues
(STAGNANT HYPOXIA)

This is generally due to failure of the heart to pump the blood adequately to the tissues (e.g. from a heart attack or air embolism). Poor circulation to the extremities in cold conditions can cause localised hypoxia to these areas without generalised hypoxia.

Inability of the Blood to Carry O_2 in the presence of Adequate Circulation
(ANAEMIC HYPOXIA)

This is generally due to inadequate amounts of circulating functional haemoglobin, usually from blood loss or carbon monoxide poisoning (see Chapter 23).

Inability of the Cells to Use the O_2 Delivered to the Cells
(HISTOTOXIC HYPOXIA)

This is caused by certain poisons including carbon monoxide (see Chapter 23).

HYPOXIA IN BREATHHOLD DIVING

Hyperventilation

As explained in Chapter 4, hyperventilation before a breath-hold dive reduces the urge to breathe during the dive and may cause the diver to lose consciousness from hypoxia while still underwater (see Case Histories 33.2, 33.3). Drowning frequently results from this.

Hypoxia of Ascent

The partial pressure of O_2 in the lungs falls as they expand during ascent from a breath-hold dive. In some circumstances, this can cause loss of consciousness from hypoxia during ascent. Details are explained fully in Chapter 4.

HYPOXIA IN COMPRESSED AIR DIVING

Scuba

Exhaustion of the air supply, equipment malfunction, regulator resistance or loss of the demand valve will leave the diver with nothing but water to breathe – inevitably resulting in hypoxia due to salt water aspiration or drowning. Panic and poor dive techniques are often precursors to these problems.

Asthma, pneumothorax (from pulmonary barotrauma) and decompression sickness (chokes) can also interfere with breathing sufficient to cause hypoxia.

Rebreathing Equipment

This type of equipment shares the same causes of hypoxia as scuba equipment, but has some additional hazards.

A hypoxic gas mixture can be breathed if the **wrong gas** or **wrong mixture** is used (ie. a gas mixture containing insufficient O_2). A specific example of this is when a gas mixture intended for use at great depth (e.g. one containing 5% O_2) is breathed near the surface. With O_2 rebreathing equipment, a **flow of O_2** sufficient for the energy needs of the diver must be maintained. This must increase with heavy **exertion**.

Dilutional hypoxia is a particular problem with this type of equipment. When the diver first begins to breathe from the circuit, a significant amount of nitrogen may be produced from the lungs and body into the counterlung (breathing bag) of the equipment. If this is not vented after a few minutes breathing, the diver is likely to rebreathe almost pure nitrogen from the rebreathing bag. Oxygen is consumed by the diver and the carbon dioxide produced is absorbed by chemicals used in the equipment. Because the counterlung will still contain gas (mostly nitrogen) the diver will be unaware of the danger.

CLINICAL FEATURES

In most cases of hypoxia, the diver is unaware that there is anything wrong and therefore can lose consciousness without warning.

Mild hypoxia starves the brain of O_2, causing confusion, impaired judgement and clouding of consciousness. The diver is frequently unaware that there is a problem and may even become over-confident. An observer may note a deterioration of performance.

More **profound hypoxia** causes unconsciousness and in some cases, muscular jerking and spasms or epileptic type fits. **Severe hypoxia** results in rapid death.

Hypoxia makes the blood blue in colour. Hypoxic blood in the body capillaries gives the skin a blue appearance, and is termed **cyanosis**.

There is a form of localised cyanosis (stagnant hypoxia) associated with **cold** which does not denote generalised hypoxia. This is seen in the fingers, ears and lips due to (peripheral) blood vessel constriction causing inadequate circulation in these areas, in response to cold. It can be distinguished from the cyanosis of generalised hypoxia (hypoxic hypoxia) by looking at the colour of the tongue. The tongue is blue only in generalised hypoxia.

TREATMENT

If hypoxia is due to insufficient O_2 in the cells, treatment should clearly aim to reverse this. The basic resuscitation principles should be applied first (see Chapter 42).

> **A.** Clear the airway.
> **B.** Establish or maintain breathing.
> **C.** Establish or maintain circulation.

Give the patient the highest possible O_2 concentration to breathe at all times (see Chapter 40).

PREVENTION

Avoid prolonged, deep breath-hold dives. **Never hyperventilate** before a breath-hold dive.

Most diving deaths are ultimately caused by the hypoxia associated with drowning, regardless of the initial problem. In many cases this can be prevented by the **buddy system** and use of positive **buoyancy.** A good buoyancy vest should keep even an unconscious diver's face clear of the water.

Maintain equipment adequately and check it before a dive.

Monitor the air supply carefully, using a contents gauge and do not rely on a J valve.

Chapter 21

OXYGEN TOXICITY

Oxygen (O_2) is toxic when breathed at a partial pressure in excess of 0.4 ATA (40% O_2 at atmospheric pressure). The two common forms of O_2 toxicity affect the lungs and the brain.

When O_2 is breathed at partial pressures between 0.4 and 1.8 ATA it is toxic to the lungs. At partial pressures in excess of 1.8 ATA, O_2 is toxic to the brain as well as the lungs. The effects are more pronounced and more rapid as the inspired partial pressure of O_2 increases.

MECHANISM

The exact cause of O_2 toxicity is unknown. It is generally considered that hyperbaric O_2 interferes with the activity of enzymes in the cells and that this disrupts the biochemical functions, particularly in the brain and lungs.

In the lungs, damage to the cells lining the alveoli causes a general thickening and stiffening of the lung tissues.

In the brain there is a reduction in the amount of certain nerve transmission chemicals as well as generalised damage to the nerve cells. If cerebral O_2 toxicity is allowed to develop, convulsions eventually follow.

PREDICTION OF O_2 TOXICITY

To calculate the inspired partial pressure of O_2, multiply the percentage of inspired O_2 by the ambient pressure in atmospheres absolute and divide by 100.

e.g. the partial pressure of O$_2$ in room air is :

$$21\% \times 1ATA \div 100 = 0.21 \text{ ATA}.$$

The risks of O$_2$ toxicity increase with increasing partial pressure. In general it is usually possible to breath 100% O$_2$ for 18–24 hours without developing significant pulmonary O$_2$ toxicity. If therapeutic recompression is contemplated, a period of 12 hours breathing 100% O$_2$ may only be possible since the therapeutic recompression will generally involve the use of hyperbaric O$_2$, and this will summate with existing O$_2$ toxicity. The amount of pre-treatment of diving casualties with O$_2$ will preferably be discussed with the diving physician responsible for the therapeutic recompression.

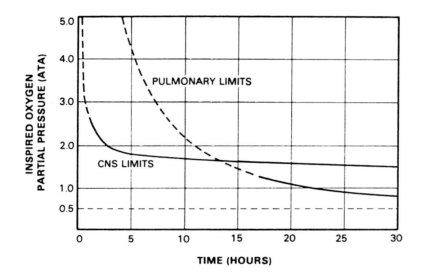

Fig. 21.1
This graph shows the predicted pulmonary and cerebral toxicity limits of exposure to varying partial pressures of oxygen. It can be noted that oxygen can be tolerated for much longer periods at lower partial pressures.

CAUSES OF O$_2$ TOXICITY

In **Resuscitation,** 100% O$_2$ should be used for hypoxic diving casualties without any fear of O$_2$ toxicity. As mentioned above, the treatment of decompression sickness and air embolism cases includes 100% O$_2$, preferably in consultation with the diving physician regarding the long term toxic effects.

Oxygen Re-breathing equipment should be restricted to military use and diving with this should not be attempted by recreational divers. O$_2$ diving sets have an absolute depth limit of 9 metres for resting dives and 7 metres for working dives in order to reduce the risk of convulsions. Re-breathing and scuba sets employing nitrogen/O$_2$ (**nitrox**) mixtures are limited to depths which produce an inspired O$_2$ partial pressure of no more than 1.6 atmospheres.

In **deep diving** operations, gas mixtures of helium, nitrogen and O_2 should have the composition adjusted so that the inspired partial pressure of O_2 never reaches the toxic range.

Therapeutic recompression using O_2 tables often involves the compression of the diver to 2.8 atmospheres while breathing 100% O_2. There is a significant risk of both pulmonary and cerebral O_2 toxicity and these tables should only be employed by diving medical experts.

CLINICAL FEATURES

Cerebral Effects

In this case the earliest symptom may be a convulsion which can develop without any warning signs. It may sometimes be preceded by a variety of symptoms such as visual disturbances, tunnel vision, faintness, or facial twitching – which may warn of an impending convulsion. Nausea, retching and even vomiting are common with cerebral O_2 toxicity. There is considerable individual variation in susceptibility to cerebral O_2 toxicity and an individual may even vary in tolerance from day to day.

During therapeutic recompression using O_2 tables, any convulsion in a diver due to cerebral O_2 toxicity must be distinguished from a convulsion due to cerebral decompression sickness or air embolism.

Pulmonary Effects

The early symptom is an irritation deep in the central part of the chest, progressing to pain which is aggravated by respiration and later accompanied by coughing. As the condition continues, shortness of breath develops and a pneumonia type illness supervenes.

TREATMENT

Cerebral Effects

Whilst undergoing therapeutic recompression, if warning signs of cerebral toxicity develop, the patient should be encouraged to hyperventilate and then be given air to breath until the symptoms abate. Modification to the O_2 treatment table may then be necessary.

If the patient convulses he should be placed on his side to protect the airway from aspiration of stomach contents and protected from injuring himself on nearby solid objects. A padded mouth piece may be placed between the teeth to protect the tongue. After the convulsion has ceased the patient may be unconscious. His airway should be protected and he should be managed according to the principles outlined in Chapter 42.

Pulmonary Effects

These effects will usually resolve spontaneously if the O_2 administration is ceased as soon as symptoms develop. If it is essential to continue O_2 therapy however, a reduction in the partial pressure of O_2 given will slow the development of toxicity. Short periods of 'air breathing' (or Heliox) are often used by experienced doctors to delay oxygen toxicity during O_2 therapy.

CONCLUSIONS

1. Recreational divers should not usually use O_2 diving equipment.

2. Resuscitation training with O_2 equipment is of great value to divers. In this case, the risks of O_2 toxicity are outweighed by the benefits of treating the hypoxic diving casualty

3. The use of O_2 in the first-aid treatment of decompression sickness and pulmonary barotrauma should always be undertaken whilst bearing in mind the prospect of eventual pulmonary oxygen toxicity. Breathing air for 5 minutes after 25 minutes of O_2 is one way of reducing the risk of pulmonary toxicity, but this should be discussed with the diving physician who will ultimately manage the case.

4. During therapeutic recompression using O_2, the use of short air or Heliox breaks during the treatment reduces cerebral and pulmonary O_2 toxicity.

5. There are other logistical problems with the use of oxygen, and some of these are discussed in Chapter 40.

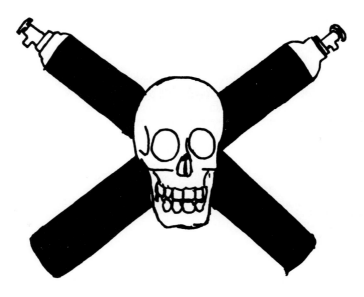

Fig. 21.2

Chapter 22

CARBON DIOXIDE PROBLEMS

Carbon dioxide (CO_2) is the gaseous by-product produced when the body consumes oxygen to fuel its metabolic processes. The body has an efficient way of disposing of CO_2, mainly through buffering systems in the blood and exhalation from the lungs.

CARBON DIOXIDE INSUFFICIENCY (HYPOCAPNEA OR HYPOCAPNIA)

Hypocapnea refers to a blood carbon dioxide (CO_2) level below normal. The CO_2 partial pressure in the blood is normally maintained within narrow limits by a biological feedback mechanism. Voluntary or involuntary hyperventilation (overbreathing) will overcome this regulatory mechanism and lower the blood CO_2 level. The most common cause for this is the rapid sighing respiration associated with hysterical and anxiety states – the feeling one experiences on confronting a great white shark during a dive.

A number of divers (fewer each year, due to natural selection) deliberately lower their blood CO_2 level before a breath-hold dive by hyperventilation, in order to prolong the dive. They often succeed beyond their wildest dreams. The lethal consequences of this practice are explained in Chapter 4.

Clinical Features

A person hyperventilating from anxiety is not usually aware of an altered breathing pattern, although it is often evident to an observer. Hyperventilation causes increased resistance to breathing with scuba, and this causes more anxiety.

Symptoms include tingling or "pins and needles" (parasthesiae) of the fingers, dizziness and light headedness, an altered conscious state or confusion. Muscular twitching or spasms can occur in extreme cases.

Treatment

The simplest treatment for hypocapnea is to reduce the breathing rate and depth. This restores the blood CO_2 level and cures the symptoms. On land, doctors often advise the patient to breathe in and out of a paper bag (rebreathing), but underwater most divers are not prepared to replace their regulator with a soggy paper bag.

Alternative Diagnoses

It is important to exclude other serious conditions such as decompression sickness, air embolism, carbon monoxide poisoning and salt water aspiration, whenever a diver presents with these symptoms. These illnesses can in themselves, also cause apparent hyperventilation and can mimic anxiety states.

CARBON DIOXIDE TOXICITY (HYPERCAPNEA)

CO_2 toxicity is due to accumulation of CO_2 through excess production or inadequate ventilation.

The effect of depth on inspired partial pressure is important. While 3% inspired CO_2 may be tolerated at atmospheric pressure without significant symptoms, the same percentage at 20 metres (3 ATA) is the equivalent of 3×3 or 9% at the surface – a level which will cause serious toxicity.

Re-breathing exhaled CO_2 is the most common cause of CO_2 toxicity in divers. Hence, CO_2 toxicity is most commonly encountered with rebreathing equipment, but it can sometimes occur in diving helmets, compression chambers, saturation complexes (habitats) or even scuba.

Causes of CO_2 Toxicity

❑ Rebreathing equipment.

Some types of military diving equipment conserve gas and reduce bubble formation by allowing the diver to rebreathe his exhaled gas. A canister of CO_2 absorbent (soda lime) is included in the circuit to remove the CO_2 which the diver exhales (see Chapter 5)

This mechanism can fail due to exhaustion of absorbent material, salt water contamination, improper packing, excessive CO_2 production due to exertion, or improper assembly of the circuit.

❑ Diving helmet problems.

With a standard-dress helmet or with some helmets used in deep diving, the diver can partly rebreathe his exhaled gas if the fresh gas flow in the helmet is insufficient to flush out exhaled CO_2.

❑ Chambers and habitats.

CO_2 which is exhaled by chamber occupants must be removed by constant flushing of the chamber or by the recirculation of the chamber gas through a CO_2 absorbent (scrubber). If either of these mechanisms is inadequate, the occupants can develop CO_2 toxicity by rebreathing their own exhaled CO_2.

❑ Scuba.

Since rebreathing is not possible with scuba equipment, CO_2 toxicity is not generally a problem for scuba divers unless there is resistance to breathing (regulator resistance, increased gas density at depth) or a reduced respiratory response of the diver to CO_2 (possibly due to adaptation, nitrogen narcosis, or high oxygen levels).

Clinical Features

These depend on the rate of onset and the actual partial pressure of the inspired CO_2.

A rapid accumulation of CO_2 may cause unconsciousness before any symptoms are experienced. A slower build-up causes a variety of symptoms, including :

- **a splitting or throbbing headache**, usually at the front of the head. This may be severe and often lasts for hours after the CO_2 levels have been corrected.
- **shortness of breath**, or air hunger.
- **flushing of the face** and **sweating** (sweating is not easy to detect underwater).
- **light headedness**, muscular **twitching**, jerks, tremors or **convulsions**.
- **impaired vision, unconsciousness**.
- **death**.

CO_2 toxicity may increase the likelihood of decompression sickness, oxygen toxicity, nitrogen narcosis and resistance to breathing (because of increased respiration).

Treatment

Any diver using rebreathing equipment who experiences symptoms of CO_2 toxicity should immediately **cease exertion, flush** the rebreathing system with fresh gas, return to the surface by a **buoyant ascent** and **breathe air**.

Attendants of a diver suffering from CO_2 toxicity should isolate him from the source of CO_2 rebreathing, give **100% oxygen** by mask, and administer cardiopulmonary **resuscitation** where appropriate. Other causes of headache and breathing difficulties such as decompression sickness, carbon monoxide toxicity etc. should also be excluded.

The severe headache which follows CO_2 toxicity should be treated with a simple analgesic such as paracetamol (acetaminophen).

Chapter 23

CARBON MONOXIDE TOXICITY

Carbon monoxide (CO) is a gas produced by the incomplete combustion of carbon containing compounds. It is a component of the smoke from **engine exhausts**, slow combustion **stoves** and **cigarette** smoke. It is also produced in divers' air compressors (see Chapter 24).

CO breathed in anything more than trace amounts is lethal. It binds avidly to the oxygen (O_2) binding sites of haemoglobin (Hb) in the blood, preventing the haemoglobin from carrying O_2. CO bound to haemoglobin forms carboxyhaemoglobin (HbCO). If a sufficient number of the O_2 binding sites are occupied by CO, death from hypoxia ensues (see Chapter 20).

CO also binds with components of the energy-producing biochemical pathways in the cells, interfering with fundamental cellular function.

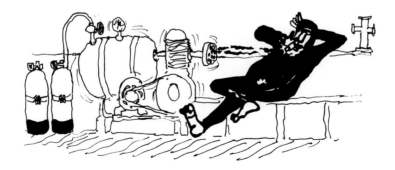

Fig. 23.1

CLINICAL FEATURES

Symptoms are those of progressive hypoxia due to the reduction in the oxygen transport by the blood. They vary with the **carboxyhaemoglobin** content of the blood as shown in the following table :

Concentration of CO in Breathing Gas	% Carboxy-haemoglobin	Effects on a Diver
400 parts per million (ppm)	7.2%	nil
800 ppm	14.4%	headaches dizziness, breathlessness with exertion
1600 ppm	29.0%	confusion, vomiting, collapse
3200 ppm	58.0%	paralysis, or loss of consciousness
4000 ppm	72.0%	coma
4500 ppm	87.0%	death

Table   23.1

The effects of CO are cumulative and are related to the concentration breathed and the duration of exposure. A concentration of 400 ppm will produce symptoms in an hour while 1200 ppm will need only 20 minutes. As the carboxyhaemoglobin (HbCO) level falls, following removal of the CO contamination, the clinical state may lag due to tissue CO, enzyme or protein damage. The classical "cherry pink" colour is only seen in the acute and early cases, before respiratory failure develops.

The effects of CO poisoning are greatly increased by increased pressure at **depth,** if the oxygen pressure is kept consistent. A 400 ppm contamination which would not produce clinical effects at atmospheric pressure will be equivalent to 4×400 ppm (or 1600 ppm) at 30 metres depth (4ATA), a concentration sufficient to cause serious toxicity. Because the oxygen partial pressure reduces with ascent, the symptoms of mild CO poisoning may only become manifest during or after ascent.

Serious **brain damage** is a frequent complication of significant CO toxicity due to prolonged hypoxia of the brain. (See Case History 24.1)

TREATMENT

The diver should be rapidly **isolated** from the contaminated gas and have **100% O_2** administered by mask. The ABC resuscitation principles (see Chapter 42) should be applied where appropriate.

Hyperbaric O_2 (HBO) is the treatment of choice. The high partial pressure of O_2, which occurs in a hyperbaric chamber, will dissolve enough O_2 in the blood plasma to meet the bodies needs without participation of the haemoglobin system. Oxygen is breathed at a partial pressure of 2.5–3 ATA to sustain life while the CO slowly detaches from the haemoglobin and is breathed out through the lungs, allowing the haemoglobin to resume its normal O_2 transport role.

If hyperbaric O_2 is to be of value it should be instituted within a few hours of poisoning. A significant delay allows irreversible brain damage in severe cases.

PREVENTION

The major danger to any diver is from carbon monoxide contamination of the compressed air supply. Sources of contamination include :

❑ Direct contamination by CO from gasoline engine exhausts.

This may emanate either from the compressor motor itself, or from other nearby motors or gas exhaust outlets. The classic case occurs where the compressor air inlet hose is located downwind from the compressor motor exhaust.

❑ Contamination produced by the breakdown of unsuitable lubricants.

The incorrect use of hydrocarbon-based lubricants used to lubricate an air compressor is a common cause, however it may also result from overheating of the compressor. Both carbon and nitrogen oxides can be formed.

❑ The intake of polluted atmospheric air to fill air cylinders.

It is important for suppliers of compressed air to regularly check the quality of the air being compressed, to ensure that this and other pollutants are not included in divers' air supplies. Adequate filtration systems are necessary on all compressors, and these should always be properly maintained.

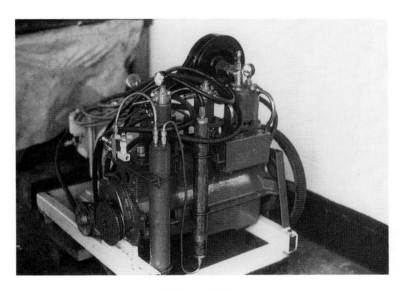

Fig. 23.2
Water lubricated compressor made from a motor vehicle engine.

Chapter 24

BREATHING GAS CONTAMINATION

The supply of uncontaminated breathing gas (air) is of vital importance to the diver because of the magnifying effect on contamination by the partial pressure rise with increasing depth. For example, 5% contamination of gas at atmospheric pressure is equivalent to 20% at 30 metres depth (4 ATA).

Contamination usually arises either from impurities in the air taken into the compressor or from contaminants generated by the compressor itself.

PREPARATION OF COMPRESSED AIR

Atmospheric air is taken into the compressor and is compressed by one of two methods. Most dive shops use a piston and cylinder compressor which raises the pressure of the gas in several stages. A more advanced compressor uses a diaphragm pump similar in principle to that in a refrigerator.

Ideally the compressed air should be treated by passing it through several purifying cartridges (or filters) to remove contaminants. Silica gel is used to remove **water** vapour, activated charcoal removes **oil** and **hydrocarbons**, a molecular sieve removes **water droplets and dust particles** and a catalyst removes **carbon monoxide**. Less scrupulous air suppliers have been known to substitute women's sanitary pads, instead of filters.

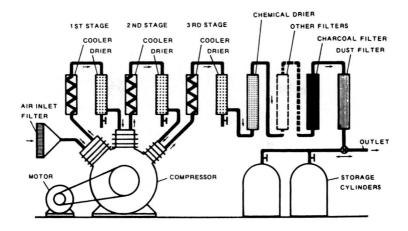

Fig. 24.1
Schematic diagram of a compressor system with filters.

GAS PURITY STANDARDS

Authorities such as the US Navy, NOAA and Standards Australia specify minimum standards of purity for breathing gas.

Case History 24.1 In an area subject to tidal currents an experienced diver planned to dive at slack water. He anchored his boat at low tide. The hookah compressor he used was correctly arranged with the air inlet upwind of the exhaust and the dive commenced. After 90 minutes at 10 metres the diver felt dizzy and lost consciousness but was fortunately pulled aboard by his attendant and resuscitated.
Diagnosis — Carbon monoxide poisoning.
Explanation — as the tide turned, so did the boat. This put the compressor **air inlet downwind of the motor exhaust** and carbon monoxide from the exhaust was breathed under pressure by the diver.

Compressors can also generate some lethal contaminants internally. The compressor piston requires lubrication and this is usually achieved by the use of special **oils**. In some circumstances, such as where there is excessive wear of the compressor, high temperatures can be generated and this may decompose the lubricating oil into toxic products such as **oxides of nitrogen** or **carbon monoxide**, which are then pumped into the diver's air tank. Poor maintenance of the compressor can also lead to an **oil** and **hydrocarbon** mist escaping into the air supply.

If the compressor is operated in an unclean environment, **dust** can find its way into the diver's air causing abnormal wear on the moving parts of both the compressor and the regulator.

Water vapour must be removed from the air delivered from the compressor or it can condense in the scuba cylinder causing rust, or allowing the regulator to freeze up during diving in cold conditions.

Most compressors have a **filtration system** both on the inlet side to prevent the intake of dust, and on the outlet side to filter out oil and water vapour. Their efficiency depends on regular maintenance and the absence of over-loading.

Occasionally contamination comes from the destruction of the filters and lubrication systems. Non-hydrocarbon based lubricants with high "flash points' are preferable. The problems of oil lubrication can be overcome by using a compressor which is lubricated with water (see Fig 23.2) or dry teflon materials. Unfortunately the expense of these is beyond the reach of most air suppliers. Diaphragm pumps also avoid the problem of oil lubrication but are also very expensive.

CLINICAL FEATURES

Contaminated air may have an unusual taste or smell, or alternately, it may appear quite normal.

• **Oxides of nitrogen** cause lung damage which is likely to present as coughing, wheezing, shortness of breath and tightness in the chest.

• **Carbon monoxide** causes headache and unconsciousness – a detailed discussion can be found in Chapter 23.

• **Oil** can cause chest pain, shortness of breath, coughing and pneumonia.

TREATMENT

If a diver is affected by breathing contaminated air he should be managed according to first-aid principles outlined in Chapter 42, and gas from his scuba cylinder sent for analysis to a chemical or gas testing laboratory.

PREVENTION

The diver should breathe from his equipment before entering the water and should not use air which has an unusual taste or smell.

As the expertise of compressed air (and other breathing gases) suppliers vary, divers are well advised to obtain air fills only from a reputable supplier. Regular checks by local authorities on the quality of the air are advisable, and in many places are now mandatory. It can be tested by chemical detector tubes that determine the level of each specific contaminant. Drager (a gas and medical equipment company) supply these tubes in a Drager Gas Detection Kit.

Following any diving accident, suspect air can be tested by commercial gas suppliers and State Health authorities.

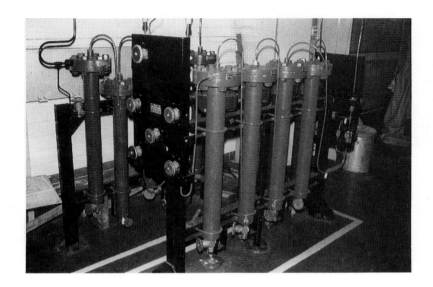

Fig. 24.2
A system of filters used for a recompression chamber "air supply bank".

Case History 24.2

A diving club had for many years been filling their cylinders from an air bank made up of large cylinders, the source of which had been lost in the mists of time. It was decided to return the bank of cylinders to a major industrial gas supplier for testing. The cylinders had their original paint in good condition – black cylinders with a white collar. The gas company tested the cylinders, found them to be sound and refilled them according to the colour code on the cylinders. Unfortunately, this was the standard colour code for pure oxygen and that is what the company filled them with, having no idea that they would be ultimately used to fill scuba tanks.

A member of the dive club took delivery of the cylinders and reinstalled them in the bank. He did not know the significance of the colour coding and assumed that because he was using the cylinders to store air that the company would refill them accordingly. Because they were already full there was no need to fill them from the compressor and the bank was immediately used to fill several sets for a dive the following day. Two divers used tanks from this source on a dive to 20 metres. One abruptly convulsed 10 minutes into the dive and was fortunately rescued by his buddy before he too convulsed.

Some clever detective work performed by the rescuing diver, and the diving physician they consulted, established the cause of the problem as oxygen toxicity. Swift action by the police to round up all the contaminated scuba tanks before they could be used, averted a major disaster. In this case, breathing from the cylinder at the surface before the dive would not have disclosed any detectable difference from air.

Chapter 25

DROWNING

Near-drowning is the correct term used for a severe aspiration of water, which does not have a fatal outcome. If it is fatal, it is called **drowning**. Minor aspiration is described in Chapter 26.

It is vital for divers to understand the management of near-drowning because it is the final outcome of a large number of diving accidents.

PHYSIOLOGY OF DROWNING

Early animal experiments showed a distinct difference between fresh and salt water drowning. **Fresh water** drowning was associated with a massive osmotic uptake of fluid from the lungs, diluting the blood, overloading the heart and causing rupture of the red blood cells.

Salt water drowning led to large amounts of fluid being drawn into the air sacs of the lungs, and depleting the blood volume, because salt water is more concentrated than blood.

It is now thought that these animal experiments represented extreme cases since the volume of fluid which was poured experimentally into the animals' lungs was the equivalent of 1 – 1.5 litres in a human. In human near-drowning cases, spasm of the airway makes inhalation of such large volumes of fluid uncommon.

Studies in human near-drowning cases have shown little difference between fresh or salt water inhalation — the extreme fluid and electrolyte changes described in animals, are usually not seen. The common **feature in** human cases is a marked increase in **stiffness** of the lungs. This impairs the **oxygen exchanging ability** of the lungs while increasing the **effort of breathing.**

Fresh or salt water entering the alveoli (air sacs of the lung) appears to damage the **surfactant** lining them, causing **alveoli to collapse** and become unavailable for gas exchange. Damage to the walls of the alveoli also causes the **capillaries to leak blood and protein into the lungs.** This interacts with air and water producing a foam which the victim may cough up in copious amounts. This is called **pulmonary oedema.**

The **sequence of events** in a near-drowning incident often goes as follows :

The degree of **panic** behaviour is variable, and may be reduced by such factors as personality, training, drug intake and nitrogen narcosis. If some air is still available from the regulator, the diver may persist with attempting to breathe from this (even at the cost of aspirating some water), and request assistance. Even if an alternative air supply is made available, **hypoxia** may still develop because of the water aspirated. Coughing and gasping may be voluntarily suppressed until the diver reaches the surface. If the diver is totally deprived of his air supply for some reason, he initially breath-holds until the "break point" is reached and then takes an involuntary breath. The resulting inhalation of a bolus of water usually provokes **coughing** and **closure of the larynx** producing involuntary breath-holding followed by unconsciousness. It is unusual for large amounts of water to enter the lungs after the victim loses consciousness as the tongue and loose tissues in the throat tend to close the airway.

CLINICAL FEATURES

When first rescued the condition of the near drowned victim may vary from fully conscious to unconscious, with normal, laboured or absent respiration.

If the victim is breathing, the stiff lungs cause laboured respiration and it is common for foam, often copious and blood stained, to be coughed up or to exude from the nose or mouth. Cyanosis (bluish coloration of lips, ears) from hypoxia is frequent.

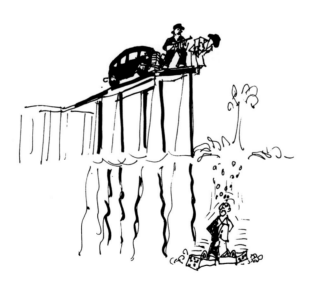

Fig. 25.1

TREATMENT

In exceptional circumstance, near drowned victims have fully recovered after periods of total immersion of over 40 minutes (especially children in cold waters), so it is worth attempting resuscitation even in apparently hopeless cases.

The resuscitation principles of airway management, restoration of respiration and circulation (**A–B–C** as outlined in Chapter 42) should be employed immediately. **Oxygen** in the highest concentration available should be given by mask to offset hypoxia.

Near drowned cases are liable to deteriorate many hours after making an apparent recovery, so all near drowned victims should be taken to **hospital** and must remain there for at least 24 hours for observation.

Chapter 26

SALT WATER ASPIRATION SYNDROME

This condition was first described in Royal Australian Navy divers in the late 1960's. Some divers were repeatedly presenting for treatment with a brief condition characterised by shortness of breath, sometimes a pale or bluish (cyanosis) skin colour, mild fever accompanied by shivering, malaise and anorexia, and generalised aches and pains. Chest X-rays sometimes showed an appearance similar to a patchy pneumonia and blood gases consistently verified hypoxia.

Close questioning of the divers revealed that nearly all the cases had aspirated a fine mist of seawater from a leaking or flooded demand valve. "Volunteer" experiments confirmed the association between aspiration of sea water and the development of the syndrome.

CLINICAL FEATURES

There is often a delay of one half to 12 hours between aspiration of the water and the major symptoms. The onset in mild cases is often provoked by exercise, movement or cold exposure.

The diver has some or all the following symptoms :

- Initial coughing, sometimes with expectoration, after surfacing
- fever with shivering (induced by cold exposure),
- malaise with anorexia, nausea or vomiting,
- shortness of breath, coughing, cyanosis
- headache and generalised aches and pains.

TREATMENT

The condition is self limiting and resolves without treatment within 24 hours. **Rest** and the administration of **100% oxygen** by mask for several hours until the symptoms have abated, is of considerable value. The oxygen not only relieves the hypoxia but produces dramatic resolution of the symptoms of this syndrome.

Because of the nature of the symptoms, it is necessary to distinguish the salt water aspiration syndrome from other serious conditions such as decompression sickness (chokes), pulmonary barotrauma (burst lung), severe infection and pneumonia – which can all present with some or all of the features of this condition.

PREVENTION

The condition can be prevented by avoiding situations which will result in the aspiration of seawater. Buddy breathing can be a fruitful source of the syndrome if the shared demand valve is not adequately cleared of water. Others include a towed search, poor regulator performance, exhaustion of air supply and free ascent practise. Proper maintenance of the demand regulator and its exhaust valves, is important.

DISCUSSION

Some of these cases are based on hyperactive airways, with a history of hay fever or asthma. In respiratory laboratories, aerosol inhalations of hypertonic saline (sea water) are used to provoke these breathing difficulties and demonstrate susceptibility to the syndrome.

Chapter 27

COLD & HYPOTHERMIA

A diver is usually immersed in water which is considerably colder than the normal body temperature of 37°C. Unfortunately, water is particularly efficient at removing body heat, having a conduction capacity 25 times that of air and a specific heat (the amount of heat necessary to raise a given volume by a certain temperature) 1000 times that of air.

Without insulation, a diver will lose body heat much faster in water than in air at the same temperature. This can cause **hypothermia**, a harmful drop in body temperature to below 35°C.

The body can reduce temperature loss by generating heat through metabolism, exercise and shivering, and by restricting blood flow to the skin. The rate of heat loss also depends on factors such as the temperature of the water, the thickness of body fat, presence a wetsuit or other insulation, and the posture of the diver.

Recognition of the early clinical features of hypothermia may convince a diver to leave the water before a serious problem arises.

CLINICAL FEATURES

All divers will have experienced the early features of cold — numbness, blueness or pallor of the skin (especially in peripheral areas such as the fingers, toes and earlobes), and shivering.

If the body temperature falls by about 2°C, loss of co-ordination and uncontrollable shivering may impair the ability to swim and render the performance of finely co-ordinated movements (like manipulating equipment and assisting buddies) impossible.

After a body temperature drop of 3–4°C, the diver may become weak, apathetic, confused and helpless. Drowning is a real risk at this stage. A body temperature less than about 30°C results in unconsciousness. This may be confused with other causes of unconsciousness in divers. Often the diver appears to just lose consciousness without other obvious clinical manifestations.

A victim who is unconscious from severe hypothermia may have a very slow respiratory rate, and a barely detectable pulse, and may appear dead to the inexperienced observer. It is important to not assume the worst in this situation. Do not presume that he is dead, unless he is warm and dead.

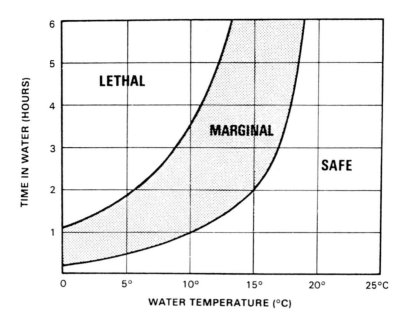

Fig. 27.1
This graph gives an indication of approximate survival times of an uninsulated human in water of various temperatures. These figures are overestimates – a diver would be severely incapacitated well before he reached the limits of survival. It is obvious that survival times of less than one hour can be expected without insulation in water temperatures found in many countries.

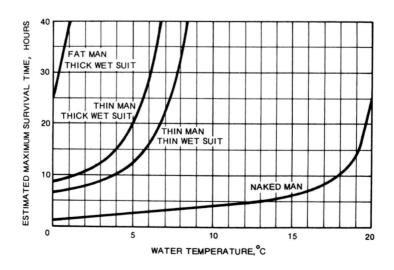

Fig. 27.2
Graph illustrating survival times in varying water temperatures for divers.

TREATMENT

Always clear the airway, check for any evidence of heartbeat or respiration, and begin resuscitation if necessary.

The basic first-aid principles of management of airway, breathing and circulation, (**A–B–C** : see Chapter 42), take precedence. It is recommended that expired air resuscitation (**EAR**) and external cardiac compression (**ECC**) be performed at half the normal rate in cases of hypothermia because body metabolism is slowed. However, unless the rescuer is confident that hypothermia is the sole cause of the victim's collapse, the usual resuscitation techniques are probably indicated.

The aim of management is to keep the victim alive, while returning the body temperature to normal. This is most simply achieved by **immersing the victim in a warm bath at a temperature of 38–40°C.** A warm shower is a less efficient alternative. A pleasantly warm bath or shower is approximately the right temperature.

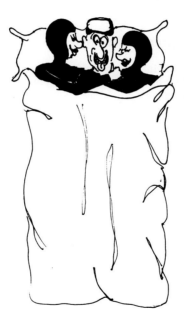

Fig. 27.3

Some workers recommend that only the torso (trunk) should be immersed in a bath initially, and the limbs kept out of the water, warming the torso first while allowing the limbs to stay cool. The reason for this is that the limbs will have restricted blood flow in response to the hypothermia, and this will be reversed by warming. Increased blood flow to the limbs at this critical stage may lower the blood pressure as well as divert heat from the vital organs to the less important periphery. In an emergency, this ideal may not be necessary or practical and it is reasonable to immerse the whole body.

Facilities to warm a diver are usually limited at a dive site and improvisation may be required. **Wrapping the victim in blankets with other divers** is an efficient and often acceptable way of transferring body heat to a mildly hypothermic diver. Warm diver buddies, especially of the opposite sex, may be sought after by some unscrupulous divers!

A reflective **survival blanket** over normal blankets improves their efficiency. Blankets used alone without a heat source are less effective, as they do not generate heat and the victim's heat output is very slow. Wrapping in a **plastic (garbage) bag,** or even **newspapers**, may also help with insulation by reducing air flow over clothes and skin.

The **engine room of larger vessels** is often warm enough to be of value in the management of hypothermia and engine cooling water may be a source of warm water in an emergency. Treatment can be suspended when the patient reaches 37°C, or starts to sweat.

Although **alcohol** produces a warm inner glow it actually worsens hypothermia by increasing blood flow to the skin, accelerating heat loss. It must never be given to severely hypothermic patients.

PREVENTION

Even in tropical waters, loss of body temperature during a dive is likely if the diver is not insulated.

The most popular and convenient insulator is the **wet suit** (see Chapter 5). Air bubbles enclosed in synthetic rubber provide an insulating barrier between the diver and the water without the need for the suit to be waterproof – hence the term "wet suit". They are available in various thicknesses depending on the expected water temperature. Wet suits have the disadvantage of compression of the air cells at depth which reduces their insulation and causes inconvenient changes in buoyancy.

This problem is overcome in deep professional diving operations by the use of a **"dry suit"** which uses air as the insulating material. Other variations include electrical, chemical or hot water warming procedures, or even an inflatable air pocket enclosed in a wetsuit, .

In a survival situation, heat loss in an uninsulated person can be minimised by floating in a curled-up posture ("foetal" position) with the knees near the chest and the arms by the side, so covering the body areas which lose heat the most (axilla and groin). This can obviously be done only if the diver has a flotation aid. Huddling together with other survivors may be of value. Limitation of movement will also minimise heat loss.

To reduce heat loss, it is best not to swim more than a short distance, as although swimming generates some metabolic heat, this is more than offset by heat lost the water during movement.

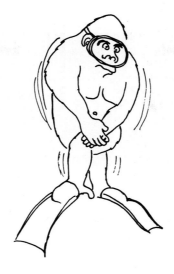

Fig. 27.4

Chapter 28

INFECTIONS

There are a variety of both exotic and mundane infections to which divers are exposed. Some are terrestrial and are the same as for non-divers. These infections represent either local extensions or spread from other divers. Others are caused by specific marine organisms and require special methods of identification.

ABRASIONS AND INFECTED CUTS

Divers are frequently subjected to minor injuries including cuts and abrasions. These injuries are more prone to infection than those encountered in terrestrial pursuits because of the unusual bacteria encountered in the aquatic environment and because cuts and abrasions frequently remain moist for long periods of time.

Cuts and abrasions which are not due to coral or other marine life do not require aggressive cleaning unless they are obviously contaminated. Bleach, antiseptic or antibiotic cream or powder should be applied as soon as possible. When out of the water they should be kept dry and loosely covered to prevent further contamination.

Coral Cuts

Coral frequently causes minor cuts and abrasions in unprotected divers in tropical waters. These cuts are particularly prone to infection, probably because of the large numbers of marine bacteria on coral and the retention of coral particles and slime in the wound.

They frequently becomes infected within hours. Even minor cuts or abrasions can become red, swollen, tender and painful. Later there may be a discharge of pus from the area.

A severe infection may spread to the blood stream, with fever, chills and tender swollen lymph glands in the groin or armpit, depending on the site of the injury.

❑ Treatment.

All coral cuts should be washed with bleach or soapy water as soon as possible and the surface of the cut or abrasion should be thoroughly cleaned by gentle rubbing with gauze or a soft brush. This removes foreign material which may be the source of inflammation. All cuts should then have local antibiotic powder, cream or ointment applied every 6 hours until healed. The senior (elderly) author, who has a tendency towards cowardice, relies more on the antibiotics than the cleansing. Suitable topical antibiotics include neomycin or bacitracin.

Early attention to every coral cut in this way will usually prevent serious infections. If treatment is delayed, or if systemic effects occur, oral broad-spectrum antibiotics may be needed. The development of a chronic inflammation causes severe itching over the next few weeks, but this usually responds to local steroid (cortisone) ointments.

❑ Prevention.

It is wise when diving on coral reefs to always wear protective clothing or a wet suit, gloves and booties. Modern lightweight "lycra suits" afford some protection and may be worn in very warm tropical waters. These provide no flotation or thermal insulation properties, and diving must be adjusted for this.

EAR INFECTIONS

Otitis Externa
(Swimmer's or Tropical Ear")

This outer ear infection is one of the most common and troublesome problems in divers. It is especially likely to occur in **hot humid conditions** (e.g. tropical climates, standard diving dress, compression chambers) or when **water is retained** within the ear after immersion, especially if **contaminated water**. Small bony outgrowths (**exostoses**) are commonly found in the ears of swimmers and divers, and these may be large enough to cause retention of water, wax, debris and organisms. **Local injury** induced by scratching the ear canals (with a match or hair pin), or by clumsy attempts to remove **wax** (often using cotton-tipped utensils) frequently precipitates the infection. Sometimes an underlying **skin disorder** is present such as eczema or dandruff. Many bacterial organisms have been incriminated, as well as fungi.

❑ Clinical features.

Mild infection causes **itching** of the ear which encourages the diver to scratch the ear canal, further breaking down the protective barrier and aggravating the infection. This has prompted the good advice that 'nothing smaller than the elbow' should be inserted into the ear canal.

Serious infection may appear as a local boil in the ear canal, or as a diffuse inflammation with narrowing of the canal and an offensive smelling discharge. **Pain** with movement of the jaws or pulling on the ear is common. Occasionally a **mild hearing loss** or **dull feeling** in the ear may be noticed, and **dizziness** during diving is a possibility if one canal is completely blocked.

❏ **Treatment.**

The condition may be difficult to cure and treatment should be supervised by a doctor. Mild cases may only require careful cleansing of the ear canal followed by local (topical) **antibiotic + steroid** ear drops three times per day. More severe cases will need pain killing tablets such as paracetamol — two tablets four hourly as required, along with packing of the canal with special antibiotic + steroid ointments e.g. "Kenacomb" . Oral antibiotics may be required in severe cases. Diving, along with further exposure to any water, should cease until the infection resolves.

❏ **Prevention.**

This can be achieved by the use of olive oil drops in the ears prior to diving, or the application of a few drops of a solution of 5% acetic acid in 85% isopropyl alcohol in each ear after a dive to ensure adequate drying. Commercial solutions include "AquaEar" and "Otic Domeboro". Scratching the ear canal with matches, hair pins, cotton buds and the like, although tempting, should be avoided.

Otitis Media
(Middle ear infection")

Middle ear infection is not very common in adult divers, but may occur after **middle ear barotrauma** or following upper respiratory tract infections (**URTIs**) or allergies. It may also follow an uneventful dive. Most infective organisms enter the middle ear cavity via the Eustachian tubes, which lead from the throat to the middle ear cavity, during middle ear equalisation. Occasionally a **perforation** in the ear drum will allow direct entry of contaminated water.

❏ **Clinical features.**

Clinically there may be **pain in the ear, fever**, **ringing** noises (tinnitus) and often a slight **hearing loss**. In this case the ear will not usually be tender to touch.

❏ **Treatment.**

Treatment is urgent and will include oral broad spectrum antibiotics, pain relieving tablets such as paracetamol and decongestants (such as pseudoephedrine). No diving or flying in aircraft should occur until resolution — usually 5-7 days.

NAEGLERIA –
AMOEBIC MENINGITIS

This lethal condition is encountered by divers or swimmers bathing in fresh water lakes, streams, hot springs, spas or hot tubs. It is caused by a microscopic amoeba which usually enters water through **sewage** contamination. It may survive in **warm fresh water** (not in sea water).

The amoeba enters the body through the nose from where it burrows through the olfactory nerve to enter the brain. After an incubation period of about a week it causes meningitis and encephalitis, which is difficult to treat and is usually fatal.

❑ Clinical features.

The condition is usually manifest by a progressively worsening headache, fever, vomiting, discomfort on looking at bright light, neck stiffness, confusion and finally, coma. Death usually follows after 5-7 days.

❑ Treatment.

There is very little that can be done to treat this dangerous condition apart from intensive nursing care in a major hospital and aggressive intravenous therapy with several antibiotics – none of which are very effective.

❑ Prevention.

Because the organism enters through the nose, infection can be prevented by not immersing the head in warm fresh water, which is at risk from contamination. Such waters should be avoided if possible, however if diving is essential in these areas (police underwater searches, mining or drainage assessments etc.) then only diving equipment incorporating helmets which totally enclose the head and face should be used, and these rinsed off thoroughly prior to undressing after the dive. Heavy chlorination will kill the organism as will seawater eventually.

SINUSITIS

Because air passes into the sinuses during descent (see Chapters 2 and 10), if the diver has an **upper respiratory tract infection** and goes diving with this, then organisms will be transferred to the sinuses as he equalises pressures. Because of the overwhelming infection that is then produced, it is common to develop symptoms within hours or days of the dive exposure.

As a general rule, the more descents carried out, the greater the infective material which passes into the sinuses. Also, if there is any sign of **sinus barotrauma** (especially on descent) then there is blood and fluid in the sinus at body temperature, which makes an ideal medium for the growth of organisms.

❑ Clinical features.

With sinusitis there is not only a feeling of **fullness over the area of the sinus** (usually maxillary, frontal, ethmoid, sphenoid or mastoid), but there is **pain** which is likely to increase in severity. If there is any significant obstruction of the sinus ostium, then pressure develops within the sinus as infection flares. There may be severe systemic signs – similar to that of an abscess, thus the diver may be **feverish**, feel ill and may look sick.

❑ Treatment.

This usually involves oral broad spectrum antibiotics, pain relief (paracetamol) and decongestants (pseudoephedrine). Sometimes a fluid level can be seen on X–Ray and rarely, surgical drainage is necessary.

Because infections tend to produce scarring, sinusitis must be avoided as much as possible by divers – otherwise the openings of the sinuses can become scarred and narrowed. This means that the diver is much more likely to develop sinus barotrauma in the future – thereby limiting his diving future.

❏ Prevention.

Avoid sinus barotrauma (see Chapter 10). The rapid and effective treatment of infections that do develop in the sinuses will be of some preventative value. Of more importance is the avoidance of diving during times in which there is any inflammatory disease of the upper respiratory tract (nose, throat), such as hay fever, rhinitis or upper respiratory tract infection.

SWIMMER'S ITCH

Swimmer's itch is a localised skin infection caused by a bird parasite (Schistosome cercaria) which can be encountered by persons swimming or wading in lakes or lagoons frequented by water birds. The parasite, which is present in the water, burrows through the skin and then dies, causing an inflammatory reaction under the skin. It causes multiple small, raised, red itchy lumps, which may last for a week or so.

The lesions usually resolve without treatment. Occasionally, more severe reactions may follow in individuals who are allergic to the parasites and may require medical attention by way of oral antihistamines and even topical or oral steroids (cortisone).

SWIMMING POOL GRANULOMA

Also called **Swimmer's Elbow**, this infection is due to an organism (marine *vibrios*) entering the skin via an underwater abrasion from a swimming pool, ship's hull etc. **Red swellings** covered with fine scales may develop 3–4 weeks after injury over bony prominences such as the elbows or knees. Thick pus may be found if the swelling is incised and spontaneous resolution may take up to a year or more. **Diagnosis** may only be confirmed by microscopic examination of a piece of the ulcer or lesion, and culture of the organism involved.

TINEA PEDIS – "TINEA" (or "ATHLETE'S FOOT")

This is a common fungal infection which affects the feet of divers and swimmers exposed to repeated wet and warm conditions. It causes itchy, scaly or raw areas between the toes and on the feet.

Many divers suffer from this infection, and are the source of cross-infection to others. The fungus can be found in many areas and makes the condition difficult to prevent because of repeated exposures.

Fortunately it responds readily to modern topical anti-fungal agents such as imidazole derivatives, (tolnaftate or undecylenic acid). The solution or cream should be applied twice daily and continued for two weeks after the condition appears to be cured. Attempts should be made to keep the feet as dry as possible, and drying with tissues between the toes after bathing or swimming is helpful. A light application of an anti-tinea powder (e.g. econazole dusting powder) daily may also be beneficial in preventing recurrence. In severe or resistant cases, oral anti-fungal medication such as ketoconazole or griseofulvin may even be necessary. Towels and footwear should not be shared.

PITYRIASIS VERSICOLOR (or "TINEA VERSICOLOR")

This mild fungus infection of the skin may either cause itching or no symptoms at all. With exposure to the sun however, a diver will notice large spotty areas which do not tan on the chest, back and arms. A fine scaliness of the skin will be seen on close inspection. It is best treated with topical anti-fungal lotions or creams such as clotrimazole or econazole applied twice daily. An alternative is 20% sodium thiosulphate (or photographer's 'Hypo' solution – but this stains clothing).

A.I.D.S.

There is currently world-wide concern regarding this disease. The risks in the diver's situation are not known with certainty. The following is a general discussion based on the current information.

AIDS (Acquired Immune Deficiency Syndrome) is a virus infection which in western countries is most frequently contracted by homosexual (anal) intercourse and by shared needles for intravenous drug use. It can also be contracted from organ and tissue transplants or transfusion with infected blood, although in developed countries blood donations are now screened to prevent this. The virus can be spread by heterosexual intercourse – and this type of transmission, once uncommon, is now increasing at an alarming rate.

An estimated 20 million people are infected world-wide. In Western countries most infected people are either homosexuals, bisexuals, intravenous drug users, or recipients of blood transfusions. In Africa, the disease is now rampant and is predominantly spread by heterosexual intercourse, the use of contaminated needles in hospitals, or transfusions of non-screened contaminated blood.

The disease primarily attacks a group of white blood cells which are essential to the immune system, making the body susceptible to infections and certain tumours. It would appear that death from the disease is inevitable in most people infected by the virus (especially in 'full blown infections'), but the time to fatal outcome varies from 3–12 years.

The virus must gain entry to the bloodstream to produce infection and is generally unable to enter through intact body surfaces such as skin or mouth lining. It can gain entry through small breaks in tissues such as cuts, abrasions or ulcers. Tissue fluid oozing from breaks in the skin or mouth lining can contain viruses in infected individuals. The virus is present in blood and saliva, making transmission a possibility (albeit probably only slight) in some situations encountered during diving.

AIDS Risks to Divers

❑ Sexual.

This is the most common mode of transmission. It can be eliminated by celibacy and reduced by using condoms ("safe sex" practices), avoidance of both promiscuity and anal intercourse. A wet suit should prove an effective barrier if worn at all times.

❑ Blood.

Blood from infected people can transmit the virus to others. This usually follows the sharing of needles or transfusions of infected blood, but there have been a few reports of transmission by infected blood splashing onto the skin — usually skin which has been broken in some way. In diving, infection in this way could theoretically follow the first-aid treatment of an injured diver after trauma, cuts or marine animal injury. The sharing of demand regulators which have not been adequately cleaned after each individual use could pose a potential risk of infection from oral abrasions.

Unless the victim belongs to a high risk group, the chance of being infected is very low. Nevertheless, it is best to avoid contact with others' blood wherever possible, especially if the skin is broken by dermatitis, cuts, abrasions or injuries. Wear gloves if they are available. Wash blood from the skin as soon as possible with soap and water, or preferably alcoholic chlorhexidine 0.5% ("Hibicol"). Viruses on the skin can also be killed by most antiseptics, pure alcohol or methylated spirits, sodium hypochlorite solution (often used to sterilise babies bottles) and household bleach. In the absence of these, motor fuel may possibly kill the virus. Obviously, where available, disposable gloves should be worn by any persons treating wounds of any type.

❑ Resuscitation.

Expired air resuscitation usually requires mouth-to-mouth or mouth-to-nose contact. There is a theoretical risk of transmission of the virus during resuscitation, especially if either the victim or rescuer has ulcers or bleeding in the mouth. The risk is probably small but it would be wise, if a known AIDS carrier was involved, to use a mouth-to-mask or resuscitation tube technique. If the rescuer is trained in its use, an O_2 or air resuscitator bag would be even better.

❑ Sharing equipment.

It is common for equipment to be shared in diving schools. Since the virus is known to be present in the saliva of infected people, there is a theoretical risk of transmission of the disease from the sharing of demand valves (including buddy breathing practice) and snorkels. The risk is probably slight and there have not been any cases of such transmission yet reported.

Until the risk is excluded it would seem wise to disinfect shared equipment between use by soaking in a solution known to be lethal to the virus. These solutions are described above. Check with the manufacturer beforehand to ensure that the chosen solution will not damage the equipment.

❑ The HIV positive or AIDS infected diver.

These individuals could pose a risk to their fellow divers in the situations outlined above. It would be considerate for them to take care to avoid situations which might bring their blood or other body fluids into contact with others. Breathing equipment should not be shared.

HIV positive cases (those with the virus infection but no obvious symptoms) have recently been shown to have neuropsychological abnormalities, and these could be detrimental to the normal intellectual functioning and judgement needed for scuba diving.

Infected divers may be exposing themselves to added risks by diving. Depression of the immune system makes them more susceptible to infection from coral cuts and abrasions, from exotic marine bacteria, and possibly to infections acquired from shared breathing equipment. It is claimed by some researchers that hyperbaric environments and hyperbaric oxygen (as occurs with diving and diving treatment respectively) may reduce the efficiency of the blood brain barrier and allow the extension of the virus into the brain, causing the dreaded neurological AIDS. The influence of some of the other physiological effects of increased pressure on AIDS infected divers is unknown.

❑ Prevention.

Avoid contamination of the skin by other people's blood where possible, and use disposable plastic or latex gloves whenever possible. If this is unavoidable, wash the blood off as soon as practicable with soap or antiseptic solutions, described above.

If medical attention is sought in **underdeveloped countries**, try to ensure that only new or disposable syringes (i.e. totally unused) and needles are used, and that re-used instruments have been properly sterilised. Transfusions of blood and blood plasma in some of these countries carries a significant risk of AIDS or hepatitis infection. Artificial blood expanding solutions such as polygeline ("Haemaccel") should be used whenever available in such countries.

Conclusions

With the above information in mind, resuscitators or first-aid deliverers would probably be concerned about risks to themselves in giving appropriate assistance to an injured diver.

• Firstly, the incidence of AIDS in the community is probably still quite small – especially in divers.

• Secondly, the chances of contracting the infection through first-aid or resuscitation, although not known for sure, are probably quite low – especially if reasonable precautions are followed. Health care workers who look after AIDS patients have a very low incidence of cross infection.

• To be balanced against the apparently small risk to a rescuer is the alternative of leaving injured or near drowned casualties to fend for themselves.

HEPATITIS

This is a highly contagious viral condition which infects and damages the liver. There are three or more variants of the virus but hepatitis-B probably poses the greatest potential threat to divers.

Hepatitis-B virus can cause a fatal initial infection in up to 10% of cases and fatal liver cancer or cirrhosis may develop after many years in apparent survivors. It is usually transmitted by infected blood.

There is potentially a small risk of infection in divers by sharing breathing equipment (as mentioned previously for AIDS), but the greatest risk comes from contamination of the skin by the blood of an infected person. In this regard it is similar to, but far more infectious than, AIDS. The virus is also far more "hardy" than that which causes AIDS, and can remain infectious for some time (eg. old dried blood in syringe needles found lying about can still infect anyone 'pricked' several weeks after being used by a carrier or actively infected person.

Prevention is along similar lines to AIDS.

INFECTIONS IN HYPERBARIC ENVIRONMENTS

Underwater habitats and compression chambers are humid areas which have a high concentration of oxygen.

This favours the growth of certain types of organisms, both in the chamber and on the skin of inhabitants. Outer ear infections (otitis externa), described earlier, are particularly common in underwater habitats because of these environmental conditions, and divers occupying these environments are frequently given prophylactic ear drops to prevent these infections.

Should severe infections occur, treatment may prove difficult within such environments. These infections include sinusitis, bronchitis, pneumonias and skin infections. An acute attack of appendicitis occurring in a diver whilst decompressing from a saturation dive will require surgery within the compression chamber. The administration of general anaesthesia, along with the sterility necessary for such surgery, render this normally simple procedure much more difficult.

Chapter 29

DANGEROUS MARINE ANIMALS

There are many marine animals which are dangerous to eat, to be eaten by, or to touch. The diver who is content to observe or photograph the creatures of this undersea environment will rarely have his safety threatened by them. Of necessity, this chapter is an oversimplification, with many significant omissions. Readers are strongly advised to obtain and read Dr Carl Edmonds' text on Dangerous Marine Creatures (see Appendix A).

SHARKS

Although encounters with sharks are commonplace in diving, shark attacks on skin and scuba divers are rare. Many of the attacks recorded have been associated with spearfishing, abalone diving, situations in which vibrations and chemicals given off by the wounded marine animal are likely to attract sharks. In one recent attack, the diver deliberately provoked a feeding frenzy before becoming a reluctant participant.

In a large proportion of attacks on divers the victim was unaware of the presence of the shark until he was actually bitten. Several behaviour patterns preceding shark attacks have been documented. In some cases the **shark circles** the victim and occasionally bumps him (presumably to gain some sensory information about the nature of this unfamiliar but potential food source), before attacking.

In many tropical species, **sharks may exhibit a threat display**, apparently in response to a territorial invasion. This is characterised by the shark swimming with an irregular jerking motion, accompanied by an arched back, head up and pectoral fins pointed downwards. This type of behaviour is the signal for the diver who wishes to experience old age, to depart the area.

The Great White shark has a **"bit and spit" technique** in which a single sudden powerful attack is made, with the shark then retreating until the victim (seal, dolphin, diver) haemorrhages in the water and loses consciousness. The shark can then feed without fear of damage from a counter attack.

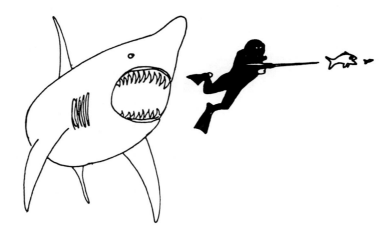

Fig. 29.1

Clinical Features

The seriousness of the injury depends on the size of the shark and the ferocity of the attack. Sharks larger than 2 metres in length have extremely powerful jaws equipped with razor sharp teeth which are easily capable of severing limbs or biting large pieces out of the torso. In spite of this, there have been many instances of divers surviving bites from sharks in excess of 4 metres in length. In some of these, the divers sustained severe lacerations from the puncture wounds of the teeth but no further injury. A shark of this size could easily bite a diver in two, so it appears that in some cases the shark will maul a victim and then not persevere, perhaps due to distaste for wet suit material or other items of the divers paraphernalia. Some divers may be as distasteful to sharks as they are to non-divers.

The blood loss from the massive lacerations accompanying shark attack is severe and immediate. Major blood vessels are frequently torn while generalised bleeding issues from the tissue laceration. Blood loss is often torrential from severed arteries.

The victim will display clinical features of severe blood loss — pale clammy skin, a rapid weak pulse, low blood pressure and rapid respiration. Consciousness may be lost, and death is not uncommon.

Treatment

The principles of successful management of shark attack victims were first described by Australian and South African authorities following their experience. They are :

❏ Stop the blood loss.

This must be done by rescuers **at the site** of the attack. Bleeding which is oozing or welling up from a wound can be stopped by applying a clean cloth pad to the wound and pressing firmly with the hand or applying a tight bandage. Spurting arterial bleeders up to about 3 mm in size can also be stopped by a pressure bandage or pad. Larger arterial bleeders can be stopped by the application of pressure by a finger or thumb. Bleeding from major blood vessels (the size of a finger) can be stopped by pinching the end of the vessel between finger and thumb, or a tourniquet if a limb is involved. Tourniquets have to be released every 10–20 minutes to let blood return to normal tissues.

It is important that pads used to stop bleeding, have pressure applied to them to force the blood vessels closed. It can be disastrous when rescuers merely cover bleeding areas with a dressing, without any pressure application. This soaks up and conceals the blood loss, without stopping it. Any clean material such as towelling, clothing or handkerchiefs are satisfactory in the first-aid situation.

❏ Resuscitate the victim at the site of the attack.

Immobilisation is vital. Once the victim is in a place of safety, (boat or shore) it is vital that he not be moved further. Bundling a victim into the back of vehicle for a bumpy ride to hospital has resulted in death of the victim on many occasions.

The victim should be kept lying horizontal at the rescue site and resuscitation equipment and personnel brought to him (see Chapter 42 for **A–B–C** of resuscitation).

Resuscitation involves replacing the patient's blood loss by the **intravenous infusion** of blood or blood substitutes such as plasma, saline or other intravenous fluids. It is not safe to move the victim until a satisfactory circulating volume has been established. Evidence for this is a relatively normal pulse (rate less than 100) and blood pressure.

This management principle is sometimes difficult to accept by rescuers who understandably wish to dispatch the victim to hospital (anywhere!) as soon as possible. However, once the victim reaches there, exactly the same management as should have taken place at the shark attack site will be needed. i.e. arrest of the blood loss accompanied by the administration of intravenous fluids.

Major hospitals in shark attack prone areas have a shark attack protocol along the lines mentioned above. Equipment may be available for immediate transportation to a shark attack site. Shark attack is so rare, however, that practice at implementing this protocol is sometimes neglected.

In spite of the severity of the injuries, it is common for the patient not to experience significant pain for some time after the attack. This phenomenon is frequently seen in other forms of severe injury such as motor vehicle and war injuries. If the patient is suffering significant pain or shock, the rescuing medical team will administer morphine in an appropriate dose.

Nothing should be given by mouth to the victim, as an anaesthetic may be required.

Prevention

Since vibrations and chemicals given off by speared fish and other forms of marine life commonly attract sharks, the avoidance of fishing should lessen the risk to the diver. The carrying of speared fish near the diver's body underwater invites a close inspection by an interested shark.

The well publicised practice of diving with a buddy should, on statistical grounds alone, reduce the likelihood of a shark attack on oneself by at least 50%.

Swimmers are protected by swimming in enclosed or shark meshed areas. They are advised not to swim where shark attacks have occurred or where fish or meat products are ditched (fish markets, abattoirs etc.). It is also safer to swim with groups of people and to avoid swimming at dusk (feeding time for sharks) or in areas of low visibility. Urine and blood are claimed to attract sharks and thus should not be released into surrounding water. Women who are menstruating, produce haemolysed blood which is not an attraction to sharks.

Divers are given the same advice, with the additional recommendation to avoid deep channels and drop-offs, and if diving with sharks, to carry an implement that can be used to fend them away (shark billy). A chain mail suit gives good protection, but it very heavy and thus dangerous for recreational divers. Ultrasonic, electrical, chemical and bubble deterrents are not effective.

BOX JELLYFISH OR SEA WASP

This deadly stinging creature is found in the tropical waters of the Indian, Pacific and Atlantic oceans during certain seasons. The season for North Australia is October to March, but local variations occur. The animal is an active swimmer which may be found even in very shallow water around beaches.

Its numerous tentacles may trail for up to 3 metres behind the body. The tentacles cling to the victim's skin and contain thousands of microscopic stinging cells (nematocysts) which can inject venom. The innumerable tiny doses of venom injected combine to form a large injection of toxin into the victim. The amount of venom injected depends on the length of tentacle in contact with the victim, and the area stung, as well as the thickness of skin.

The venom has its most serious effects on the heart and the respiratory system. It paralyses the respiratory muscles leading to death. Weakening of cardiac contraction, as well as cardiac rhythm disturbances, compounds the problem.

The venom also exerts a local effect producing agonising pain.

Clinical Features

The victim experiences **immediate agonising pain** on contact with the tentacles. With a large sting, sudden **collapse, cessation of breathing, cyanosis, unconsciousness** and **death** may follow rapidly. These effects are particularly dangerous in small children or old frail swimmers.

If the victim recovers, severe pain still persists for many hours, and **scarring** is common in the stung areas due to local tissue destruction.

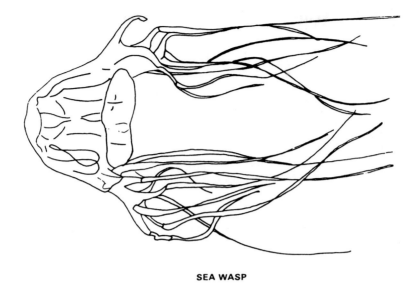

SEA WASP

Fig. 29.2

Treatment

Rescue the victim from the water and prevent drowning. This takes immediate precedence.

The first-aid principles of **A–B–C** (airway maintenance, breathing support and circulation maintenance) as described in Chapter 42 should be applied.

Apply copious amounts of ordinary **household vinegar** to the tentacles and gently remove the tentacles from the victims skin. The tentacles cannot sting effectively through the thick skin of the palm of the hand and fingers so this may be safer than it sounds. It is important not to rub or damage the tentacles as this will encourage the injection of further venom into the victim.

Alcohol application is no longer advised, as there is some evidence that this may cause the discharge of further venom into the victim. If it is of good quality, the alcohol may be more beneficial to the rescuer, once the victim has been taken safely to hospital.

The cause of death in box jellyfish sting is usually respiratory arrest. However, this may be transient if the victim is kept alive by **expired air resuscitation (EAR)** or other artificial ventilation during this period. The victim should be transported to hospital urgently.

An **antivenom** against the Chironex box jellyfish neutralises the venom present in the victim's body. It has been developed by the Commonwealth Serum Laboratories (CSL Australia) and should be used in severe cases or where significant local scarring is threatened. It may not be effective against other sea wasp species.

Prevention

The practice of covering as much exposed skin as possible by the wearing of a face mask, wet suit and hood, overalls, or a Lycra suit, prevents the access of tentacles to the skin. This protection also reduces the risks of stings from other jellyfish and injuries from corals.

OTHER JELLYFISH STINGS

Several other stinging jellyfish such as the **Portuguese Man-of-War, fire coral** and **stinging hydroids** can produce painful and sometimes incapacitating stings, although they are unlikely to be lethal.

The same technique of general management as described for box jellyfish should be followed. However, different local applications seem to work for different species. Some degree of pain relief can be afforded by the application of **local anaesthetic** (e.g. lignocaine ointment) to the stung area. Other preparations which have a variable effect, include "Stingose", "Stop-Itch", Tannic Acid Spray, etc. Any **anti-burn** preparation, including ice packs, may give some relief.

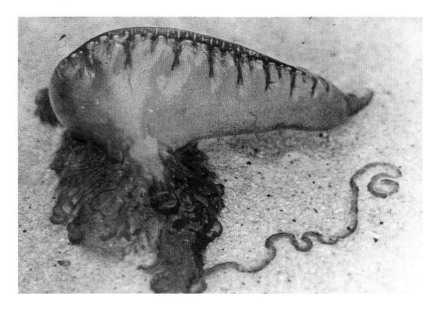

Fig. 29.3
"Bluebottle" or Portuguese-Man-of-War.

VENOMOUS CONE SHELLS

A small number of the cone shell family are capable of delivering a lethal venom. This is injected by a tiny dart shot from a tubular appendage which the animal can direct to any part of its shell. This apparatus is normally used by the animal to kill its prey (usually small fish), but it will use it as a weapon against a human who is careless enough to handle it.

Expert knowledge is required to differentiate venomous from harmless cone shells, and divers are advised to avoid handling them at all. Reef walkers, being less valuable than divers, may do as they wish.

Clinical Features

The initial sting may or may not be painful. The toxin affects the heart, skeletal and respiratory muscles. Muscle spasm develops. Death is usually from respiratory arrest.

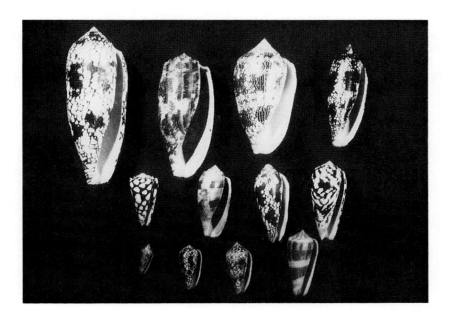

Fig. 29.4
A collection of venomous cone shells.

Treatment

The application of a **pressure bandage and immobilisation** (see later) should delay the spread of venom from the wound, although there have been no clinical case reports to verify this.

The **A–B–C** resuscitative measures (see Chapter 42) may keep the patient alive until the respiratory paralysis has worn off. This may involve many hours of artificial respiration.

BLUE RINGED OCTOPUS

This attractive little animal is found in rock crevices along the water's edge of many islands in the Pacific and Indian oceans, as well as in deeper water. If annoyed it will display a colourful array of blue or purple rings on its skin. This may arouse the curiosity of a potential victim, especially a child.

Unfortunately it can inflict a small, relatively painless, bite and inject venom through a beak at the base of its tentacles. The bite may go unnoticed by the victim until the major effects of the venom are felt.

The injected venom can produce muscular paralysis within minutes, leading to cessation of breathing. The victim will normally remain fully conscious but will be unable to communicate with bystanders due to the paralysis. Death is due to the respiratory failure, unless treatment is given.

Treatment

Artificial respiration must be continued until recovery (**6–12 hours**). This is necessary because of the respiratory muscle paralysis.

A **pressure bandage** and **immobilisation** (see later) should be applied to delay spread of the venom, until full resuscitation measures have been prepared.

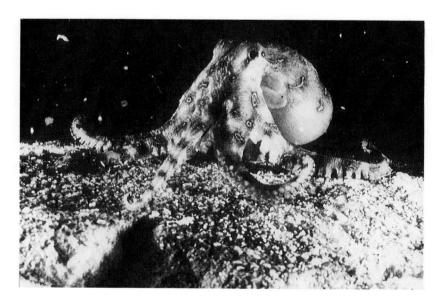

Fig. 29.5
This dangerous little animal should not be handled.

Case Report 29.3. A diver found a small octopus with attractive iridescent blue rings - hiding in a shell. He placed it under his wet suit vest, intending to show it to his companion later. After the dive he complained of double vision and respiratory difficulty. When he showed the octopus to his buddy, the buddy correctly diagnosed the problem and kept the victim alive by mouth to mouth respiration until hospital was reached. The victim later pointed out that he was not encouraged by comments such as "it looks as though he is not going to make it " from bystanders who had not realised that he was fully conscious, in spite of being paralysed.

SEA SNAKE

Sea snake bites are not uncommon in the Indo-Pacific ocean waters. In certain areas, sea snakes will approach divers underwater. These advances may be inspired by curiosity, as it is rare for sea snakes to bite divers without provocation. They will retaliate if grabbed.

The venom of sea snakes is more potent than that of the cobra. Even when bites occur, the presence of short fangs at the back of the mouth deprives many sea snakes of an efficient way of delivering this venom into humans. Often venom is not injected, despite the biting.

Clinical Features

If envenomation occurs, **symptoms may become evident within minutes to hours after the bite. Muscle weakness leading to paralysis, including **respiratory muscle paralysis** and **asphyxia**, and finally **cardiac failure** may follow the bite.

Occasionally the sea snake bite itself results in severe **lacerations** and **blood loss.**

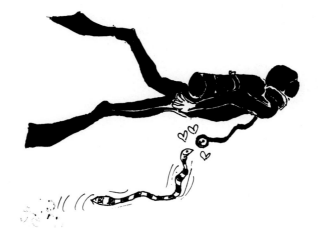

Fig. 29.6

Treatment

The **pressure bandage — immobilisation** technique (see later) will delay the symptoms until medical assistance, resuscitation facilities and antivenom can be acquired.

A–B–C first-aid measures should be instituted where necessary (see Chapter 42). Mouth to mouth respiration is the major requirement. The victim should be taken to hospital as soon as possible. Serious cases should be treated with sea snake **antivenom** (made by CSL – Australia).

STONEFISH

This is the most venomous fish known. It is extremely well camouflaged and may not move away when approached, as is implied by its name.

It is capable of inflicting severe stings by means of 13 poisonous spines along its back. The spines are able to penetrate rubber soled shoes or neoprene boots. At the base of each spine is a venom sac which empties its contents into the victim's wound.

Clinical Features

Envenomation results in severe **agonising pain at the site** of puncture. Extreme **swelling** and **local paralysis** develops rapidly. The venom can lead to **respiratory distress, cardiac disturbances** and syncope (**fainting**) with a reduction in **blood pressure**. Death is uncommon except in children or the infirm.

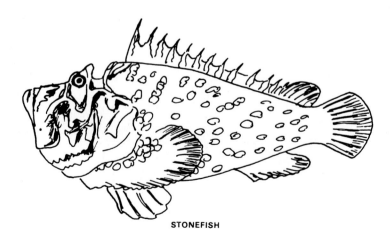

STONEFISH

Fig. 29.7

Treatment

Immersion of the stung area in hot water about **45°C** (first tested by the attendant's hand, to ensure against scalding) often gives significant pain relief and should be employed as soon as possible as a first-aid measure. Elevating the wound may reduce swelling.

The severe pain of the sting can be relieved by the **injection of local anaesthetic** (with no added vasoconstrictor agent such as adrenaline) **into the puncture sites.** This treatment may need repeating several times before the pain ceases to recur as the effects of the local anaesthetic injection wear off. A physician may prefer to block the nerve supply to the region with local anaesthetic as an alternative. Cleansing of the wound and antibacterial treatment is required.

Resuscitation (A–B–C supportive measures, see Chapter 42) should be instituted if necessary. **Antivenom** from the Australian CSL Laboratories is now available and its use may be necessary in severe cases.

OTHER SCORPION FISH

Other members of the scorpion fish family such as the **fortescue, lionfish** (or **butterfly cod**) and **bullrout,** produce painful stings similar to that of the stonefish, although both the local and generalised effects are usually not as severe. **Cat fish** have a similar effect.

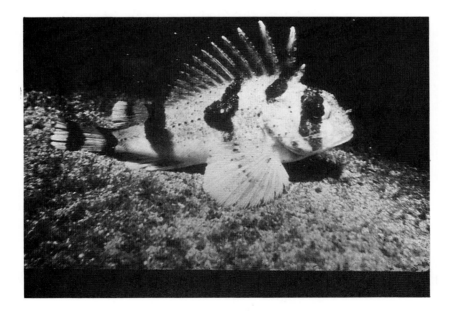

Fig. 29.8
Fortescue.

Pain relief can be obtained by **immersing the area in hot water** at about **45°C** (previously tested by immersing an unaffected limb in the water) as for the Stonefish sting (above), while more sustained relief can again be obtained by **injecting the punctures with local anaesthetic.** Cleansing of the wound and antibacterial treatment may be required, and the wound should be elevated.

STINGRAY

These flattened relatives of the shark have one or more long bony spines, which are intended for self defence, at the base of the tail.

The animals often bury themselves in the sand where they can inadvertently be stood upon, or otherwise disturbed, by an unsuspecting diver. The stingray defends itself by swinging its tail quickly over the top of its body, driving the spine into anything which happens to be above it.

The spine may produce a puncture and deposit venom. Its serrated edge can cause serious or even lethal lacerations. Parts of the spine, marine organisms and a toxic slime may be left in the wound to cause infections and local inflammation.

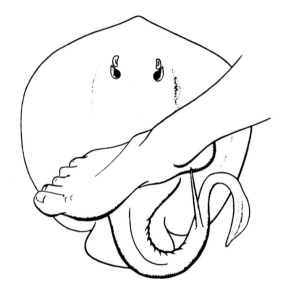

Fig. 29.9
Typical manner in which a stingray injury occurs.

Clinical Features

Pain caused by the toxin is **immediate** and **very severe. Swelling** is rapid. Toxin may be absorbed into the body producing **generalised symptoms** of syncope (**fainting**), weakness, palpitations, low blood pressure and disturbances of cardiac rhythm. **Death** is rare – except in cases where a vital organ such as the heart have been pierced by the spine.

Treatment

The **hot water** immersion treatment and the use of **injected local anaesthetic**, as described for stonefish injury, is useful. The wound should be **cleaned** to remove any foreign body or venom. An X–ray may demonstrate an embedded spine, which needs to be removed surgically. Local antibiotic cream, and often oral antibiotics (such as doxycycline), are needed. Swim well above the sea bed.

Prevention

Shuffling the feet while wading in areas frequented by stingrays will usually cause them to move away. Footwear may not be adequate to protect the feet or lower legs from these injuries. Diving into shallow waters where these animals are seen could be dangerous.

OTHER MARINE ANIMALS

Many other marine animals may cause major or minor injuries, and require different first-aid treatments. These, together with more detailed descriptions of the potentially lethal animals and those poisonous to eat, are fully discussed in the companion text "Dangerous Marine Creatures" by Dr. Carl Edmonds (See appendix A).

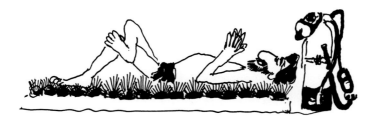

Fig. 29.10

PRESSURE BANDAGE — IMMOBILISATION TECHNIQUE

This is used to delay the absorption of venom from a wound. A bandage (preferably elastic) is applied over the bite and then wrapped around the limb (preferably from above downwards) tight enough to block the drainage vessels (lymphatics). The pressure is approximately the same as that used to treat a sprained ankle.

Care must be taken not to put the bandage on so tight that it causes pain and cuts off circulation. For this reason the technique is not applicable to painful, swollen bites that already have circulation restrictions.

The limb should then be immobilised with a splint to prevent any local muscle movement (this spreads the venom despite the bandage).

The pressure bandage — immobilisation of a limb should be continued until the victim has knowledgeable medical personnel and facilities available to cope with the envenomation. This happens as the bandage is released and the venom moves into the bloodstream. The doctors may well administer antivenom (if available), before removing the bandage.

The technique is especially applicable to sea snake, blue ringed octopus and cone shell bites. A variant may be used if the bite is on the torso, with a pad and bandage to produce the pressure.

Chapter 30

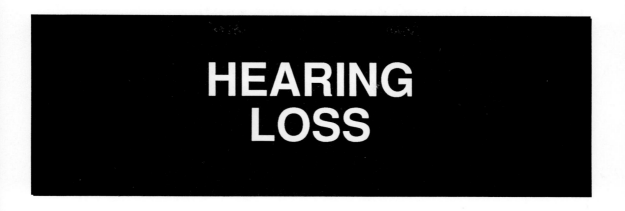

HEARING LOSS

This chapter may be easier to understand if the structure and function of the ear, as outlined previously in Chapter 9, is reviewed. All cases of hearing loss should be reviewed by a diving physician.

Divers frequently complain of a sensation of hearing loss which cannot be verified when hearing tests (pure tone audiometry) are performed. It is likely that currently available hearing tests, such as speech discrimination, are not sophisticated enough to detect such subtle alterations in the sensation of hearing.

The **causes** of demonstrable hearing loss fall into two categories :

- **Conductive hearing loss** – where there is some impediment to the conduction of sound vibrations (usually in the external and middle ear) en route to the hearing organ.

- **Sensorineural (nerve) hearing loss** – where sound vibrations reach the hearing organ (cochlea) in the inner ear, but the sound is not perceived due to damage of the cochlea or its nerve.

CONDUCTIVE HEARING LOSS

The likely causes of conductive hearing loss are in the external or internal ear.

External Ear Obstruction

Any obstruction to the outer ear such as wax accumulation, plugs or hoods, outer ear infections (see Chapter 28) or exostoses (see Chapter 32) can cause this.

Tympanic Membrane Damage

This membrane can be torn by :

- **Excessive stretching** during descent (middle ear barotrauma)
- A **shock wave** passing down the ear canal
- An **underwater explosion** or a **pressure wave from a fin** passing close to the divers ear
- An excessively forceful **Valsalva** manoeuvre has also been known to rupture the tympanic membrane.

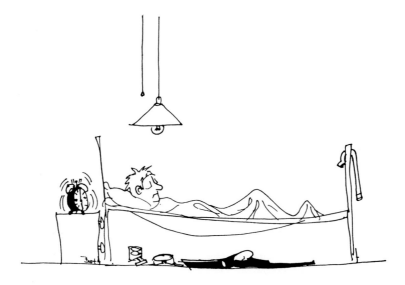

Hearing loss.

Fig. 30.1

Case History 30.1. A diver swimming closely behind his buddy suddenly felt pain in his left ear as his buddy's fin swept past his ear. Dizziness followed but soon settled. He surfaced and noticed a small amount of blood coming from his ear.

Diagnosis: Rupture of the ear drum caused by a pressure wave from a fin. The dizziness was due to cold water entering the middle ear through the ruptured ear drum. The blood was extruded by gas expanding in the middle ear, during ascent.

Middle Ear Disorders

Disturbances of the middle ear impair conduction of sound vibrations from the ear drum, through the bony chain to the cochlea. Causes include :

• **Middle ear barotrauma** which produces bruising and swelling of the middle ear tissues and bleeding into the middle ear space. Both factors dampen sound transmission (see Chapter 9).

• **Middle ear infection (otitis media)** which causes swelling and inflammation. This fills the middle ear space with pus, which impairs sound conduction (see Chapter 28).

SENSORINEURAL HEARING LOSS

Noise Induced Deafness

Repeated exposure to loud noise may produce a progressive hearing loss which usually affects high frequency perception first. This loss may be noticed by hi-fi enthusiasts who will complain that music has lost its sparkle. It is often insidious and may not be noticed for many years. Occasionally, a single exposure to loud noise can cause noticeable hearing loss immediately. Rock concerts and discos are also incriminated.

Noise induced hearing loss may be transient in the early stages but repeated exposure leads to permanent deafness, which worsens with more exposure. Industrial noise, usually affects the ears symmetrically, but other noise such as gunfire, commonly affects only one ear (the one exposed to the noise or blast).

The diving environment is often a noisy one. Recompression chambers, compressors, boat engines and compressed air leaks are often loud enough to present a threat to the hearing of those in their vicinity. Divers should take care to protect their ears when necessary by the use of industrial protective ear muffs or ear plugs (but not when diving).

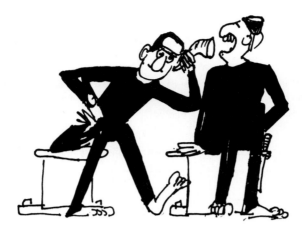

Fig. 30.2

High frequency hearing loss also renders consonants such as "S" or "CH" difficult to hear – hence the story of the yacht owner who was delighted when the curvaceous blonde diver with sensorineural deafness accepted his invitation to "crew" on his yacht.

Barotrauma

Inner ear barotrauma or associated round window fistula may lead to temporary or permanent hearing loss (see Chapter 9).

Decompression Sickness

Inner ear damage is an uncommon complication of decompression sickness (see Chapter 15) in air breathing divers. It is more common in deep Helium or mixed gas divers.

OVERVIEW OF HEARING LOSS

• **All prospective divers must have their ears examined to exclude ear problems** likely to predispose to barotrauma.

• **All divers should have a baseline audiometry** performed, to enable the physician to detect early hearing loss, to make assessment of future hearing problems much easier and to allow early and more knowledgeable treatment to be administered in the (not uncommon) event of a diver presenting with hearing loss.

• **Any case of hearing loss in a diver should be seen as soon as possible by a diving physician.** The doctor will take a history of the condition, examine the ears, test the hearing by pure tone audiometry at least, and possibly perform other specialised investigations such as bone conduction, speech discrimination, impedance audiometry, diving tympanogram, electro-nystagmograms and brain stem evoked auditory responses.

The cause is usually fairly obvious and **management** of the specific conditions are covered in other chapters.

• **Divers with pre-existing hearing loss** should realise that any deafness arising from barotrauma will be added to the loss they already have. It is also believed that people with hearing impairment are more susceptible to further damage than others. Divers who are aware of hearing loss should discuss the implications with a diving physician.

• **Occupational implications are raised.** Those who need excellent hearing for their livelihood, such as musicians, cardiologists, sonar operators and airline pilots, should consider whether the small but real risk of hearing damage associated with diving is worth taking.

• **Hearing loss is sometimes associated with abnormalities of the body's balance mechanism**, which might have safety implications with diving (see Chapter 31).

Chapter 31

DISORIENTATION

Accurate orientation whilst underwater is important for the diver so that he can find his way back to the surface. On land the diver uses a combination of vision, the feeling of gravity on his body, and the balance organs to tell him which way is up.

When underwater, the diver becomes virtually weightless, depriving him of the sensation of gravity and making him reliant on vision and his balance organs for spatial orientation. With poor visibility, even the visual cues are lost, leaving the diver almost totally reliant on his balance organs for this orientation. A sensation of disorientation requires investigation by a diving physician.

The experienced diver can acquire some cues about his body position from :

- the way heavy objects such as the weight belt or other metal objects hang,
- the direction his bubbles are going,
- the direction of a life-line or hookah hose.

Inexperienced or panicking divers are often unable to use this subtle information. If the diver becomes disoriented he is likely to experience anxiety. Panic can easily ensue.

VERTIGO — OR "DIZZINESS"

This is a false sensation of spinning or moving. The diver may either have a sensation of himself spinning or the environment spinning about him. It happens because the balance organ (**vestibular system**) can be unreliable underwater – it was designed to work on land. Under certain circumstances it can supply the brain with misleading information which is falsely interpreted as movement.

The sensation of vertigo is bad enough, but it is often accompanied by **nausea** and **vomiting** which can threaten a diver's life. These symptoms may vary from mild to very severe. Vomiting into, and then breathing from, a demand valve is not easy underwater.

Function of the Vestibular System

The balance or vestibular system comprises two marble-sized structures located in the skull above and behind the middle ear space on either side of the head. Each vestibular apparatus has two parts. Abnormalities of either cause vertigo and disorientation. They are :

❏ A system of three interconnecting tubes (semi-circular canals).

These are aligned at right angles to each other and filled with fluid. They detect movement in all three planes. If the body rotates, the fluid in these three canals tends to lag behind, due to its inertia. The differential movement of the body and the fluid is detected by nerve endings – hair like projections into the fluid (hair cells) at the base of each canal.

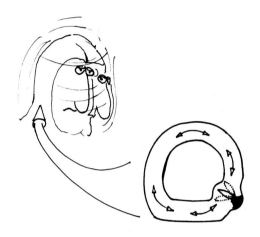

Fig. 31.1

❏ The Otolith organ.

These other fluid-filled structures have a viscous base which contains minute calcium granules. Hair like projections of nerve cells penetrate this gel and detect any movement of the granules. Because of their weight, the granules tend to move in response to **gravity** and **acceleration**. The hair cells detect this and continuously inform the brain about which way is up and the direction of any acceleration.

The semi-circular canals are located close to the ear canal. Cold water entering the ear canal can cool them slightly, causing convection currents in the fluid. The movement of the fluid is detected by the hair cells and with ascent and descent causes vertigo. This is termed **caloric** induced vertigo and is usually associated with the diver being in a horizontal position. Pressure changes can cause **barotrauma** induced vertigo, and it is possible that this could be due to stimulation of the otoliths or the semicircular canals and is usually associated with the diver being in a vertical position.

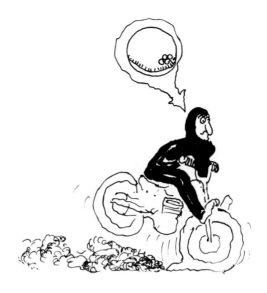

Fig. 31.2

CAUSES OF VERTIGO

Problems arising from the vestibular system fall into two principle categories :

- unequal vestibular stimulation and
- unequal vestibular response.

Unequal Vestibular Stimulation

If both vestibular systems are equally sensitive but are stimulated unequally, then vertigo may result due to the unequal responses received by the brain.

Any condition causing more cold water to enter one side than the other causes unequal **caloric** stimulation. Wax blocking one ear, an air bubble, otitis externa, exostoses, ear plugs or a ruptured ear drum will all have this effect.

With middle or inner **ear barotrauma** (see Chapter 9) affecting one side, or **decompression sickness** (see Chapter 15) on one side, unequal vestibular stimulation may result in vertigo.

Failure of the ears to equalise pressures to the same degree can stimulate the vestibular system unequally. This is not uncommon on ascent, as the pressure of the expanding gas in the middle ear spaces can become greater on one side than the other due to differences in patency of the Eustachian tubes. This is termed **Alternobaric Vertigo** (see Chapter 9). It is very common and is often noticed as the diver ascends a metre or so, from depth. He may even be aware of the sensation of one Eustachian tube opening before the other, or of the expansion of air in the other middle ear.

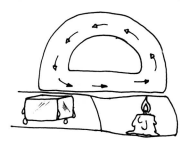

Fig. 31.3
Caloric stimulation producing "convection" current flows in inner ear fluids.

Case Report 31.1. A diver using hookah apparatus on a training dive at night lost contact with the bottom. He was unable to see his bubbles and had no idea which way was up, but by feeling the direction of his air hose, he was able to establish where the surface was.

Diagnosis: disorientation due to the reduced sensory input (decreased vision) of night diving.

Case Report 31.2. An inexperienced diver had difficulty equalising his middle ear during descent. He continued to descend in spite of this. The pain was abruptly relieved and he became aware of a hissing sound and cold sensation in his ear as his ear drum perforated. Seconds later he developed a severe sensation of spinning which was accompanied by nausea. He clung onto his shot line and was relieved when the vertigo gradually passed off after several minutes.

Diagnosis: Vertigo due to one sided vestibular stimulation (caloric) from cold water entering the middle ear. As the water warmed to body temperature, the cooling effect to the vestibular system subsided.

Unequal Vestibular Response

The two vestibular systems are normally equally sensitive to any stimulus such as movement. In some people, they have unequal sensitivity. This can be due to a slight imbalance (either overactive or underactive function) which has been present from birth or to damage to one side from causes such as ear barotrauma or some medical conditions. In this situation, the same stimulus causes a greater response from one side than the other, and is experienced by the person as vertigo.

People with this problem unconsciously adapt by avoiding sudden movements of the head or body. They learn by experience to avoid gymnastics and roller coaster rides, but are usually not aware of the dangers posed to them by the extreme stimuli which are commonplace in diving.

Water entering the ear canals is a potent cause of vertigo in these people. As mentioned above, this water can cool the fluid in the semi-circular canals setting up convection currents (**caloric stimulation**). If the vestibular systems on each side are not equally sensitive, a stronger response will be produced from one side. The brain will interpret this information as indicating movement, and the diver will experience vertigo and feel disorientated.

During ascent or descent, **pressure changes** in the middle ear can also produce vertigo and disorientation in those with unequal vestibular response.

Other Causes of Vertigo

If the diver is deprived of normal visual cues in conditions of **poor visibility** or at night, it is possible for the resulting disorientation to culminate in vertigo, especially in inexperienced divers.

Nitrogen narcosis may aggravate vertigo. Vertigo has also been recorded as a symptom of other conditions not commonly encountered by recreational divers. These include **oxygen toxicity, carbon dioxide toxicity, carbon monoxide toxicity,** and **high pressure neurological syndrome**.

CONCLUSIONS

While **disorientation** under water can be unpleasant and dangerous, **vertigo** can be life threatening because of the risk of vomiting or panic.

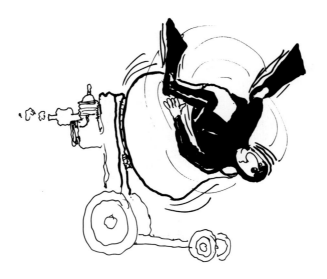

Fig. 31.4

A thorough diving medical examination before a prospective diver undertakes training can exclude some of the factors predisposing to vertigo, and is mandatory for all divers.

A diver experiencing vertigo under water should avoid unnecessary movement and hold onto a fixed object if one is available. Fortunately, in most cases, the vertigo is frequently short lived. If the vertigo fails to abate and there are no obstacles above him, ditching of weights, along with cautious inflation of a buoyancy compensator, should return the diver to the safety of the surface.

Any diver who experiences vertigo under water and survives should abandon the dive, **consult a diving physician** to investigate, identify and correct the cause before diving again.

Chapter 32

MISCELLANEOUS DISORDERS

CONTACT LENSES

Contact lenses are a convenient alternative to spectacles but can be a source of problems to the diver. The most common of these is **loss** of the expensive lens during removal of the face mask. The eyes should be shut while removing the mask underwater or on the surface!

In certain circumstances, especially during long or deep dives or in compression chambers, it is possible for **gas bubbles** to form behind the contact lens (particularly with hard, non gas-permeable lenses) causing pressure and damage to the cornea of the eye. If this happens, the diver may experience discomfort in the eye, blurred vision and the appearance of halos around bright lights. Long term effects could include scarring of the cornea.

Gas bubble damage can be overcome in the hard contact lens by drilling a small hole in the centre of the lens (a **fenestrated** lens) which allows gas bubbles to escape. This has no effect on the visual performance of the lens. Soft contact lenses are usually not a problem because of their gas permeability and flexibility.

It is now relatively easy to have corrective lens ground into or attached to the diver's face mask, as an alternative to contact lenses.

MUSCULAR CRAMPS

Cramp is a painful spasm of a muscle group. It is common in divers and can cause dangerous behaviour or incapacity. The muscles most commonly affected are those in the sole of the foot, the calf and the thigh but other muscles can also be involved.

Unusual exertion of the muscles, due to changes in fins or equipment, makes cramp more likely, especially if the diver is generally unfit. Cold water is another predisposing factor.

Cramp is managed by slowly stretching and maintaining tension on the muscles involved. Sometimes this may require the diver to actually stand and push down onto some firm underwater surface in order to allow the muscle to be stretched. Ditching of weights underwater or inflation of the buoyancy vest on the surface may be helpful in an emergency, avoiding the need to continue swimming.

This condition can be inconvenient or even dangerous if the diver is simultaneously coping with environmental problems such as white water or strong currents or tidal flows.

It is best **prevented** by maintaining a high level of physical fitness, using familiar and comfortable fins and having adequate insulation from cold water.

EAR PROBLEMS

Wax (Cerumen)

Ear wax (cerumen) is a protective substance which coats and waterproofs the external ear canal. Occasionally the ear produces excessive wax which accumulates and obstructs the ear canal, or contributes to water retention with subsequent otitis externa (see Chapter 28). Divers often try to remove this wax with cotton-tipped "buds", but unfortunately this usually results in the wax being compacted even tighter in the canal, often precipitating total obstruction. This may produce curable hearing loss, or caloric induced vertigo if water is able to enter only one ear (see Chapter 31).

The excessive wax is easily removed by a diving physician using an instrument or syringe. This leaves the ear canal somewhat open to infection however (otitis externa – see Chapter 28), and therefore should not be done unless the wax totally occludes the canal. Ear drops are readily available (Cerumol, Waxsol, olive oil etc.) which help to soften wax so that the normal self cleaning function of the canal can proceed more easily. Diving itself helps in wax removal.

Exostoses

The inner part of the external ear canal passes through bone. People who swim or dive regularly, especially in cold water, sometimes develop outgrowths of this bone, known as exostoses, into the ear canal. These can cause partial obstruction which may lead to the accumulation of wax and the retention of water causing infection or hearing loss.

Large troublesome exostoses can be removed surgically, however this is not usually necessary.

Others

Infections (otitis externa, otitis media) are discussed in Chapter 28, hearing loss in Chapter 30, vertigo and disorientation in Chapter 31, barotrauma in Chapter 9 and decompression sickness in Chapter 15.

HEADACHE

Headache during or after a dive is a frequent complaint and can be caused by conditions ranging from trivial to life threatening. It always requires careful assessment.

The most likely cause of the headache can usually be deduced from the past medical history, location of the pain, dive history, mode of onset and progression.

Details of clinical and diagnostic features can be found in the relevant chapters elsewhere. Although most headaches are not serious, the more serious causes will be dealt with first.

Decompression Sickness and Pulmonary Barotrauma

Air emboli and bubble development in the brain cause brain injury and swelling which is often heralded by headache. This may start within a short time after surfacing, or may be delayed for several hours. Headache followed by confusion or loss of consciousness is very suggestive of this dangerous disorder. The dive profile is helpful in diagnosing headaches of this type (see Chapters 15 and 11).

Sinus Barotrauma

This condition usually affects the various sinuses located around the eyes, or the maxillary sinuses in the cheek bones. Sharp pain in the affected sinus may be experienced during descent or ascent, or a more dull pain in the region of the sinus may be felt after the dive (see Chapter 10).

Pain may be referred from the sinus to the upper teeth or behind the eyes. After minor barotrauma, an infection (**sinusitis**) can develop hours or days after the dive causing a headache in similar sites to those mentioned (see Chapter 28).

Migraine

This condition can be a worrisome problem in divers. It is common in the general population.

❑ Clinical features.

These may include an "aura" before the onset of the headache, with visual effects ranging from flashes of light, shimmering lines, partial loss of a visual field to mild blurring of vision. A severe headache aggravated by bright lights, usually accompanied by nausea and vomiting, and sometimes numbness, tingling, weakness or paralysis of the limbs, most often follows the visual aura.

Migraine headaches can be trivial or can be associated with vomiting, severe incapacity and neurological symptoms (visual disorders, numbness or 'tingling sensations' in arms or legs etc.). These more severe symptoms lead to diagnostic confusion with air embolism and decompression sickness and may result in an emergency evacuation and inappropriate treatment.

A severe migraine developing during a dive can incapacitate the diver or induce vomiting underwater with subsequent drowning.

For reasons which are not well understood, mild migraine sufferers can sometimes have very severe and unusual migraine attacks precipitated by diving. It may be that this is a response to bubbles within the cranial extravascular system. Migraine may also result from excessive exercise and carbon dioxide – oxygen pressure variations. Cold and exertion are also possible causes.

For these reasons migraine sufferers are not encouraged to dive. Nevertheless, some have no "neurological" features and are very infrequent and mild. Then if they do dive, they are usually **restricted to non-decompression dives** and to **less than 18 metres** (i.e. dives that do not typically produce intra-arterial bubbles or cerebral decompression sickness).

Tension Headache

Diving and training for diving can be a stressful experience which can cause headaches in susceptible individuals from excessive muscular tension. These individuals will often recognise the headache as similar to those associated with other stressful experiences. Most are frontal or involve the neck and back of the head.

Mask Strap Tension

Inexperienced divers often tighten their mask strap excessively in the hope that the alarming prospect of loss of the mask underwater can be avoided. Excessive tension of this strap interferes with blood supply to muscles around the skull causing a headache similar to tension headache. The pain is prevented by slackening the strap. As the diver gains confidence in his ability to deal with a flooded or displace face mask, the need to keep the strap excessively tight disappears. Some headaches are related to the design of the strap (ie. wide single straps verses narrow split straps.) Trial and error may sort out this type of problem.

Other Types of Headache

Cold water entering an ear canal can cause headache (or earache) when it comes into contact with the ear drum. This is easily prevented in swimmers by the use of ear plugs. These cannot be used by divers. The best prevention is a neoprene hood, which allows the trapped water to warm to body temperature.

There are many other causes of headache, including neurological, barotraumatic, thermal, orthopaedic and vascular mechanisms, that are too complex to be assessed here. Any headache associated with diving deserves investigation, before its consequences during future diving become more serious than those occurring while on land.

SUNBURN

Sunburn, especially in tropical areas, is a common problem for divers. It is caused by ultraviolet radiation from the sun. This radiation is scattered by the atmosphere and reflected from water so that even sheltering in shade does not provide complete protection.

The **clinical features** of sunburn have been experienced by almost all divers and do not require elaboration.

❏ Treatment.

This is essentially symptomatic. Further exposure to sunlight (even indirectly) should be avoided. A soothing or cooling lotion is often of value in relieving the pain, and steroid (cortisone) creams may be beneficial in severe cases. Blisters should not be ruptured as this invites secondary infection.

❏ Prevention.

Protection can be afforded by covering the skin by clothing, by wearing a hat and by the use of a broad spectrum UV screening cream or lotion. Snorkel divers are advised to wear one of the lightweight protective Lycra suits, which also give protection against marine stingers and coral cuts.

Ultraviolet screening agents are now coded by a SP number which gives an approximate indication of the degree of protection compared with unprotected skin e.g. SP 10 cream will protect the skin from burning for at period 10 times longer than unprotected skin. Unprotected skin can begin to burn in 15 minutes in strong sunlight so that a sun screen with this level of protection can be expected to protect for 2.5 hours if an adequate thickness is maintained by repeated application and the screen is not washed off. SP 15+ creams are even more effective and are advised.

Prolonged exposure to sunlight is associated with an increased incidence of skin cancer and premature skin ageing.

SEASICKNESS

This is a distressing and potentially hazardous problem for divers. It usually develops in susceptible individuals in the dive boat but can also develop underwater, during decompression on a shot line in rough conditions or with underwater surge. On the boat, less attention is paid to dive planning and equipment preparation, by the sea sick diver.

The associated vomiting causes dehydration on the boat and requires considerable skill to cope with underwater, if the diver is to continue breathing through his demand valve. It does have the advantage of attracting all sorts of fish homing in for a free feed.

Another potential problem relates to the sedating effect which is produced to some degree by most of the available anti-seasickness medications. This will affect judgement and aggravate nitrogen narcosis.

❏ Prevention.

General measures to be taken include :

- remain in the centre line of the boat, but not near the bow (reduce spatial movements),
- positioning in the boat so that head movement is minimised, remain still (lie down),
- either keeping eyes closed or focussing on the distant horizon (avoid reading),
- if in an enclosed cabin, ensure air circulation with a fan if possible.

If mildly seasick, swimming or snorkelling around on the surface of a sheltered area for a short while will often settle symptoms. The diver can then reboard the boat to don gear and start the dive.

Short acting anti-seasickness tablets such as cyclizine are effective if taken 1 or 2 hours before boarding the boat. These last about 4 hours.

Another effective preventative measure is to take promethazine tabs (a well known oral antihistamine), 25 mg. at bed time the night before. This will cause sedation during the night but corresponds to the normal sleep time. One dose at night will provide some resistance to sea sickness for the early part of the following day, with minimum sedation. The **depth** of diving should be **limited to less than 30 metres** (100 ft.), maximum, and preferably less than 18 metres (60 ft.). A cup of coffee (caffeine) beforehand reduces seasickness and counters sedation in some.

In all cases, medication should have been tried previously (a "dry run") to ensure adverse side effects are not produced. It should not be taken if alcohol has been consumed because of additive effects.

Transdermal ("Scop") skin patches are not recommended for diving due to side effects, but may be effective for sailors.

Acupuncture (via acupressure pads) and ginger, although currently fashionable, are really only of psychological value.

TEMPORO-MANDIBULAR ("JAW JOINT") DYSFUNCTION OR ARTHRITIS

Novice divers tend to be apprehensive underwater, especially about the reliability of their air supply. They therefore clamp their jaws tightly on the mouth piece, causing excessive stress on the joint between the upper and lower jaw. This can cause minor injury to the joint, manifested by spasm of the jaw muscles, pain, tenderness over the joint (in front of the ear), and inability to fully open the jaw.

In recreational divers this condition is usually temporary and is reversible by correcting the cause. The diver is encouraged to grip the demand valve less tightly with the jaws. Some older demand valves are heavy and bulky, placing undue stress on the jaw, while other types may be positioned so that the air hose pulls the jaw to one side, causing uneven and excessive strain.

In some older divers, permanent arthritic changes to the joint can occur, from this cause. Individually mouldable lugs on the mouthpieces of snorkels and regulators may help minimize these effects in some cases.

EXPLOSIONS – UNDERWATER BLAST

This topic is included only as a warning for recreational divers not to use explosives underwater. Military divers are particularly at risk from these hazards, even in training – because of the use of "scare charges" which are designed to discourage underwater saboteurs and are sometimes used in the vicinity of trainee divers to toughen them up.

When an underwater explosion is observed from the surface, a sudden explosive projection of water and foam into the air can be seen immediately after the explosion. This is the effect of the pressure wave emanating from the blast when it meets an air–water interface.

A similar effect is produced at air–tissue interfaces in the body as the shock wave travels through them. This can shred tissues such as lungs, intestines, sinus cavities and the middle ear spaces, which are in contact with air – all gas containing spaces within the body can be affected.

❑ Clinical features.

The organs worst affected are the lungs and intestines. Rupture and bleeding of the tissues in the lungs and bowel cause :

- chest pain
- shortness of breath
- vomiting or coughing up of blood
- passage of bloody or black bowel motions.

Damage to the ears and sinuses causes features similar to barotrauma. Ruptured ear drums and deafness are particularly common.

If a diver is caught in the water where an explosion is inevitable, some protection can be afforded by attempting to float on the back on the surface – this will remove some of the air containing tissues from contact with the water.

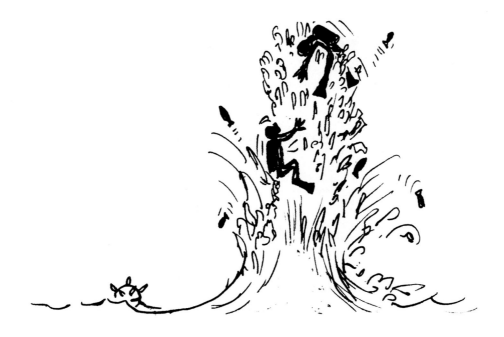

Fig. 32.1

Chapter 33

UNCONSCIOUSNESS IN DIVERS

There are many causes of a diver losing consciousness in the water but the final outcome is very often the same – **drowning**. This chapter provides an overview of the causes and treatment.

Unconsciousness on land rarely leads to death. Underwater, it frequently does. Because of the hazardous nature of diving in a state of impaired consciousness, great care must be applied to ensuring divers are medically fit and have no increased propensity to loss of consciousness. Also, once loss of consciousness does occur, the adherence to a genuine "buddy system" is of demonstrable value.

When an unconscious diver is rescued and the first-aid measures necessary for all these cases are then instituted (see Chapter 39, 40 and 42), the remainder of the management depends on the cause of the unconsciousness. It is therefore important to be able to identify the likely causes.

They are best classified according to the type of diving being performed, and the equipment used. More information can be found on each topic elsewhere in this book.

CAUSES OF LOSS OF CONSCIOUSNESS

The causes **common to all types of diving** are :

- Hypoxia (from a diversity of causes)
- Salt water aspiration or near drowning
- Cold
- Marine animal injuries
- Vomiting and inhalation of vomit or sea-water
- Miscellaneous medical conditions
- Underwater explosions

In addition to these the causes associated with **scuba diving** are :

- Hypocapnea
- Decompression sickness

- Air embolism from pulmonary barotrauma
- Nitrogen narcosis
- Carbon monoxide toxicity
- Hypoxia due to faulty equipment or gas contamination

In addition to these, causes associated with **rebreathing** or **mixed gas diving equipment** (not commonly used by recreational divers) include :

- Hypercapnea
- Oxygen toxicity
- Hypoxia due to ascent, dilution or excessive consumption.

The more **common causes** of unconsciousness are as follows :

HYPOXIA
(SEE CHAPTER 20)

Hypoxia of the brain associated with near-drowning is the final event in many diving accidents and is the most common cause of unconsciousness in divers. It may follow events as diverse as inadequate air supply, salt water aspiration, equipment faults or misuse, inhalation of vomit, pulmonary barotrauma, gas contamination, etc. It is frequently associated with panic and physical exhaustion.

Case History 33.1 A diver breathing from a semi-closed breathing apparatus lost consciousness shortly after leaving the surface. He was brought back to the surface and revived with 100% oxygen. His slightly bluish face turned red later on when it was discovered that he had filled his cylinders with pure nitrogen.

Diagnosis: Hypoxia due to inadequate (i.e. nil) inspired oxygen.

HYPOXIA DURING BREATHHOLD DIVING
(SEE CHAPTER 4)

❏ Hypoxia of ascent.

A diver can lose consciousness from hypoxia of ascent during deep breathhold dives. The partial pressure of O_2 in the lungs can fall dangerously low during ascent or immediately after surfacing.

❏ Hyperventilation.

Hyperventilation before a breathhold dive makes hypoxia more likely because the urge to breathe is suppressed. This technique was used by some divers to increase the duration of dives. The practice is gradually dying out, along with the divers who use it.

Case Report 33.2. A young diver was attempting to beat a local swimming pool underwater distance record. He was seen to hyperventilate before the dive. Midway through the second lap, he ceased to swim and sank to the bottom. Luckily, he was quickly pulled from the water and revived my mouth to mouth respiration. He was discharged some weeks later, with only minor brain damage.

Case Report 33.3. An experienced diver taking part in a spear fishing competition was found dead on the bottom with a speared fish nearby. Post-mortem revealed no abnormality apart from drowning. He was known to practise hyperventilation.

NEAR DROWNING
(SEE CHAPTER 25)

This is the consequence of many diving accidents. The hypoxia associated with near drowning can render a diver unconscious, or the diver can become unconscious first, and then drown.

COLD OR HYPOTHERMIA
(SEE CHAPTERS 4, 27 AND 35)

Exposure to cold water can cause an excessive fall in body temperature which can make a diver initially confused (at a body temperature of around 34°C) and then unconscious (below 30°C). A diver suddenly entering cold water can sometimes develop cardiac rhythm disturbances which can produce unconsciousness immediately.

MARINE ANIMAL INJURIES
(SEE CHAPTER 29)

Venomous animals can cause unconsciousness either from the direct effect of the venom on the brain, from hypoxia due to respiratory paralysis, or due to inadequate cerebral circulation from a lowering of blood pressure. Shock from blood loss after shark attack can also cause unconsciousness.

Case History 33.4. A group of divers on their first dive on a tropical reef eagerly took to the water. They returned later with speared fish, coral and shells among which were several varieties of venomous cone shells which they had handled, and in some cases, carried under their wet suits. A member of the boat crew recognised the cone shells and advised the divers of their narrow escape.

Diagnosis: potential loss of consciousness, or "accidents looking for somewhere to happen".

DECOMPRESSION SICKNESS
(SEE CHAPTERS 14–16)

Cerebral Decompression Sickness can lead to unconsciousness. It is more likely after deep dives and repetitive diving.

AIR EMBOLISM FROM PULMONARY BAROTRAUMA OF ASCENT
(SEE CHAPTER 11)

Cerebral arterial gas (air) embolism (CAGE) can cause abrupt loss of consciousness either during or immediately after ascent. It is sometimes associated with pneumothorax, which needs special management.

Case Report 33.5. A 26 year old diver undertook a 55 metre (180 foot) dive with a bottom time of 8 minutes. He returned rapidly to the surface when his contents gauge indicated an almost exhausted air supply. While climbing into the boat, he complained of numbness down one side, and developed slurred speech. He then had a convulsion and lost consciousness. He died en route to a recompression chamber 600 km. away.

Diagnosis: the probable diagnoses would include cerebral decompression sickness or air embolism (CAGE) from pulmonary barotrauma (burst lung). Autopsy verified the diagnosis.

CARBON MONOXIDE TOXICITY
(SEE CHAPTER 23)

Divers breathing compressed air are vulnerable to this problem if the air source is contaminated, often from the exhaust of a nearby internal combustion engine.

OXYGEN TOXICITY
(SEE CHAPTER 21)

Military divers using oxygen equipment, or professional divers breathing mixed gases, are at risk from convulsions due to oxygen toxicity under certain circumstances. A convulsion can be followed by confusion or unconsciousness.

GENERAL MEDICAL CONDITIONS

A variety of medical emergencies including hypoglycaemia (low blood sugar) in diabetics, heart attack, stroke, epileptic fit, drug overdose, head injury, severe infection and shock can cause unconsciousness. Many conditions with the potential to cause unconsciousness require exclusion in a diving medical examination and people with these conditions would normally be advised against diving.

Case Report 33.6. A 30 year old diver using scuba at 10 metres (33 foot) became unconscious ten minutes after the start of the dive while swimming strenuously on the bottom. He was brought rapidly to the surface by his buddy. He remained unconscious on the boat and was pale and sweaty with a rapid pulse. He was breathing adequately and 100% Oxygen breathing on a mask produced no improvement. Those present were at a loss for a diagnosis until the diver's wife informed them that he was a diabetic taking insulin. He was successfully treated in hospital by intravenous glucose.

Diagnosis : Hypoglycaemia (low blood sugar level) due to unexpected exertion, even though the diver took a reduced Insulin dosage. He was advised that diving and diabetes requiring medication was a suicidal combination and he agreed to take up a sport less dangerous to diabetics

---

RESCUE AND FIRST AID
TREATMENT
(SEE CHAPTERS 39–42)

First **ditch the diver's weight belt.** The **diver must be brought to the surface and then removed from the water** as **rapidly** as possible. Emergency buoyant ascent takes precedence over concern for burst lung (pulmonary barotrauma) when the recreational diver is unconscious. These unconscious divers will usually exhale passively during ascent.

After surfacing the airway must be cleared and if there is no breathing, expired air resuscitation commenced. Details of the rescue and resuscitation technique are explained in Chapters 39 and 42. After securing the essential **A–B–C** (airway, breathing and circulation) the cause must be sought and **specific treatment** started. Medical advice should obviously be sought as soon as possible.

Diagnosis of the cause is made by a logical process of elimination taking into account the medical history of the diver, the equipment used, the type of diving, the dive profile, the events leading to the unconsciousness and the appearance of the diver. Assume the most serious and treatable diagnosis.

Administer 100% O_2, if needed or if in any doubt about the diagnosis. Keep detailed records and ensure that these accompany the patient. Retain the equipment for future assessment.

Chapter 34

WHY DIVERS DIE

INTRODUCTION

Experience of life suggests that anything which is fun tends to be either illegal, immoral, fattening, or dangerous. Recreational diving partly conforms to this universal law, ranking below hang gliding and parachuting but above most other sports as regards the risk of a fatal accident.

Diving statistics show diving death rates of 16–20 per 100,000 divers per year, with the statistical chance of a fatality being about 1 in 95,000 dives (Monaghan)

These figures tend to contradict the misinformation issuing from some sections of the diving industry (fatalities of <4 per 100, 000) which would have us believe that diving is a very safe recreation. It is not, but then we accept risks every day. Even driving an automobile to a dive site carries an appreciable (but less) risk of death - a possibility which we generally regard with equanimity.

This chapter will show that many diving deaths should be preventable and that a diver ought to be able to minimise his chances of becoming a statistic by understanding and influencing the factors which are now known to be associated with diving deaths.

STATISTICAL EVIDENCE

The information presented here is mainly based on data gathered by two valuable studies involving recreational diving fatalities. One included over 2500 cases covering 20 years, documented by John McAniff, Director of the National Underwater Accident Data Centre (NUADC), University of Rhode Island (USA), and the second is by Drs Carl Edmonds and Douglas Walker — based on a much more detailed analysis of a smaller number of diving accidents in Australia and New Zealand (Australasia) during the 1980's. Deaths in Hawaiian divers were also described by Carl Edmonds and Roy Damron.

The NUADC study detailed diving activity and the Australasian study had more detail of the conditions contributing to the accident. The statistics from both studies correlated with surprising closeness, probably reflecting that the diving equipment and affiliated instructional organisations are common to both countries.

The following is a review of the important factors involved in diving deaths related to recreational divers. Figures have been rounded off, for simplicity.

OVERVIEW

The average age of victims was 33 years, but 10% were over 50 years.

- **90% died with their weight belt on.**
- **86% were alone when they died.**
- **50% did not inflate their buoyancy vest.**
- **33% were inexperienced, 33% had some experience and 33% had considerable experience.**
- **25% encountered their difficulty first on the surface, 50% actually died on the surface.**
- **10% were under training when they died.**
- **10% were advised that they were medically unfit to dive.**
- **5% were cave diving.**
- **1% of rescuers became a victim.**

❏ Gender.

1 in 10 of the casualties were women. The actual percentage of women in the overall diving population is difficult to gauge, but is probably about 1 in 3, suggesting that women are safer divers than men.

❏ Major causes of death seen at autopsy.

Most divers ultimately drowned (86%), but a number of factors usually combined to incapacitate the diver before this terminal event. These are referred to in the following sections. The other common causes of death included pulmonary barotrauma (13%) and heart disorder (12%).

CONTRIBUTING FACTORS

Deaths usually followed a combination of difficulties, which alone may have been survivable. The factors contributing to deaths are easier to understand when classified, and we have categorised them into the following groups :

- **Diving Techniques** (Inadequate air supply, buoyancy, buddy system)
- **Human Factors** (medical, psychological, physiological)
- **Equipment Factors** (misuse, faults)
- **Environmental Factors.**

DIVING TECHNIQUES

Inadequate Air Supply

In **half the deaths (56%), critical events developed when the diver was either running low or was out-of-air (OOA).** When equipment was tested following deaths, few victims had an ample air supply remaining.

Most problems arose when the diver became aware of a low-on-air (LOA) situation. Some divers then died while trying to snorkel on the surface, attempting to conserve air (8%).

Concern about a shortage of air presumably impairs the diver's ability to cope with a second problem developing during the dive, or causes the diver to surface prematurely and in a stressed state of mind, where he is then unable to cope with surface conditions. In many cases the LOA diver faced these difficulties alone, as his buddy who had more air, continued the dive oblivious to the situation (see later). LOA situations should be avoidable by adequate dive planning, using a cylinder with ample capacity for the planned dive, and frequent reference to a contents gauge.

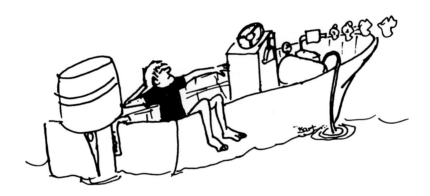

Fig. 34.1

In some cases the diver was using a smaller cylinder than the usual 2000 litre (72 cu.ft.). An 1400 litre (50 cu.ft.) cylinder has much less endurance than a conventional cylinder, and allows only a few breaths once a LOA situation develops at a significant depth. Also, a diver using a smaller cylinder will usually run out of air sooner, encouraging separation from his group.

Buoyancy

Half the diving victims (52%) encountered buoyancy problems. Most of these were due to inadequate buoyancy, but some (8%) had excessive buoyancy.

The **buoyancy changes peculiar to wet suits** were a significant factor. The considerable buoyancy offered by a wet suit at the surface needs to be compensated by weights. An approximate formula for this is :

- 1 kg for each 1 mm thickness,
- 1 kg for "long john" extensions and a hood,
- 1 kg for an aluminium tank,
- ± 1–2 kg for individual body variations in buoyancy.

Based on the above formula, **40% of divers who perished were found to be grossly overweighted** at the surface. This factor would have been greater at depth.

When weighted according to this formula, a diver should be neutrally buoyant at or near the surface. In this state, descent or ascent are equally easy.

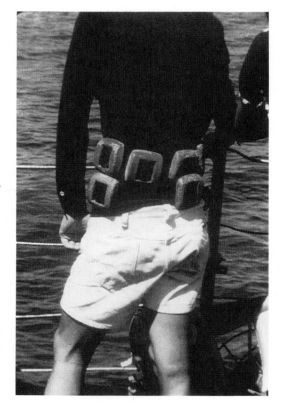

Fig. 34.2
A potential "human anchor".

During descent, the wet suit becomes compressed, making the diver negatively buoyant. This is where the **buoyancy compensator (BC)** comes in. It is inflated just sufficiently to restore neutral buoyancy. This is why it is called a buoyancy compensator.

Evidently, **some divers deliberately overweighted on the surface**, using this excess weight to descend more easily and were then using the BC to maintain depth and then later to return to the surface. This places excessive reliance on the BC.

This dangerous practice is unfortunately promoted by some instructors. It has advantages from a commercial point of view, as it expedites training. Groups of divers can be quickly taught to descend with minimum skill. The technique is less advantageous in terms of longevity of the diver.

In spite of being heavily reliant on their BC, **many divers then misused them.** Examples of this include accidental inflation or overinflation causing rocket like ascents ("polaris missile effect"), confusion between the inflation and dump valves, and inadequate or slow inflation due to being deep or LOA. The drag induced by the inflated BC (needed in many cases to offset the non-discarded weight belt) was a factor contributing to exhaustion in divers attempting to swim to safety on some occasions.

There are other unpleasant consequences of buoyancy problems. The American Academy of Underwater Sciences, in a symposium in 1989, reported that **half the cases of decompression sickness** were **related to loss of buoyancy control.**

In an emergency requiring either ascent or buoyancy, to keep the diver afloat on the surface, several kilograms of flotation are immediately available by simply discarding the weight belt.

Ditching of Weights

This was omitted by most victims (90%). This compelled them to swim towards safety carrying several kilos of unnecessary weight, and made staying on the surface impossible in many cases. This critical and avoidable factor should be easily remedied by restoring the traditional weight belt ditching drills.

Earlier diving instructors taught that the weight belt was the last item put on, the first taken off. It was to be removed and held at arm's length in the event of a potential problem. The diver then had the option of voluntarily dropping the belt if the situation deteriorated, or replacing it if the problem resolved. When problems did develop, the belt was dropped automatically! Some present diving students now question the validity of dropping these lead (?dead) belts – perhaps the high cost of replacement is worth more than their lives. "Lead poisoning" is a frequent contribution to fatalities.

When ditched, the belt is held at arms length to avoid falling and fouling on other equipment. This entanglement occurred in some of the reported fatalities. In other cases, the belt could not be released because it was worn under other equipment (e.g. BC, backpack harness, scuba cylinder etc.), or the release buckle was inaccessible because a weight had slid over it ,or it had rotated to the back of the body. In some cases the belt strap was too long to slide through the release buckle. Other fatalities have occurred where release mechanisms have failed, due to the use of knotted belts (which could not be untied), or lead balls contained within a backpack.

Buddy Diving System

The value and desirability of the buddy system is universally accepted in the recreational diving community. Two maxims have arisen in diving folklore from this concept :

- "Dive alone – die alone"
- "Buddies who are not in constant and direct communication are not buddies,
    — merely diving in the same ocean".

In spite of this, **only 14% of divers who perished in the ANZ series still had their buddy with them,** and in the Hawaiian series it was 19%. In 33% of the ANZ cases, the deceased diver either dived alone or voluntarily separated from his buddy beforehand, 25% left their buddy after a problem developed, and 20% became separated by the problem.

A common cause of separation was one diver (the subsequent casualty) having inadequate air, OOA or LOA. In this case, the buddy often continued the dive alone, or accompanied the victim to the surface, before abandoning him and continuing the dive.

There were many misapplications of the buddy system. In some cases more than two divers 'buddied' together, leading to confusion as to who was responsible for whom. A particular variant of this is a training technique in which a group of inexperienced divers follows a dive leader. When one becomes LOA, he is paired with another (also usually inexperienced diver) in the same situation, and the two instructed to return to the surface together. Often the heaviest air consumers are the least experienced and are overbreathing through anxiety. Two such inexperienced, anxious divers, both critically low on air, are then abandoned underwater by the dive leader and left to fend for themselves!

In others, the buddy was leading the victim and therefore not immediately aware of the problem. Generally, the more experienced diver took the lead, affording him the luxury of constant observation by his buddy, while he gave intermittent attention in return. In this situation, unless a **"buddy line"** is used, the following diver (upon developing a problem such as LOA or OOA) has to expend precious time and energy and air, catching his buddy to inform him of the difficulty. Often this was impossible, and the first indication the leading diver had of the problem was the absence of his buddy, who by this time was unconscious on the sea bed or well on the way to the surface.

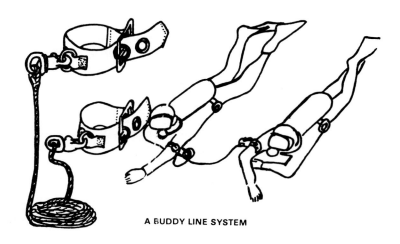

A BUDDY LINE SYSTEM

Fig. 34.3

❑ Buddy rescue.

In only a minority of cases was the buddy present at the time of death. Most divers ultimately died alone, usually because of poor compliance with the principles of buddy diving. In only 1% of cases did the buddy die attempting rescue, indicating that adherence to the buddy principle is reasonably safe for the would-be rescuer.

❑ Buddy breathing.

4% of fatalities were associated with failed buddy breathing. In a study of failed buddy breathing conducted by NUADC, more than half were attempted at depths greater than 20 metres. In 29% the victim's mask was displaced and the catastrophe of air embolism occurred in 12.5% of cases.

One in 8 victims refused to return the mouthpiece, presumably to the righteous indignation of the donor. In one reported instance, knives were drawn to settle the dispute! Nevertheless, donating a regulator rarely results in the donor becoming the victim.

The use of an **octopus rig** or (more sensibly) a complete **separate emergency air supply** (e.g. "Spare Air") would appear to be a more satisfactory alternative, having the added advantage of providing a spare regulator for the owner in the (not so rare) event of a failure of the primary air supply.

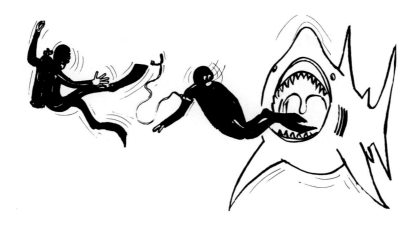

Fig. 34.4

HUMAN FACTORS
MEDICAL, PSYCHOLOGICAL
AND PHYSIOLOGICAL

In at least **25% of cases, the diver had a pre-existing disease which should have excluded him from diving** (compared to 8-10% in the potential diver trainee population). The diseases either killed the diver or predisposed to diving accidents in the vast majority of these cases.

In assessing the cause of scuba fatalities, is too easy to ignore the disorders which have no demonstrable pathology, such as panic and fatigue, but to do so results in less appreciation of the incident. Drowning obscures many other pathologies and some, such as asthma or the sudden death syndrome, may not show up at autopsy.

Panic

39% of deaths were associated with panic. Panic is a psychological stress reaction of extreme anxiety, characterised by frenzied and irrational behaviour. It is an unhelpful response which reduces the chance of survival. This topic is covered in detail in Chapter 7.

Evidence of panic was derived from witness accounts of the diver's behaviour, contained mainly in the Australasian series. Other studies suggest a 40–60% incidence of panic.

Panic was usually precipitated when the diver was confronted by unfamiliar or threatening circumstances such as LOA, OOA, poor visibility, turbulent water, unaccustomed depth, buoyancy problems (usually insufficient buoyancy), or separation from diving companions.

After panicking, the diver frequently behaved inappropriately by actions such as failure to ditch weights or inflate the BC, rapid ascent, or abandoning essential equipment such as the mask, snorkel and regulator.

Fatigue

In 28% of cases fatigue was a factor. Fatigue is a consequence of excessive exertion, and limits the diver's capacity for survival.

It commonly arose from a variety of circumstances including attempting to remain on the surface while overweighted, long swims in adverse sea conditions or swimming with excessive drag from an inflated BC.

The fatigue factor was not restricted to unfit divers — under special circumstances any diver will become fatigued. In some cases the fatigue was associated with salt water aspiration syndrome, cardiac complications or asthma.

Salt Water Aspiration

This factor was present in 37% of cases. It refers to inhalation of small amounts of sea water by the conscious diver.

In many cases this was the result of a leaking regulator, while in a small percentage, buddy breathing was the cause. In most cases salt water aspiration was a pre-terminal event as the situation became critical. It frequently predisposed to the development of panic, fatigue, respiratory and other complications.

Pulmonary Barotrauma

13% of deaths had autopsy evidence of pulmonary barotrauma (burst lung). In some cases it was a complicating factor rather than the initial cause. Factors promoting the barotrauma were diverse, including panic, rapid buoyant ascents, asthma and regulator failure.

Cardiac (Sudden Death Syndrome)

In at least 12% there was either gross cardiac pathology or an excellent clinical diagnosis of cardiac disease (See Chapter 35). Victims tend to be older, experienced divers in cold water, often with a history of cardiac disease (3%) or high blood pressure (4%), under control with medication (especially beta blockers). They die quietly, soon after entry or at the end of an otherwise uneventful dive. Resuscitation is difficult or impossible under these environmental conditions.

The trigger factors producing the very rapid ineffective heart beat (ventricular fibrillation) include the following — exercise, drugs, hypoxia from salt water aspiration, respiratory abnormalities from breathing under dysbaric conditions through a regulator, cardio-respiratory reflexes and cold exposure.

Asthma

In at least 9% of deaths the diver was asthmatic, and in at least 8% of cases asthma contributed to the death.

Asthmatics should normally be excluded by a competent medical examination. Even so, surveys have shown that between 0.5 and 1% of divers are asthmatics. When this figure is contrasted with the 9% of fatalities who have the condition, it implies that **asthma is a significant risk factor.** As medical histories were only available in half the deaths, this figure is certainly an underestimate.

There was often a series of adverse contributors to death in this group, including panic, fatigue and salt water aspiration. The ultimate pathology was usually drowning or pulmonary barotrauma.

The risk of pulmonary barotrauma is predictable, considering that asthma narrows and obstructs airways. Added to this is the possibility of an incapacitating asthmatic attack during the dive. A considerable number of divers in the survey died this way, some as they were returning to get their medication (aerosol inhalers). Others took it before the dive!

The diving environment can aggravate asthma in several ways :

❑ Salt water aspiration.

Respiratory physicians use nebulised salt water to provoke an asthmatic attack in cases of questionable asthma. Divers immerse themselves in such a solution and often breathe a fine mist of seawater through regulators.

❑ Cold dry air.

Breathing this air precipitates attacks in some asthmatics. Divers breath this type of air continuously. It is carefully dried by the filling station before being used to fill scuba tanks, and cools as it expands in the regulator.

❑ Exertion.

This aggravates many attacks. Even the most routine dive can require unexpected and extreme exertion, due to adverse environmental factors such as rough water or currents.

❑ Hyperventilation.

The effects of anxiety causes hyperventilation and changes in respiratory gases. This will have little effect on normal lungs. It provokes asthma in those so inclined.

❑ Breathing against a resistance.

Many of the cases first notice problems at depth or if there is increased resistance in the regulator – such as with a LOA or OOA situation.

Vomiting

Apart from the cases that vomited during resuscitation – and there were many – in 10% vomiting initiated or contributed to the accident. It was often produced by sea sickness or salt water aspiration.

Nitrogen Narcosis

This was an effect of depth, and contributed in 9%, but was never the sole cause of death in these series.

Respiratory Disease

A further 7% of casualties had chronic bronchitis, pleural adhesions, chest injury or other respiratory conditions. Because divers with these conditions are in a minority, they appear to be over represented in the deaths.

Drugs

Alcohol and cannabis (marijuana) are well known contributors to drowning. Cocaine is an established cause of sudden death in athletes. What surprised us was the apparent association between drugs taken for hypertension and the deaths from the sudden death syndrome. Anti-asthma drugs seemed to have the same association.

Decompression Sickness

The dread of DCS is prominent in the minds of most divers. Perhaps this is why there are no deaths due to this condition in the ANZ studies, and less than 1% in the NUADC. Hawaiians reached 4%, due to deep diving for black coral.

While DCS is an important cause of serious disability (such as paraplegia) in recreational divers, it is not a significant cause of mortality. This is not, however, true with professional divers.

EQUIPMENT PROBLEMS

A significant proportion of deaths were associated with equipment malfunction (35%) or misuse (35%). There was some overlap in the equipment faults and the equipment misuse categories. In spite of the advanced technology available, modern equipment still frequently fails and divers need to be prepared for this possibility (see Chapter 5).

Regulator

In 14% of deaths the regulator failed, and in 1% it was misused. Subsequent testing of the regulators showed the majority of problems were due to leakage allowing inhalation of salt water, but in some cases there was excessive breathing resistance following a mechanical dysfunction. In a few cases, the regulator failed catastrophically, or the hose 'blew out'.

The difficulty of obtaining useable air from the regulator was often complicated by other factors such as panic or exhaustion.

Fins

13% of cases lost one or both fins. In some cases this was due to defective or ill fitting fins, but in the majority of instances the cause was not obvious.

A likely explanation is that the fin(s) was lost because of vigorous swimming efforts during attempts to stay afloat with inadequate buoyancy, or during an attempt to swim to safety. Once a fin is lost swimming efficiency is drastically impaired. Panic and fatigue probably had a significant role in these situations.

Buoyancy Compensator

In 8% of cases the BC malfunctioned. Usually this was due to failure of the inflation system, but some BCs did not remain inflated.

In 6% of deaths, the BC was misused. Some divers confused the inflation and dump valves, usually causing over-inflation of the BC and precipitating an uncontrolled ascent. Others pressed the wrong button and sank when they wanted to float.

Scuba Cylinder

12% of deaths had problems with the cylinder, usually from misuse. These included under-filling, using a cylinder too small for the dive, the cylinder falling out of the harness, and failure to turn on the cylinder valve.

Other Equipment Problems

In 5% or less of deaths, problems were experienced due to failure or misuse of :

- **weight belt** – usually inability to discard it (see Chapter 5)
- **harness** – design faults or covering the weight belt
- **mask** – loss, flooding, and broken straps
- **protective suit** – ill fitting, usually too tight
- **lines** – entanglement
- **gauges** – faulty readings, blow offs
- **J-valve** – usually misuse.

ENVIRONMENTAL PROBLEMS

Environmental factors contributed to 62% of deaths (see Chapter 6).

Deaths near the Surface

25% of the accidents commenced on the surface, and 50% of the divers died at the surface. This may seem surprising as most divers would regard the surface as a safety zone. In many cases they were compelled to surface because of exhaustion of the air supply.

Turbulent (White) Water

Difficult water conditions caused problems in 36%. These included excessive **current, rough** water, **surf** and **surge** around rocks, **underwater surge** from wave movement, and impaired **visibility** caused by these conditions.

These unfavourable conditions often assailed the diver who was forced prematurely to the surface, OOA or LOA, and who was also frequently overweighted and hampered by the drag of his inflated BC. Exhaustion or panic then resulted in drowning.

Depth

Excessive depth was a factor in 12%. Often the fatal dive was the deepest ever for the victim. Deep water is a more gloomy and dangerous environment.

The dangers of excessive depth are predictable. They include — increased air consumption, impaired judgement from nitrogen narcosis, colder water, reduced visibility, slow or failed response to BC inflation, excessive air consumption and resistance to breathing, and a prolonged ascent in the event of problems.

Other Environmental Problems

Factors which contributed to less than 10% of fatalities included :

- **cave** dives – sometimes causing multiple deaths
- **marine animal injury** – including shark and other animal bites, marine stings (3–6%)
- **difficulties entering** and **exiting** the water
- **cold**
- **entanglements** with ropes, lines and kelp
- **entrapment** – under caves, ledges, or boats
- **night** diving.

DEATHS IN PROFESSIONAL DIVERS

Professional divers have a much higher death rate than recreational divers, especially when operating from oil rigs. Death rates up to 4.8 per thousand divers per year have been reported.

The causes of death are different from recreational divers. DCS and CAGE account for up to 28% of deaths. These divers not only frequently develop DCS, but sometimes die from the disease.

Because of the inhospitable environment in areas like the North Sea, cold and heavy seas were a significant factor in deaths.

Other important factors were equipment failure (saturation divers are highly dependent on equipment integrity for their survival), and panic.

Surprisingly, in spite of legislation requiring careful medical supervision, 6% of deaths had a contributing medical factor.

SUMMARY

Diving fatalities generally arise from a combination of factors, none of which alone would have caused disaster.

The contributing factors show an emerging pattern which needs to be addressed by diver education and training. For example, the majority of deaths were in divers who were medically unfit to dive or had a **LOA or OOA element.**

These should be largely preventable by **adequate dive medical examinations** prior to commencing diving, and proper planning and air supply monitoring. Most of these were preventable.

The most significant factors in diving fatalities are :

- **diving with disqualifying medical conditions**
- **panic**
- **fatigue**
- **water movement**
- **buoyancy problems**
- **LOA or OOA**
- **adverse sea conditions**
- **failure to ditch the weight belt when in difficulty**
- **ignoring or misapplying the buddy system**
- **improper use of equipment**
- **failure of equipment.**

Case Report 34.1 A typical diving fatality might unfold as follows :

A young, inexperienced, slightly overconfident, indifferently trained, male diver undertakes a dive in open water under conditions with which he is relatively unfamiliar. He is healthy but does no regular exercise apart from occasional diving. He has a vague dive plan which he does not discuss with his equally casual buddy. He is mildly anxious because of the unfamiliar conditions. He follows his usual practice of using a generous number of weights, initially inflating and then deflating his BC on the surface, to allow his weights to help him descend. Fascination with the environment leads him and his buddy to descend to 40 metres, deeper than they originally intended. He checks his contents gauge and is alarmed to find he is close to his reserve. His anxiety is increased by the realisation that there may be a decompression requirement for this dive, but he may have insufficient air to complete even a safety stop. He is unsure of the decompression requirement, if any, and he did not bring any tables with him.

He activates the inflation valve on his BC but gets so little response that he swims for the surface. He heads for the surface alone with some urgency, unable to communicate with his buddy who is some distance away and preoccupied with other marine life. His air supply runs out during the ascent and he arrives at the surface in a state of panic.

He has extreme difficulty staying afloat but in his frenzied state, neglects to ditch his weight belt or orally inflate his BC. His predicament is aggravated by inhalation of sea water and the loss of one of his fins. He becomes exhausted trying to remain on the surface, because of his negative buoyancy and reduced propulsion.

A search team later find his body on the bottom – directly below where he surfaced. They have difficulty in surfacing the body, until they release the weight belt.

PREVENTION

Many of the factors associated with diving deaths are avoidable.

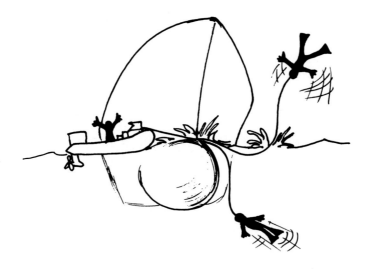

Fig. 34.5

Ways of achieving this include the use of adequate **medical examinations** of prospective divers by doctors with training in diving medicine, **safer diving techniques**, maintenance of **good physical fitness**, a thorough **knowledge of equipment** and its limitations, and an appreciation and **respect for adverse environmental conditions.**

Some changes in the emphasis of teaching, aimed at better education concerning the high risk areas of diving would be helpful. Divers who are extremely knowledgeable of decompression theory and practice, are running out of air and drowning in solitude, with their excessively laden weight belts still firmly attached.

Chapter 35

SUDDEN DEATH SYNDROME (Cardiac Death)

PATHOLOGY

Sudden death in divers, especially middle aged divers, is not a rare event. The usual cause is cardiac — either a fatal disturbance of cardiac rhythm (arrhythmia), heart muscle death from a blockage of a diseased coronary artery (coronary occlusion causing myocardial infarction or "heart attack"), or a disease of the heart muscle itself (myocarditis, cardiomyopathy).

Statistical studies on deaths in diving show a disturbingly high incidence of death attributed to heart disease, the figures ranging from 12% to 21% depending on the diagnostic criteria.

Cardiac Arrhythmias

The heart normally beats in an orderly and regular way (see Chapter 3). The atria contract, first propelling blood into the ventricles which then in turn contract, ejecting blood into the major arteries.

If this rhythmic contraction is disturbed (an arrhythmia or "irregular heart beat"), the efficiency of cardiac function is impaired and the heart has to work harder, requiring more oxygen and blood flow of its own. Impaired efficiency may also cause lowered blood pressure, which can reduce blood flow to the brain causing unconsciousness. The arrhythmia which causes sudden death is called **ventricular fibrillation,** and this usually results in unconsciousness within a few seconds.

Coronary Artery Disease

The heart receives its own blood supply from the coronary arteries. Its requirement for blood increases when it has to perform more work, for example during exercise. For a given level of exercise, the heart has to work even harder if the blood pressure is elevated, if the heart has to beat too rapidly, or if the resistance to blood flow is increased. Arrhythmias also increase the cardiac workload.

The heart is less able to cope with extra demands for work if the coronary arteries are obstructed, since the blood flow to the heart is reduced. When the coronary arteries do not supply sufficient blood and oxygen to the heart muscles, the latter becomes painful and produces central or left sided chest pain ("angina"). This may be temporarily remedied by reducing the exercise and the demand for oxygen , by resting. If this deprivation of oxygen to the heart muscle is severe enough, heart muscle dies, and this is then called a myocardial infarction ("heart attack"). In divers, the first sign of this may be at autopsy.

Heart Muscle Disease

Some forms of heart muscle disease (cardiomyopathy – hereditary, alcoholic, or toxic) may affect its function. In non-divers who become aware of these diseases, heart transplants are often the only successful treatments. In divers who may be unaware of the effects on the heart, they may be discovered first at autopsy. Viral infections often involve the heart muscle (myocarditis), often without the patient being aware of this, and these infections predispose to cardiac deaths.

CONTRIBUTING CAUSES

There are a number of ways death or incapacity from cardiac diseases can come about and they are usually precipitated by one or more **trigger factors**. Some of these are :

Exercise

Severe exercise can cause sudden death by a number of mechanisms. Probably the most well known example was the death of the first marathon runner who dropped dead after running from Marathon to Athens to deliver the news of the Greek victory over the Persians. In reality, his death was probably due to heat stroke or heat exhaustion. Usually exercise will cause cardiac deaths only in those with some cardiac disease or malfunction.

A diver is at a disadvantage in some ways during exercise. During exertion on land, the cardiac output increases to meet the metabolic demands of the exercising muscles. In doing this, the work of the heart is made easier by blood vessel dilatation in the peripheral circulation, reducing the resistance to blood flow. In an exercising diver however, the skin blood vessels do not dilate because of a heat conserving response to the surrounding cold water. The diver's heart has to pump against an increased resistance and so work harder for a given amount of exercise, compared to a land athlete.

One of the limitations to exercise on land is the inability to disperse the metabolic heat of exercise. With the diver, much of this heat is conducted away by the water. As a result, it is possible to exercise in the water to a greater degree without the "hot and sweaty" discomfort.

It is therefore possible to exercise to a great degree in the water, with less discomfort but at a greater strain on the heart. In a trained athlete with a healthy heart this probably is only of academic interest. In a middle aged (i.e. over 35 years) diver with some degree of coronary artery disease ("narrowing of the arteries") the diver can overload the heart without realising it. This can result in sudden death.

Exercise, even in fit healthy divers has been shown to cause significant arrhythmias with diving. It is much more likely to cause incapacitating or fatal arrhythmias in divers with cardiac disease.

Psychological and Personality Factors

Some personalities are more susceptible to cardiac disease than others. The so called **Type A personality** is believed to be most prone to cardiac disease. These individuals are intensely competitive, aggressive and as a result, by society standards, usually successful. They drive themselves hard and do not give up. They are twice as likely to develop coronary artery disease than others, and when they develop it they are likely to push their diseased heart beyond its limitations.

Traditionally this has been a **male personality trait**, but in a more competitive and equal society it is probable that a similar disease pattern will emerge in women competing in previously male dominated areas. Sudden death is not uncommon in Type A personalities.

Anxiety can have threatening cardiac consequences. Anxiety typically causes internal release of adrenaline, one of the stress hormones, which stimulates the heart to contract more forcefully, beat faster, and makes it more prone to arrhythmias. A fast beating heart has less time to replenish its own blood supply and becomes relatively starved of blood.

In the peripheral circulation, adrenaline causes constriction of blood vessels to the skin and internal organs, increasing the resistance to blood flow and the work of the heart. The stressed anxious individual thus has a fast beating heart with a poor blood supply which is more prone to arrhythmias and which has to work harder for a given exercise load.

A condition analogous to fainting (known as **vasovagal syncope**) is commonly seen in individually threatening situations such as a blood donation or the receiving of injections. A nervous response through central stimulation of the vagus nerve causes profound slowing of the heart. The end result is inadequate blood pressure and reduced cerebral circulation causing the diver to lose consciousness.

Cold

Sudden incapacity and death of divers soon after entering cold water has been frequently reported. The body has several immediate responses to cold water which could explain this.

During **cold water immersion** there is an increased sympathetic nervous system activity resulting in the release of adrenaline. This causes the potentially deleterious cardiac effects described above. A greater sympathetic response has been described in individuals who are **not adapted** to cold water exposure or who are **unfit**.

Sudden death from **vagal stimulation** associated with the **diving reflex** can occur after immersion of the face in cold water, although it can be produced by immersion of the trunk in cold water as well.

Sudden immersion in cold water is thought to be associated with a sudden death syndrome associated with reflex **coronary artery spasm, fatal arrhythmias** or **myocardial infarction**.

Divers will be familiar with the involuntary over breathing which can accompany immersion in cold water or even a cold shower. In experimental animals, and also in man, the heart becomes more prone to arrhythmias caused by the reduction in blood carbon dioxide from this **involuntary hyperventilation**.

Hypothermia also makes the heart more prone to arrhythmias and may combine with some of the other problems mentioned above to cause sudden death.

Reflexes Associated with Diving

❑ The Diving Reflex.

Diving mammals such as whales are able to hold their breath for an hour and attain amazing depths. They are able to do this partly because of the evolution of the dive reflex. When the mammal leaves the surface there is a profound stimulus of the vagus nerve which slows the heart to about a fifth of its normal rate. At the same time, there is intense constriction of the blood supply to the skin and most organs with the exception of the heart, lungs and brain. This conserves oxygen reserves for use by the organs which need it most. The diving mammal maintains a normal blood pressure, but the output and work of the heart is dramatically reduced.

This reflex is present to some extent in humans. When a human is immersed in cold water there is vagal stimulation which slows the heart, as well as sympathetic nervous stimulation which constricts blood vessels to the skin and other organs. Because the reflex is only incompletely developed in man, there is often a rise in blood pressure but minimal or no fall in cardiac output. This increases, rather than reduces, the work of the heart.

The result of this process in man is increased work of the heart as well as the development of cardiac arrhythmias. Studies conducted on the breathhold Ama divers of Korea showed an incidence of arrhythmias of 43% in summer, and an even higher incidence in winter.

❑ Carotid Sinus Syndrome.

The Carotid arteries, on each side of the neck, are the main arteries which supply the brain with blood, and these have a pressure sensing organ – the carotid sinus – in their walls at about the level of the larynx. External pressure on these carotid sinuses causes the cardiac control centre of the brain to mistakenly assume that the blood pressure has suddenly risen. This leads to a **reflex slowing of the heart** and **reduced blood pressure**. This can cause faintness or even loss of consciousness.

A similar effect is caused by pressure from the collar of a tight fitting wetsuit or dry suit neck seal, on the carotid sinus. The problem is especially likely in wet suits without a front zip fastener or having tight "crew necks".

In a series of 100 carefully documented diving deaths in Australia, only one case was thought to be clearly due to this carotid sinus syndrome. In other cases however, distressed divers were seen to pull a constricting wetsuit away from the neck. This may have been a response to respiratory difficulty from cardiac causes, a tight neck opening in the suit, or the carotid sinus syndrome.

Hyperbaric Exposure

Studies in experimental subjects breathing air at pressures similar to those experienced by sports divers showed a significant incidence of arrhythmias caused by the hyperbaric exposure. This may be partly due to the elevated partial pressures of oxygen breathed at these depths.

Immersion and Aspiration

Simply immersing the body in water causes an increased return of blood to the heart, due to the change from a gravity influenced circulation to weightlessness. This rush of blood to the heart can rapidly double its workload until stability is returned.

Aspiration of seawater – always a possibility in diving – can cause immediate cardiac effects by a mechanism akin to the diving reflex, followed by delayed effects due to hypoxia as the lungs are involved.

Drug Effects

A large variety of drugs have arrhythmic and other effects on the heart, which may predispose to sudden death. Many can be purchased 'over-the-counter' in pharmacies or supermarkets. Some are contained in 'cold cures' and 'cough mixtures' and may be inadvertently used by divers. Some of these drugs include :

- Alcohol
- Nicotine – cigarette smoking
- Caffeine – coffee and tea, stimulant drugs to overcome sleepiness
- "Social" drugs such as cocaine, weight reducing and stimulant drugs such as amphetamines
- Blood pressure controlling drugs (e.g. calcium channel blockers, beta blockers)
- Drugs used to suppress arrhythmias (e.g. beta blockers)
- Drugs that change electrolyte concentrations in the blood – diuretics and electrolytes
- Sympathomimetic drugs (e.g. decongestants such as pseudoephedrine, anti-asthma medications such as salbutamol, and some anti-seasick drugs).
- Others that may cause arrhythmias – tricyclic antidepressants, digoxin, some anti-malarials, local anaesthetics.

Cardiac Disease

❏ Coronary artery disease or CAD.

This heart disease (causing narrowing or obstruction of the coronary arteries), while considered to be a disease of middle and older age, is probably present to some degree even in some young adults.

It would appear from post-mortem studies done during the Korean and Vietnam wars that coronary artery disease begins in early adulthood, but usually only causes symptoms and death from heart attack after 40 years of age. The older the diver, the more significant this is likely to be. Divers with this disease are more prone to sudden death due to arrhythmias or myocardial infarction secondary to impaired blood supply to the heart muscle.

❏ Coronary artery bypass grafts.

Some blockages of the coronary arteries can be bypassed by blood vessel grafts – usually using veins from the lower legs. This reduces cardiac pain and improves cardiac performance but does not cure the underlying disease. People with such grafts are still more prone to arrhythmias and cardiac dysfunction and should not dive. A similar situation exits in those people who have already suffered a myocardial infarction or "heart attack".

❏ Myocarditis.

Some viral infections which produce a flu-like illness can temporarily affect the heart muscle, impairing its performance and making it susceptible to arrhythmias. Sudden deaths from this often insidious condition (myocarditis) are occasionally reported in very fit athletes and in divers. It is unwise to dive or perform heavy exertion when suffering from a viral infection, for this reason.

Sometimes the heart is permanently and irreversibly damaged by such viruses. It is then similar to a cardiomyopathy. In terminal cases the only effective treatment is a heart transplant.

PREVENTION

All candidates should be carefully examined by an experienced diving physician before dive training. Those with known cardiac disease or a tendency to arrhythmias cannot dive safely. Middle aged divers, and those with high coronary risk factors need regular assessments.

Coronary risk factors include :

- a family history of heart disease at a similar age to the diver
- cigarette smoking
- hypertension
- obesity
- high cholesterol – hyperlipidaemia
- physical unfitness
- diseases such as diabetes and alcoholism.

Diving emergencies often require extreme physical exertion which stresses the heart. A high standard of physical fitness brought about by regular exercise will make the heart better able to cope with this exertion.

While jumping into cold water gets the discomfort over quickly, it maximises the physiological stress. Enter cold water slowly to minimise these physiological stresses.

The combination of performance anxiety, transport stress, inadequate sleep, excessive alcohol, coffee and cigarettes which often accompany a "high-living" diving holiday may be a possible contributor to cardiac arrhythmias, and some deaths in divers.

Chapter 36

PSYCHOLOGICAL DISORDERS

Psychological Traits of Successful Divers

This topic has not been extensively researched, but the few studies which have been done on the psychological make-up of divers have shown the following — successful divers tend not to be anxiety prone; they are self sufficient, intelligent and emotionally stable. Their tolerance to stress often allows them to continue to function during difficulties which would incapacitate many non divers. This may be helped by their tendency to use "denial", a mental mechanism by which they refuse to consciously acknowledge the hazards which may confront them.

In spite of their overall stability, divers, like anyone else, can suffer from psychological disturbances. (See Chapter 7 for a full description of stress and panic responses).

Anxiety States

It is quite normal for divers to feel anxious in the face of some of the very real hazards of diving – this book is full of them. Some people, however, develop an excessive and inappropriate anxiety to diving hazards which may become a **phobia** – an irrational fear. This may be the result of a previous traumatic event (such as near drowning during childhood) or may be an exaggerated reaction to some diving danger. Phobias may relate to diving in general or to a specific diving hazard (such as an excessive fear of sharks) or situation (e.g. claustrophobia with the face mask, night diving, poor visibility).

Phobias can be treated by psychological de-conditioning therapy, if the diver wishes.

Most people who are anxious about diving are aware of this early in their training and quite sensibly desist. Why continue a recreational activity which causes apprehension? Unfortunately some continue because of peer pressure, ego challenge or other personal reasons. These divers tend to have a high baseline level of anxiety (**neuroticism** or "**high trait anxiety**") when diving and are more prone to panic when confronted with real or imagined hazards.

Some divers experience a specific anxiety reaction called the **Blue Orb Syndrome**. It is an aquatic manifestation of a general medical (psychological) disorder called "agoraphobia". It usually happens to a lone diver in deep water, where there are no visual references. The diver develops an anxious feeling of being alone in the vastness of the ocean. This can lead to mounting anxiety and panic. The panicked diver may rush to the surface, omitting decompression or develop pulmonary barotrauma from failure to exhale on ascent. The symptoms usually subside if the diver can establish visual contact with concrete objects such as the sea bed, a dive boat or even another diver, or concentrating on diving instruments, such as a watch.

This syndrome can be avoided by diving with a buddy who provides reassuring company and a visual reference. Avoidance of deep water where there are no visual references, is also helpful.

Panic

This frenzied and irrational behaviour is the end result of a number of diving difficulties. It is more likely to occur in anxiety prone divers and frequently results in a diving accident or fatality. It is an important topic for divers to understand and is covered in detail in Chapter 7 and Case History 7.1

Psychological Disturbances due to Physical Causes

Brain function can be disturbed by physiological factors (such as **nitrogen narcosis, hypothermia**) and by other diving related illnesses.

Cerebral decompression sickness and **air embolism** can cause alteration of brain function during both the acute event and recovery.

Near drowning, hypoxia and the **gas toxicity diseases (oxygen, carbon dioxide, carbon monoxide**, etc.) may also cause temporary or permanent brain damage.

Symptoms include confusion, irritability and irrational behaviour. This should always be borne in mind if a victim of a diving accident is unreasonably reluctant to undergo treatment. People who know the diver well will normally be the best judges of whether the behaviour is out of character.

Dementia

This is a deterioration of intellectual capacity and memory which is common in the elderly and has a variety of causes. Alzheimers ("old timers") Disease is a severe form of dementia. Diving folklore holds that divers suffer an increased incidence of dementia. This belief has been supported by press reports and anecdotal accounts of divers suffering from the condition. Some even believe only "demented" persons take up diving!

There are plausible theoretical reasons why divers could sustain brain damage sufficient to cause dementia from conditions such as repeated subclinical, or overt, cerebral **decompression sickness, air embolism, near drowning** or **carbon monoxide poisoning,** etc. to name a few.

There are also some scientific studies which show evidence of at least transient brain damage in some divers. A study in Sweden showed 3.5% of free ascent trainees to have **EEG** ("electrical brain wave") abnormalities after free ascent training, and in another survey, EEG abnormalities were found in 43% of a group of Polish professional divers compared to 10% in a normal population.

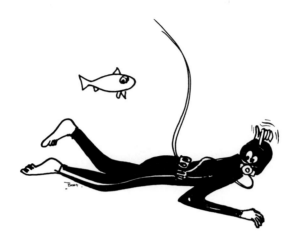

Fig. 36.1

In Australia, a group of divers studied after treatment for **decompression sickness** showed **neurological, psychological** and **EEG abnormalities** for some weeks after treatment, even in divers who had no symptoms of neurological decompression sickness.

There have been several studies worldwide which appear to show deterioration of intellectual performance and psychological disturbances in divers suffering from neurological decompression sickness or "near miss" diving accidents. Unfortunately the methodology of these studies was grossly inadequate, making the conclusions unreliable.

To clear up some of the controversy, a study of 152 professional **abalone divers** was undertaken in Australia by Edmonds and others in 1988. The divers in the study had diving exposure which would generally be regarded as extreme. On average they had been diving for 16 years and had been professional abalone divers for 12 years. They averaged 5 hours underwater per day on Hookah equipment for 105 days per year at an average depth of 50 ft. (15 metres) and admitted to being "bent" four times. Most cases of decompression sickness went untreated. Half of the divers used a dive profile which would, according to conventional dive tables, require decompression but which they omitted. Of the 69 cases of decompression sickness in this group which were actually treated, half were neurological.

It would seem that if there was any group of divers prone to brain injury after excessive diving exposure, it would be this one.

The divers were subjected to a battery of tests including **intelligence tests, psychometric** investigations to detect psychological abnormalities, **memory tests** and studies designed specifically to detect early dementia, **EEG studies** and **neurobehavioural tests**. The divers were compared with a control group taken from non-diving fishermen from the same locality.

The results showed the divers studied were within the normal range for the general population and displayed no evidence of brain damage or dementia. This implies that air divers in general, have no greater risk of dementia or brain damage than non-divers. If brain damage does occur, it is either rare or so mild that it cannot be detected by conventional testing.

Since the diving practices of this group were extreme, it seems reasonable to conclude that divers following more conservative practices, as well as other, more conventional, professional compressed air divers, have no greater risk of dementia or brain damage than non-divers, unless they suffer a major accident (such as those mentioned above).

The signs of brain damage which have been described in studies performed soon after minor diving events are presumably temporary in nature.

Chapter 37

DRUGS
AND
DIVING

It is common for divers to enter the water under the influence of drugs. These may vary from paracetamol taken for a minor headache, to alcohol or marijuana from a beach party the night before, or a therapeutic drug for an illness such as high blood pressure.

Since some drugs are innocuous while others can have potentially lethal effects with diving, it is important to know something about them.

Problems can arise from effects of the drugs themselves, but commonly the condition for which the medication is taken poses a greater threat to the diver. For instance, most antibiotics have no harmful influences on divers, but a diver being treated for bronchitis with an antibiotic, has a significant risk of developing pulmonary barotrauma until the condition resolves.

We will consider commonly used drugs under four categories :

- Drugs taken for treatment of illnesses
- Drugs taken for prevention of illness (prophylaxis)
- Recreational or social drugs
- Drugs used for diving related illnesses.

TREATMENT DRUGS

In many cases the illness can be a greater hazard to the diver than the drug.

Cardiac and Blood Pressure Medications

❑ Beta blockers.

A variety of these drugs (e.g. atenolol, metoprolol) are used to treat high blood pressure or pain from coronary artery disease (angina). Their main action is to block the effect of the cardiac stimulant, adrenaline, on the heart. Adrenaline acts on specific drug receptors in the heart known as "beta receptors", thus giving rise to the term beta blocker.

By inhibiting the action of adrenaline, beta blockers reduce the force of contraction of the heart muscle. This diminishes the work it performs which reduces angina, while the reduced output of blood lowers the blood pressure.

A diver taking beta blockers has a significant limitation of the reserve pumping capacity of the heart. If a large blood supply is required by the muscles to extract the diver from an emergency – heavy wave action or and adverse current for example – it may not be available.

Beta blockers also act on the muscle lining of the bronchi which may unmask asthma in some individuals, exposing them to the dangers of both asthma and burst lung. Even those beta blockers which are described as "cardio-selective" can still have these effects.

These drugs are often used in eye drops for the treatment of glaucoma. Significant amounts can sometimes be absorbed into the body causing generalised effects. Divers using these drops should seek medical advice to ensure that they are not affected in this way, or that their glaucoma is not worsened.

The conditions for which the drugs are taken can cause difficulties as well. For example, a diver under treatment for high blood pressure is also at high risk of coronary artery disease, and may already have a sub-clinical form of this disease. The drugs may summate with, or potentiate, other causes of heart rate reduction associated with diving, and provoke the sudden death syndrome (see Chapter 35).

❏ Other blood pressure drugs.

Apart from beta blockers, blood pressure lowering drugs fall into two broad categories — blood vessel dilators and diuretics (stimulators of urine production).

> • **Blood vessel dilators (vasodilators)** reduce blood pressure by widening peripheral blood vessels, where most of the resistance to blood flow occurs. These include prazosin and felodipine.

Some can inhibit the bodies ability to compensate for changes in posture, causing fainting on standing. This is an undesirable side effect in a diver attempting to ascend a ladder to leave the water, especially in adverse sea conditions or if he is preceding his buddy.

One of the newer drugs of this type, the ACE inhibitors, can produce a dry cough which can be troublesome in the diving environment. Others, (such as beta blockers and calcium channel blockers such as verapamil) may affect the nerve condition of the heart, making it more susceptible to the sudden death syndrome (see Chapter 35).

> • **Diuretics** stimulate the production of urine and tend to dry the body out. This reduces blood volume and so tends to lower the blood pressure, but there are probably other mechanisms acting as well. The effects on diving are not clear but there are potential problems.

Reduction of the blood volume may effect blood viscosity and the dynamics of blood flow and so increase the possibility of bubble formation. In addition, changes to regional blood flow may alter the pattern of gas uptake and elimination (decompression).

Some diuretics tend to lower the blood potassium level, making the heart more prone to disturbances of rhythm. These arrhythmias may be unmasked by the effects of cold, the dive reflex, heavy exertion and the other causes of the sudden death syndrome (see Chapter 35).

Psychologically Active Drugs

❑ Tranquillisers and sedatives.

This group of drugs includes **benzodiazepines**, of which diazepam ("Valium") is a common example, and barbiturates. A significant proportion of the population take these drugs to relieve anxiety. Excessive anxiety alone is a significant risk factor in diving, and the drugs taken to relieve it further complicate the problem.

Another class of tranquillisers, the **phenothiazines**, (e.g. chlorpromazine – "Largactil") are used to treat serious psychiatric disorders such as schizophrenia. Apart from the side effects of these drugs, people suffering from this disorder often have a tenuous grip on reality which can seriously impair their ability to make safe judgements related to diving.

Tranquillisers and sedatives cause – drowsiness, impaired judgement, slowing of thought processes and reduction in problem solving ability. These effects are intensified by nitrogen narcosis, but they are potentially dangerous at all depths.

❑ Antidepressants.

Depression is not an ideal state of mind for an active diver. Even when successfully treated with antidepressants, the diver is left with potentially harmful side effects from the drugs. Some of the antidepressants cause sedation, but the principal problem is the tendency of some of the drugs to cause potentially lethal disturbances of heart rhythm. Others can react with certain foods and other drugs to affect blood pressure and consciousness.

❑ Anticonvulsants (anti-epileptic drugs).

These have similar sedative side effects to most of the tranquillisers as well as some peculiar to these drugs. Any form of epilepsy can have disastrous effects on cerebral activity, with loss of consciousness being common. The influence of nitrogen narcosis on these drugs are unknown. Some diving conditions (stress, glare and flickering light, high or low oxygen and carbon dioxide levels) can precipitate convulsions, despite these medications. Epilepsy, and medications used for its control (e.g. phenytoin or carbamazepam), preclude safe diving.

Antihistamines

These are usually taken to treat allergic conditions. Pharmacologically, many are closely related to the psychiatric drugs and share a common side effect, sedation. They cause the same potential hazards to diving as other sedatives. In addition, if antihistamines are taken to treat hay fever, there is a strong possibility of the diver developing ear or sinus barotrauma. These drugs seldom completely cure the nose and throat congestion. Other recently developed drugs are less sedative, but may provoke cardiac arrhythmias or bronchospasm (asthma).

Antibiotics

These have a large number of side effects, but few of specific relevance to diving. Tetracyclines can occasionally cause photosensitivity, a condition resembling sunburn caused by enhancing sensitivity to sunlight. Many antibiotics increase susceptibility to **vomiting**.

The condition for which the antibiotic is taken is usually of more concern. This especially applies to respiratory tract infections which make the diver prone to barotrauma.

Analgesics

A diver suffering from pain which warrants the use of pain killers should generally not be diving. Apart from the adverse interactions some diseases can have on diving, the commonly used analgesics can have undesirable side effects. There is also the **diagnostic confusion** that may result between the painful condition and decompression sickness etc..

❏ Aspirin.

This commonly used analgesic causes an inhibition of the clotting ability of blood, with just one dose and lasting for several days.

This is usually not a problem in everyday use – in fact the blood effect is used to prevent heart attacks and strokes. However, it can have potentially serious implications if the diver develops **inner ear barotrauma** or serious **decompression sickness**. The increased bleeding tendency can result in haemorrhage into injured tissues, such as the spinal cord, with disastrous consequences. Ulcer-like erosions can also occur in the stomach, with vomiting and occasionally bleeding from the gut

It may also cause bronchospasm, like **asthma**, in some divers.

❏ Paracetamol (acetaminophen).

If a diver needs to take analgesics for minor pain (hopefully after excluding diving related illnesses as a cause), it is better to use paracetamol which has fewer side effects than aspirin. Paracetamol does not effect blood coagulation and avoids the stomach upsets, common with aspirin.

❏ Strong analgesics.

Preparations containing codeine or dextropropoxyphene (both narcotic derivatives) and other strong analgesics are sometimes prescribed for severe pain.

These drugs have comparable sedative effects to the tranquillisers and can have similar adverse interactions with diving. People with pain of this intensity should not be diving.

Insulin and Anti–diabetic Agents

People taking these drugs are prone to sudden depression of the blood sugar level which produces **anxiety, confusion** and then **unconsciousness**. This is particularly likely during exercise. This complication in the water often has a fatal outcome. Because of this possibility and other potential physiological complications (e.g. acidosis and hyperventilation), diabetics are precluded from diving.

Bronchodilators and other Asthma Medications

Asthma is an inflammatory condition of the air passages of the lungs. It causes swelling of the lining of the airways, spasm of the muscles in the airways (bronchospasm) and obstruction of airflow through them. The bronchospasm can be reduced by aerosol sprays containing drugs such as salbutamol ("Ventolin") or oral bronchodilators. These can disturb cardiac rhythm and precipitate the sudden death syndrome during diving, because of the multiple trigger factors (see Chapter 35).

While the use of these and other asthma medications will improve some of the airway flow and thus relieve symptoms, it does not cure the condition. Asthmatics have airways which are excessively sensitive to irritants, reacting with bronchospasm to stimuli such as cold dry air and sea water inhalation. There is usually a degree of obstruction in some of the airways most of the time. This makes them susceptible to pulmonary barotrauma or death from the diving sequelae of asthma - panic and drowning.

Some oral bronchodilators (theophyllines) can cause pulmonary vasodilatation – which could potentially allow asymptomatic venous bubbles from normally safe dives to enter the arterial circulation as gas emboli, even without pulmonary barotrauma. **Asthma, and these medications, are incompatible with safe diving.**

Implanted Drug Delivery Systems

Implanted **reservoirs** are now being used to deliver drugs which cannot be taken orally and which need to be used over prolonged periods. Many of the conditions for which these reservoirs are used are incompatible with scuba diving.

Implants form a potential site of bubble formation during decompression. If bubbles form inside the reservoir, expansion in response to the gas laws may lead to excessive delivery of the drug. As experience with these devices in diving is limited, divers fitted with them are advised to seek expert medical advice concerning the possible complications.

PROPHYLACTIC DRUGS

Oral Contraceptives — the "Pill"

These preparations can have serious and even lethal side effects, even without the complication of diving. In older high dosage drugs, excessive blood clotting resulted in occasional deaths from pulmonary embolus or strokes, in women taking them.

Occasionally the pill produces serious psychological sequelae, migraine, nausea and vomiting, which may make diving more hazardous.

The newer low dose oral contraceptives have a lower incidence of these disorders. The concern with diving is the possibility of more coagulable blood interacting with gas bubbles during decompression. There is no factual evidence to either confirm or refute this theoretical risk, despite a number of surveys on female divers.

Anti-Sea Sickness Drugs

See Chapter 32.

Antimalarial Drugs

Tropical countries offer some spectacular diving locations but also frequently have endemic diseases, including malaria.

The chances of contracting this potentially lethal disease are reduced by the use of antimalarial drugs such as chloroquine and pyrimethamine ("Maloprim"). Unfortunately many countries now have strains of malaria which are resistant to conventional antimalarial drugs, making their use as a preventative measure not fully reliable. As well as being fallible, these drugs can have serious side effects including suppression of white blood cell production, anaemia, and eye damage.

One of the more recently developed antimalarials, mefloquine ("Lariam") can cause coordination disturbances and vertigo which may have alarming implications and cause diagnostic problems for divers.

A diver intending to visit a malaria endemic area should seek expert medical advice regarding prophylaxis for malaria in that area, as well as other more exotic tropical diseases. A diving physician should also be asked about possible interactions of the prescribed drugs with diving.

RECREATIONAL (SOCIAL) DRUGS

Alcohol

Diving culture has traditionally included substantial use of alcohol. Like other drugs, it can have adverse interactions with diving.

There is no safe blood alcohol level for diving and few people in their right mind would consider diving while under its influence. Some may not be aware that the liver has a limited capacity to metabolise this drug, so it is possible to have an appreciable blood alcohol level on the morning after a night of heavy consumption. Traffic police are well aware of this. They frequently apprehend drivers going to work with an illegal blood alcohol level on the morning after.

The danger of alcohol consumption associated with aquatic recreations is well documented — 80% of **drownings** in adult males are associated with alcohol use. The hazards are predictable. Alcohol intoxication, as well as **impairing judgement** and **coordination**, causes **cardiac rhythm disturbances**, **impairs the pumping ability of the heart, reduces the blood volume** due to excessive urine production, and increases **heat loss** through the skin (**hypothermia**).

The disturbed physiology – otherwise known as a "hangover" – after excessive alcohol consumption is known to most divers. Used to excess, this drug is a toxin, damaging the liver, heart and brain. In divers, the vascular and metabolic dysfunction after heavy consumption is a known risk factor for the development of **decompression sickness**. Increased susceptibility to both **sea sickness** and **vomiting** is observed. Soporific effects may summate with those of **nitrogen narcosis**.

Tobacco

The gentle art of inhaling burnt tobacco leaf has some unfortunate side effects. The associated risks of lung cancer, heart and vascular disease are well known. There are more subtle effects.

A smoker inhales carbon monoxide, which binds to the haemoglobin and reduces the blood's ability to transport oxygen by up to 10%. This severely reduces the capacity for exertion and impairs the physical ability to respond to an emergency (e.g. fatigue from a surface swim). The nicotine in the tobacco also stimulates the heart, making it prone to **rhythm disturbances** (arrhythmias).

Airway narrowing caused by chronic smoke irritation impairs exercising ability and increases the risk of **pulmonary barotrauma**. A similar chronic irritation of the upper respiratory tract predisposes to **ear** and **sinus** barotrauma.

Marijuana — cannabis or "pot"

Chronic use of this drug causes many of the diving related respiratory problems attributable to cigarette smoke, and **chronic bronchitis** is especially common in heavy users. This predisposes to **pulmonary barotrauma**.

Marijuana causes altered perception, **impaired judgement**, and mood alterations which are incompatible with diving safety. As with other drugs, these effects are compounded by the effects of nitrogen narcosis. It also is said to increase the likelihood of **hypothermia** by blocking blood vessel response to cold. The allegedly "beneficial effects" of marijuana are negated by pressure!

Cocaine ("coke")

This drug has similar physiological effects to adrenaline, stimulating and irritating the heart, causing potentially lethal **cardiac rhythm disturbances**, and elevating the blood pressure. Sudden death in young people from the cardiac effects is common, especially in athletes who exercise while taking cocaine.

The mental stimulation and mood elevation **impair judgement** and encourage **risk taking**. Its use while diving, apart from being illegal, is very risky.

Caffeine

This drug is found in coffee, tea, cola, and many natural foods. Even chocolate drinks, periodically given to children at bedtime, contain it. It is one of the more innocuous drugs which is used almost universally.

When used to excess it can irritate the heart causing **rhythm disturbances** which are a potential problem in diving or other strenuous exercise. It also stimulates urine production which discourages some divers from lending their wet suit to known caffeine abusers.

Narcotics

The **sedative** and **judgement impairing** qualities of these drugs makes their use during diving even more dangerous and destructive than their use as a recreational drug.

Intravenous drug users have a significant risk of being infected with the **hepatitis** and **HIV (AIDS)** virus, which should be born in mind by their diving companions (see Chapter 28).

DRUGS FOR DIVING DISEASES

Sinus and Ear Problems

Many inexperienced divers have difficulty equalising the ears and sinuses to pressure changes. Often this difficulty is associated with congestion of the lining of the nose, generally due to allergy (hay fever) or infection (URTI). Poor technique is a contributing factor.

Nasal congestion can be relieved to some extent by the use of tablets such as pseudoephedrine ("Sudafed"), or nasal decongestant sprays such as phenylephrine or ephedrine. They all have a **disruptive effect** on the **heart's conduction system** and may thus increase the likelihood of the sudden death syndrome.

These agents used in proper doses on land have few harmful generalised effects. However their activity on the nasal tissues can be unpredictable. Prolonged use causes localised tolerance to the drug, eventually aggravating the congestion which they are supposed to relieve. This applies particularly to nasal sprays. Their effect can wear off during the dive, allowing a trouble free descent, followed by sinus or ear barotrauma during ascent (see Chapters 9 and 10).

These drugs are sometimes used by divers to overcome the temporary nasal congestion of an upper respiratory tract infection (a cold or URTI). A safer approach is to avoid diving during the course of these infections.

If the decongestant is somewhat effective, it may result in the diver avoiding barotrauma of descent (as the beneficial effect is on the nasal lining) but have little or no effect on the "internal" opening of each of the air passages (Eustachian tube, sinus ostia, etc.). Thus the diver is now vulnerable to an internal blockage which manifests during ascent and produces **barotrauma of ascent**. This disorder is far more dangerous as it prevents him ascending to safety. Barotrauma of descent merely stops him diving.

Self medication with these drugs is unwise and divers with congestion problems should seek the advice of a diving physician.

Medication for use in Decompression Sickness

In view of the relative unreliability of the decompression tables, researchers have experimented with drugs to inhibit the development of bubbles and speed gas elimination from the body. While some experimental drugs now allow laboratory animals to dive with a much greater margin of safety, no agents useful to human divers have yet been convincingly demonstrated.

Chapter 38

MEDICAL EXAMINATIONS FOR DIVERS

This chapter is not adequate to instruct a medical practitioner on the complexities of performing diving medical examinations. Special courses are available for this purpose.

Because of the unique physical and physiological conditions encountered in diving, medical standards for divers differ considerably from those of other sports. As a result it is sometimes necessary for a diving physician to advise a prospective diver against diving because of a disqualifying condition. Often the recipient of this advice is supremely physically fit, and some cases have been of Olympic standard. These individuals understandably find it difficult to comprehend how a physically fit athlete is not necessarily fit to dive, medically.

To those with some knowledge of diving physiology it becomes obvious that even the highest standard of physical fitness will not protect a diver with lung cysts or asthma from a diving death.

The examining physician must consider many factors when conducting a diving medical examination. Almost 10% fail the medical and 10–15% incur specific diving limitations or advice, for safety reasons.

PSYCHOLOGY

The ideal diver is probably the cool James Bond like character we would all like to be - stable, calm under stress, able to endure physical and mental pressure, not prone to anxiety, able to conveniently ignore danger, slightly overweight and perhaps not surprisingly, a fluent liar.

Psychological stability is difficult to evaluate during the medical examination. Some clues may be gained from the history of sporting activities and occupation. Often the diving instructor is best able to evaluate the diver's psychological make-up during the course of instruction.

AGE

Ideally the trainee diver should be aged between 18 and 35 years although exceptions can be made at both extremes of age. Divers over 45, if complying with the medical standards should be acceptable, but may require special tests such as cardiac risk assessment.

Divers younger than 16 require very careful supervision during training because of their generally smaller stature, limited strength and (most importantly) emotional immaturity. A buddy line to an experienced adult diver is recommended during the training of youthful divers. The mature and experienced buddy of an adolescent diver should take control of the dive and remember that his buddy may be an unreliable rescuer if difficulties arise. Most medical authorities will not certify divers under the age of 15–16 years, without qualification. This does not prevent younger divers being given a limited "diving experience" by qualified diving instructors under very strict and controlled conditions, and provided they are medically fit.

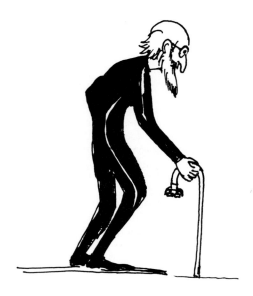

Fig. 38.1

OCCUPATION

Pilots and aircrew are advised of the risks associated with flying after diving. Musicians, sonar operators, cardiologists, pilots and others reliant on excellent hearing for their livelihood are informed of the small but real risk to their hearing, should they develop ear barotrauma.

MEDICATION

Any illness requiring drug treatment bears careful consideration because either the illness or the drug may compromise diving safety. Sedatives, tranquillisers, antidepressants, antihistamines, antidiabetic drugs, steroids, anti-hypertensives, anti-epilepsy drugs, alcohol and hallucinatory drugs such as marijuana and LSD all place the diver at risk. See Chapter 37 for specific details.

Some antibiotics may have no direct adverse effect on diving, but the condition for which they were prescribed may have.

Experimental evidence indicates that many drugs which affect the brain have unpredictable effects on a diver exposed to the very high pressures encountered in deep diving.

HEART

Most heart diseases or abnormalities of heart rhythm are incompatible with safe diving and are disqualifying conditions. They can often be detected from the personal or family history, by examination, from biochemical tests or electrocardiograms (ECGs). The blood pressure should be normal for the age of the diver.

OBESITY

The overweight person is more prone to decompression sickness and is likely to have a reduced level of physical fitness. Most physically fit obese individuals may dive safely with appropriate reductions of the allowable durations of dives.

LUNGS

Lung disease is a disqualifying condition. The diver needs normal lung function to allow a reserve of respiratory function to cope with exertion and to permit easy air flow from the lungs to prevent pulmonary barotrauma. The lungs must be very elastic to enable them to stretch during sudden volume changes on ascent. A history of asthma, chronic bronchitis, bronchiectasis, fibrosis, cysts, spontaneous pneumothorax, chest injury or chest surgery are disqualifying conditions.

The doctor may be able to detect localised airway obstruction (which can lead to a burst lung) by listening to sounds made in the chest when the diver breathes deeply and rapidly. The history, chest X–ray and **respiratory function tests** (expiratory spirometry) aid in the assessment.

There was a dramatic drop in the incidence of burst lung in Navy divers after the institution of these standards.

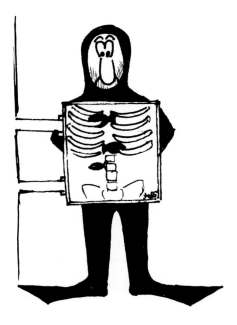

Fig. 38.2

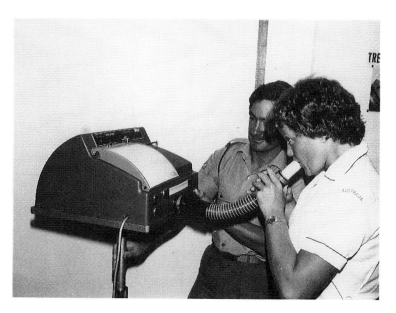

Fig. 38.3
Diving candidate blowing into a "Spirometer" to assess lung function.

EAR, NOSE AND THROAT

The ears, nose, throat and sinuses account for most diving related illnesses. Any acute infection such as a cold will temporarily disqualify a candidate. A history of chronic or recurrent allergies, hay fever, sinusitis, tonsillitis, or tooth decay need special assessment. Diving should be avoided while so affected. A deviated nasal septum (often appearing as a crooked nose) can cause obstruction of the sinus openings. All these factors can predispose to **sinus** or **ear barotrauma**.

The ears are carefully examined. The outer ear must be free from infection and not blocked with wax. The eardrum must be seen to move during the **Valsalva,** or other equalising manoeuvre. An eardrum which has been scarred from previous perforation may be weakened. The examining physician can advise on correct techniques to be used when equalising.

The hearing function test (**pure tone audiogram**) measuring hearing up to 8000 Hz is performed. Any significant hearing loss is regarded seriously since there is a risk of further hearing loss if **barotrauma** to the ears occurs during the diver's exposures.

Damage to the hearing organ may also be associated with disturbance of the balance organ. A special type of balance test is used to detect this, and investigation is by an electronic measurement (electronystagmogram) if necessary. It is important to detect any balance organ dysfunction since it can lead to **vertigo** and **vomiting** underwater.

EYES

Good **vision** is essential for the diver to see his boat or buddy, if he surfaces some distance away. A diver who has impaired vision can have **corrective lenses** included into his face mask, but should always dive with a visually fit buddy in case the mask is lost or broken during the dive.

Contact lenses can pose problems and advice is needed about these. Hard lenses can trap bubbles between them and the cornea, causing pressure damage. Soft lenses are susceptible to loss – especially during mask removal. These divers are advised to keep the eyes closed when removing the mask, either underwater or on the surface. See Chapter 32.

The operation of **radial keratotomy,** used to surgically correct short sightedness, can cause problems. With this procedure, the cornea is cut radially in a sunburst pattern to change the curvature of the cornea. These cuts weaken the cornea which is prone to burst if the eye is bumped or subjected to external pressure reduction. If such a diver develops face mask squeeze (see Chapter 12), the eyeballs may actually rupture. Anyone who has undergone this operation should not dive.

Colour vision is of lesser importance, apart from a few professional diving situations involving colour coded cylinders or wires (involving explosives).

BRAIN

Any disorder of the nervous system will complicate and confuse diagnosis and treatment of diving illnesses such as air embolism and decompression sickness.

Epileptics, even if controlled by drugs, should not dive as an epileptic fit underwater could prove fatal. The higher partial pressures of oxygen encountered during a scuba dive may render these persons more vulnerable to such attacks. Hypoxia, hyperventilation and sensory deprivation can aggravate fits. Many divers have had their first fit underwater.

Migraine is often made worse by diving (see Chapter 32). Severe migraine attacks leading to incapacity have occurred during dives in previously mild sufferers. It may also complicate recompression treatments. If certain precautions are observed some migraine sufferers can engage in limited diving in reasonable safety.

GENERAL CONDITIONS

Other diseases of the body such as **diabetes mellitus** (see Case History 33.6), severe **kidney** or **liver** disease also increase the risks of diving.

Muscle, bone and **joint** diseases or injuries can predispose to decompression sickness and make diagnosis and treatment more difficult. Fatigue may be induced more easily.

Professional divers or those who frequently undertake decompression diving may require **long bone X-rays** (see Chapter 17) to establish a baseline in the event of bone abnormalities developing, and for legal reasons. Because of the low risk of dysbaric osteonecrosis and the potential hazards posed by radiation exposure, these X-rays are not usually recommended for recreational divers.

A history of **motion sickness** is significant because it interferes with safe diving and it is difficult to vomit through a demand valve. Divers with a propensity to this condition need advice from the physician on remedies for seasickness which are compatible with safe diving (see Chapter 32).

Smoking diminishes physical fitness and can predispose to lung, sinus and ear barotrauma.

Pregnancy should preclude diving (see Chapter 8).

PHYSICAL FITNESS

This refers to the strength and speed, so necessary to athletes. It includes muscular, cardiac and respiratory capability. It is important to divers, as they are often called upon to exert themselves, to survive. One reasonable standard is to require an ability to swim, unaided, a distance of 200 metres in less than 5 minutes for recreational divers who do not subject themselves to difficult conditions. For professional or competent divers, this could be reduced to 4 minutes.

Medical fitness in this context refers to the freedom from illness likely to prejudice diving safety.

'Physical fitness' does not necessarily equate with 'diving medical fitness'.

It is not uncommon for fit young individuals to feel quite distressed when advised against scuba use by diving medical practitioners.

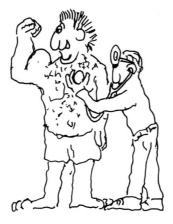

Fig. 38.4

MEDICAL EXAMINATION FORMAT

There is no doubt amongst responsible diving instruction groups and diving medical associations, that mandatory full and comprehensive medical examinations must be performed on all divers before commencing any scuba training. It is also needed before using scuba apparatus – even in such shallow and apparently safe locations as a swimming pool.

During a recent workshop on diving medical examinations, the following consensus was achieved with this advice for recreational divers :

> • All diving candidates must be examined according to an established diving medical Standard. An example is the South Pacific Underwater Medicine Society (SPUMS) Medical Format (included in this Chapter) prior to commencing any use of scuba apparatus – even if only in a pool.

> • The medical examiner must have been trained appropriately (at a recognised course) in diving medicine.

> • Should any doubt exist as to the 'fitness' of an individual, then that person must be referred to a specialist diving medical practitioner (i.e. one with extensive training and experience in diving medicine).

This textbook is not aimed at instructing medical practitioners in Diving Medicine – although it will serve as a useful primer for those interested in this type of medicine. A list of recommended courses of instruction and reading texts is included in Appendix A.

A copy of the **SPUMS Diving Medical Format** follows. It is suitable for candidates wishing to experience Scuba diving or to subject themselves for diver training. It must be performed and interpreted by a physician trained in diving medicine by an accredited body.

It comprises 3 sections :

(1) Medical history
(2) Diving [and diving medical] history
(3) Clinical examination and investigations.

Each is necessary and every item except for identification data, is of relevance to diver safety and diving limitations.

PRE-DIVE MEDICAL FORM FOR PROSPECTIVE ENTRY-LEVEL SCUBA DIVERS
The first two pages to be completed by candidate.

1	Surname Other Names		2	Date of Birth
3	Address		4	Sex: Male Female
			5	Telephone (Home)
6	Principal Occupation		7	Telephone (Work)
8	Intended Dive School			
9	Do you participate in any regular physical activity?		Yes	No
10	Description of activity			
11	Do you smoke?		Yes	No
12	Do you drink alcohol?		Yes	No
13	How many drinks a week?			
14	Are you taking any tablets, medicines or drugs? List:		Yes	No
15	Do you have any allergies? Details:		Yes	No
16	Have you had any reactions to drugs or medicines or foods? Details:		Yes	No

Have you ever had or do you now have any of the following? Tick Yes or No.

		Yes	No	Notes on History
17	Previous diving medical			
18	Prescription glasses			
19	Contact lenses			
20	Eye or visual problems			
21	Hay Fever			
22	Sinusitis			
23	Other nose or throat problem			
24	Dentures/Plates, etc.			
25	Recent dental procedures			
26	Deafness or ringing noises in ear(s)			
27	Discharging ears or other infections			
28	Operation on ears			
29	Giddiness or loss of balance			
30	Severe motion sickness			
31	Seasickness medication			
32	Problems when flying in aircraft			
33	Severe or frequent headaches			
34	Migraine			
35	Fainting or blackouts			
36	Convulsions, fits or epilepsy			
37	Unconsciousness			
38	Concussion or head injury			
39	Sleep-walking			
40	Severe depression			
41	Claustrophobia			
42	Mental illness			
43	Heart disease			
44	Abnormal blood test			
45	ECG (Heart tracing)			
46	Abnormality of your heart beat			
47	High blood pressure			
48	Rheumatic fever			
49	Discomfort in your chest with exertion			
50	Short of breath on exertion			
51	Bronchitis or pneumonia			
52	Pleurisy or severe chest pain			
53	Coughing up phlegm or blood			

		Yes	No
54	Chronic or persistent cough		
55	TB		
56	Pneumothorax ("collapsed lung")		
57	Frequent chest colds		
58	Asthma or wheezing		
59	Use a puffer		
60	Other chest complaint		
61	Operation on chest, lungs, or heart		
62	Indigestion, peptic ulcer or acid reflux		
63	Vomiting blood or passing red or black motions		
64	Recurrent vomiting or diarrhoea		
65	Jaundice, hepatitis or liver disease		
66	Malaria or other tropical disease		
67	Severe loss of weight		
68	Hernia or rupture		
69	Major joint or back injury		
70	Limitation of movement		
71	Fractures (broken bones)		
72	Paralysis or muscle weakness		
73	Kidney or bladder disease (cystitis)		
74	In a high risk group for HIV or AIDS		
75	Syphilis		
76	Diabetes		
77	Blood disease or bleeding problem		
78	Skin disease		
79	Contagious disease		
80	Operations		
81	In hospital for any reason		
82	Life insurance rejected		
83	A job or licence refused on medical grounds		
84	Unable to work for medical reasons		
85	An invalid pension		
86	Other illness or injury or any other medical conditions		
Have any near relations had			
87	Heart disease		
88	Asthma or chest disease		
89	TB		
Females Only			
90	Are you now pregnant or planning to be?		
91	Do you have any incapacity during periods?		

92   Date of most recent chest x-ray

Previous Diving Experience		Yes	No
93	Can you swim?		
94	Have you ever had any problem during or after swimming or diving?		
95	Have you ever had to be rescued?		
96	Do you snorkel dive regularly?		
97	Have you tried scuba diving before?		
98	Have you had previous formal scuba training?		
99	Year		
100	Approximate number of dives		
101	Maximum depth of any dive		
102	Longest duration of any dive		

I certify that the above information is true and complete to the best of my knowledge and I hereby authorise Dr.   to give medical opinion as to my fitness, or temporary or permanent unfitness to dive to   (Diveshop). I also authorise him or her to obtain or supply medical information regarding me to other doctors as may be necessary.

Signed:

Date:

MEDICAL EXAMINATION: To Be Completed By An Approved Medical Practitioner.

1 Height cm	2 Weight kg	3 Visual Acuity R6/ Corrected 6/ L6/ Corrected 6/		4 Blood Pressure	5 Pulse
6 Urinalysis Albumen Glucose		7 Respiratory function test (Measured by equipment capable of reading to 7 litres) Vital capacity FEV$_1$ Percentage		8 Chest x-ray (if indicated) Date Place Result	

9	Audiometry (air conduction)					
Frequency, Hz	500	1,000	2.000	4,000	6,000	8,000
Loss in DB(R):						
Loss in DB(L)						

If abnormal enter in diver's log book and on certificate

Clinical Examination/Assessment

		Normal	Abnormal
10	Nose, septum, airway		
11	Mouth, throat, teeth, bite		
12	External auditory canal		
13	Tympanic membrane		
14	Middle ear auto-inflation		
15	Neurological Eye movements Pupillary reflexes Limb reflexes Finger-nose Sharpened Romberg		
16	Abdomen		
17	Chest hyperventilation		
18	Cardiac auscultation		
19	Other abnormalities		

Notes on Abnormalities

Fit to Dive   Yes   Advice put on certificate
No   Temporary   Reason:
No   Permanent   Reason:
Printed Name: Date
Signed:

Detach the certificate below and hand to the candidate.
     Medical Benefits Refund and/or Medical Rebate is not permissible, by law, for this examination. Issue of any Item Number which allows the candidate to claim such benefit will result in the physician being guilty of medifraud.

This is to certify that I have examined
Name:
Address:

in accordance with the requirements of the Australian Standard for the training and certification of recreational divers, and have found him/her to be:
Fit   Permanently Unfit   Temporarily Unfit   (to be reviewed on   ) for diving and diving training to 18 m, undertaken using compressed air underwater. Audiogram normal/abnormal (see below).
Printed **Name**   Signed
Address:

Date
Telephone

Advice

Chapter 39

FIRST - AID KIT

Certain drugs and equipment are of value in a diving accident and a diving team could reasonably be expected to acquire and carry these on diving expeditions. Training in the use of these, as well as in resuscitation, is of great benefit.

FIRST-AID MATERIALS

For shark attack or trauma, large sized thick **cotton pads** (more than 20 cm square) with 10 cm **crepe bandages** (6 of each) are useful to make **pressure dressings** to stop bleeding and also for pressure bandages to reduce venom absorption. If obtainable, **shell** dressings of the type used by the military are ideal for this purpose. They can sometimes be obtained from army disposal stores.

A **rubber bandage** 10 cm wide ("esmarch" bandage obtainable from a medical equipment supplier) for use as a **tourniquet**. When wrapped tightly around the limb this is the best form of tourniquet. It covers a wide area, effectively stopping blood flow to the limb while minimising damage to tissues under the tourniquet.

Small adhesive skin **dressings** such as Elastoplast or Bandaids.

Surgical instruments — scissors, fine forceps, disposable scalpel blade, disposable syringes and needles.

An aluminised **thermal blanket** such as a "Spaceblanket" to protect divers suffering from hypothermia.

Heat packs — of value in treating fish stings.

Cold packs — of value in treating jelly fish sting and general muscular strains

Eye irrigation solution.

Torch, pen and paper (for recording purposes).

RESUSCITATION EQUIPMENT

• **Airways (Guedel type)** in two adult sizes are useful if the victim loses consciousness and develops airway obstruction, or if artificial respiration is needed. A positive pressure air system (such as an Ambu Bag) is of value in combination with the airway for prolonged artificial respiration.

• **Oxygen Resuscitation Equipment.** A supply of oxygen and equipment to administer it can be lifesaving in some diving accidents. Devices as described in Chapter 40 should include a complete oxygen supply and delivery system in a robust portable container.

• A **large oxygen cylinder** with appropriate adaptors should be available if diving at a distance from diving medical facilities and recompression chambers.

An **underwater oxygen** system (appendix E) for recompression therapy by more sophisticated groups, in remote areas.

MEDICATIONS FOR DIVING PROBLEMS

• Household **vinegar,** preferably in a one litre container, to neutralise adherent stinging cells of box jelly fish and some other jelly fish. Household **bleach** is useful for sterilising coral cuts.

• **Local anaesthetic spray or ointment** (lignocaine) to relieve the pain from minor stings from animals such as Portuguese man-o-war and other jellyfish stings. **Solacaine** or other anti-burn preparations such as **Tannic acid** sprays may be efficacious for this purpose.

• Topical **antibiotic powder** to prevent infection from coral cuts and other minor injuries.

• **Skin antiseptic solution** such as chlorhexidine for cleaning wounds contaminated with dirt.

• Broad spectrum **antibiotic tablets** (e.g. erythromycin) to initiate treatment for serious infections, otitis externa, otitis media, sinusitis, coral cuts etc.

• **Prophylactic ear drops** such as commercial preparations of Aqua Ear, Vosol or Otic Domoboro.

• **Therapeutic ear drops,** including antibiotics and steroids, such as "Kenacomb" or "Sofradex" for outer ear infections.

• **Local anaesthetic for injection** such as lignocaine 1% (without adrenaline) for wounds from stone fish and other scorpion fish. Up to 15 ml of this solution can be injected into the stung area in an adult and repeated every 2 hours if necessary.

• **Antivenoms** — depending on the geographical location.

GENERAL MEDICATIONS

• **Anti-diarrhoea** tablets such as diphenoxylate ("Lomotil") or loperamide ("Imodium").

• **Analgesics** (pain killers) such as paracetamol (acetaminophen). Aspirin, or drugs containing this substance, may be dangerous and are best avoided.

• **Ultra-violet** blocking sunscreen (SP15+ is best). A **1% hydrocortisone cream** is useful to treat sunburn, allergic dermatitis or itching.

• **Seasickness** tablets (see Chapter 32).

• **Decongestants** — pseudoephedrine tablets, and topical nasal sprays.

• **Topical antibacterial and antifungal** preparations, such as Cicatrin or Neosporin.

TRAINING

A diving team venturing to a remote locality should have at least one member (preferably two in case that one becomes the victim of an accident) trained in first aid relevant to divers. Training in the use of injections is an advantage, both for the administration of local anaesthetics, antivenoms and other drugs under the direction and advice of a distant medical specialist.

MEDICAL INFORMATION

Perhaps the most valuable addition to any first aid box is a source of information. This should include diving **medical texts** (see appendix A) and general **contact numbers** (see appendix B) for both medical assistance and recompression chamber availability. This should be supplemented by local contacts and phone numbers of knowledgeable divers and diving physicians.

A copy of **this book** should remain with the First-aid kit. Also in the kit should be a list of its **contents**, including purchase and expiry dates of the drugs.

Chapter 40

OXYGEN THERAPY TECHNIQUES

100% Oxygen (O_2) therapy is an essential technique in first-aid treatment of many diving emergencies. Unfortunately, the correct use of O_2 equipment is often poorly understood by divers. See Chapter 16 for details of the use of O_2 in decompression sickness.

OXYGEN BREATHING EQUIPMENT

The apparatus for administering O_2 is not unlike a scuba system. It comprises a **cylinder** which holds the oxygen at a pressure comparable to scuba tank pressure, and a pressure **reducing valve (regulator)** connected either to a **demand valve** or to a **constant flow system**. There is a need to avoid the use of flammable lubricants (such as oils and silicone grease) which can cause explosions in the presence of O_2.

For this reason, any use of O_2 requires a strict fire prevention attitude. Oxygen should not be administered near heat sources (no, you cannot smoke when O_2 equipment is in use). Nor should it be used in poorly ventilated areas. All equipment must be kept clean and the cylinder valve should be turned on slowly and the system purged before O_2 is given to the patient. If the patient is unconscious, always check that the apparatus is working by you or an attendant breathing on it first.

The O_2 can be delivered in high or low concentrations depending on the apparatus used. With a constant flow system, the O_2 can be delivered to the patient through either a cheap disposable (usually loose fitting) plastic **oxygen mask, nasal prongs, a nasal catheter** or a **bag-valve-mask resuscitator system.**

The administration of 100% O_2 means that nothing but O_2 is inhaled by the diver. Many of the O_2 masks commonly used in medicine have 100% O_2 **delivered to** the mask, but, the patient inhales only about 25-50% O_2 because the design of the mask allows this O_2 to mix with air, which dilutes the final breathing mixture. The disposable plastic O_2 masks in common use in ambulances and hospital casualty rooms are of this type.

These are **NOT** adequate for treating serious diving injuries (see photograph overleaf).

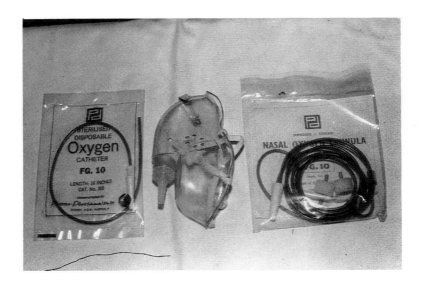

Fig. 40.1
These plastic masks, catheters and nasal prongs
are not adequate for treating divers with 100% O$_2$.

As a general rule, **decompression sickness, air embolism** (and other manifestations of **pulmonary barotrauma**) and **near drowning** cases should be given 100% O$_2$ from the outset.

Other diving accidents which produce shock or hypoxia can sometimes be helped with lower concentrations of O$_2$. In general, if the patient is cyanosed (blue) they need O$_2$ in a sufficient concentration to make them pink again. Usually, 100% O$_2$ is needed for treatment of diving accidents.

CONSTANT FLOW SYSTEMS

Such devices deliver a constant flow of O$_2$ to a mask or an alternative delivery system.

There are several types of plastic **disposable oxygen masks** available, the **Hudson** mask being typical. Each is normally accompanied by instructions which specify the correct O$_2$ flow to use, most masks using a flow of about 4–6 litres per minute. Because these masks are loose fitting, some also containing various holes, the O$_2$ flow is diluted by inspired air, the flow of which varies during inspiration and peaks at about 30 litres per minute. When the patient inhales, the O$_2$ flow is diluted by air, reducing the concentration of O$_2$ which the patient actually inhales from 100% to about 40 or 50%.

To increase the inspired O$_2$ percentage, increase the O$_2$ flow. Unless this is increased beyond 30 litres per minute an inspired percentage of 100% is not attainable. Such high flow rates rapidly deplete the O$_2$ supply.

A device known as a **nasal prong** (see above photo) is available which delivers O$_2$ by small tubes directly into the patients nostrils. An elastic head strap holds the prongs in place. This system has a similar efficiency to the common loose fitting O_2 mask but is more comfortable and more effective for long term use because it is less likely to dislodge when the patient sleeps.

A **nasal catheter** (or cannula) is sometimes used in hospitals but, as with the prongs described above, these are not recommended for most diving accidents.

These systems are acceptable when O_2 supplementation in low concentrations is all that is required. Cases in this category would include typical general medical conditions found in hospitals such as heart attack, and mild recovering cases of near drowning, salt water aspiration syndrome and shock associated with serious trauma or shark attack.

HIGH CONCENTRATION OXYGEN SYSTEMS

When near 100% O_2 delivery is required in cases such as decompression sickness, pulmonary barotrauma or near drowning, a more efficient O_2 delivery system is necessary.

This can be achieved by a **demand valve,** an O_2 circuit incorporating a **rebreathing bag,** or a bag–valve–mask device with an O_2 inlet and a reservoir bag with a very high O_2 flow rate.

Demand Valves

The simplest and most effective way to deliver 100% O_2 is via a **demand valve** like a second stage regulator.

Some demand valves have been specially designed for O_2 administration. Some, such as the Oxiden and LSP demand valves, are designated to provide O_2 only to spontaneously breathing patients. Others, such as the Robert Shaw (which is used on the Oxy Viva 3, marketed in Australia) and the Elder demand valves, can produce 100% O_2 to a spontaneously breathing patient as well as provide O_2 resuscitation to a non-breathing casualty via a manual trigger.

These demand valves are usually used with a tight fitting anaesthetic type mask. However, some can be fitted with a scuba mouthpiece to provide O_2 to a breathing diver (in this case the diver's nose should be sealed with a nose clip or by some other means).

Certain demand valves can be adapted to deliver O_2, with an adaptor connected to an O_2 reducing valve, or alternatively by connecting the diver's first stage regulator to an O_2 cylinder, using the specialised adaptor. Throughout the Pacific islands, the Bendeez was marketed for several years, however it is no longer available for purchase.

It is essential if this system is used that all components in the breathing system (including the lubricants) are O_2 compatible. Otherwise the diving illness may be complicated by fire, explosive and shrapnel injuries. When using this type of system the regulator should be tested for safety by purging it before anyone breathes from the system.

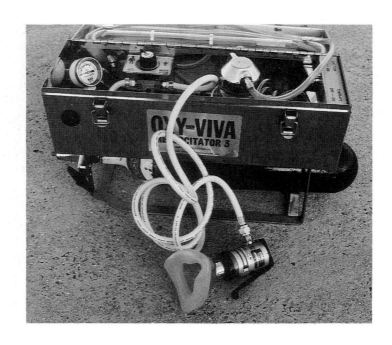

Fig. 40.2
An Australian manufactured Oxy-Viva Resuscitator with Robert Shaw demand valve fitted
to an anaesthetic-type mask. This system allows positive pressure ventilation with 100%
O_2 for a non-breathing diver, or passive demand supply for a breathing diver. A long
supply hose can be fitted to a larger cylinder containing 100% O_2 for prolonged use.

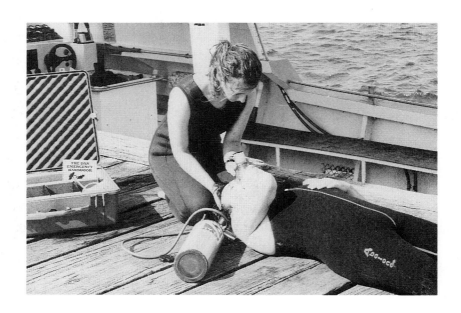

Fig. 40.3
A conscious diver breathing 100% O_2 from a demand valve with tight fitting mask.

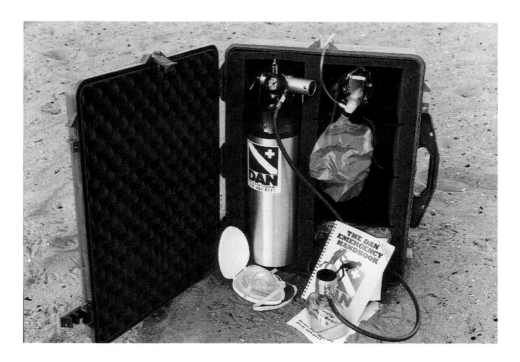

Fig. 40.4

A system designed by DAN (USA) specific for divers and incorporating a demand valve for $100\% O_2$ inhalation.

Rebreathing System

Oxygen use can be reduced if the diver breathes from a system which permits him to rebreathe some of his exhaled gas. This requires the nitrogen to be flushed from the breathing circuit after a few minutes rebreathing, and the exhaled CO_2 to be absorbed in a soda line (or similar chemical) canister. Drager has such a commercial system available.

The **Auer Superoxide system,** is a variant of the rebreathing techniques and one of the few ways of supplying O_2 without the need of an oxygen cylinder and is thus easily transportable in aircraft. It allows for many hours of O_2 supply, triggered by the interaction of CO_2 with superoxide.

Bag–Valve–Mask Respirator

These devices comprise a self inflating rubber or plastic bag and a valve system which allows the patient to be ventilated with air through a mask by squeezing the bag. Oxygen can be piped into the circuit to increase the inspired O_2 concentration. If a reservoir bag is attached to the inflation bag, the inspired O_2 concentration can be increased to almost 100% by using a large O_2 flow (approx. 12–14 litres per minute), providing a good seal is achieved and the patient's respiratory volume is not excessive. The valve system also allows the patient to breath spontaneously, with minimal inspiratory resistance, out of the circuit. Details of the operation of these devices vary between manufacturers and are outlined in the instructional manual supplied.

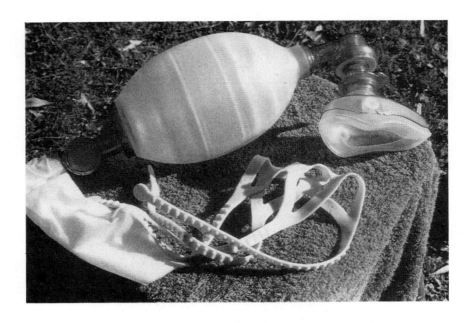

Fig. 40.5
Laerdal resuscitator showing anaesthetic-type mask, hand-squeezed breathing bag, oxygen reservoir bag and head strap to secure mask to diver's face.

Multiple Systems

Most countries have a variety of multi-purpose near 100% O_2 delivery systems available. Aga, AG, CIG, Ambu, LSP, Drager and Laerdal manufacture such units. Self-contained O_2 therapy units and resuscitation devices are now available with a demand valve allowing the patient to either breathe spontaneously out of the device, be given positive pressure ventilation by manual pressure, or use a breathing bag. A flow meter can be fitted to another part of the system, to allow O_2 to be delivered to a mask at a high continuous flow rate. The details vary slightly between resuscitators but are clearly explained in instructions supplied with them. The entire device should be contained in a sturdy rustproof metal or heavy duty plastic box which is compact, water resistant and easy to carry.

DAN market an O_2 unit specifically designed for divers. It utilises a LSP demand inhalator valve and provides 100% O_2 to a breathing diver. It also incorporates a constant flow device which can be attached to a pocket mask and administer O_2 to supplement resuscitation, or to a loose fitting mask with a reservoir to provide relatively higher O_2 concentrations to a second, breathing casualty.

Oxygen Toxicity

See Chapter 21. 100% O_2 will cause some reversible damage to lungs after 18–24 hours. This has to be balanced against the benefit of the O_2 condition being treated and this will usually be physician's decision. If medical advice cannot be obtained, in decompression sickness and gas embolism cases O_2 toxicity is generally the lesser of two evils, and it is usually best to continue giving 100% O_2 until expert advice to the contrary is given.

Oxygen toxicity is generally not a consideration with low concentration devices as they do not delivery much more than 40% O_2, which is below the threshold for toxicity.

Contraindications to O_2 Therapy

In addition to the problems of O_2 toxicity, there are some problems associated with oxygen usage in the general community.

There is a theoretical risk to premature babies (eye damage) and to sufferers of emphysema (respiratory depression). Neither of these groups are numerous in the diving population.

In recent years a problem of sensitivity to O_2 has emerged in cancer sufferers who have been treated with the drug **Bleomycin**. These people can suffer from severe, permanent lung damage if given O_2 in concentrations greater than 21% (air). This problem is not likely to be frequently encountered, as these people should be excluded from scuba diving.

Practicalities of O_2 Administration

The main disadvantage of resuscitation apparatus is the limited O_2 supply available from the contained O_2 cylinder, because sufficient O_2 must be supplied to allow for transport of the diver from the accident site to an appropriate medical facility. This can be overcome by carrying additional cylinders or by an adaptor which allows a connection to a larger O_2 cylinder. Estimate the rate of consumption of O_2, the supply available, and plan accordingly.

All divers are encouraged to undergo additional training in resuscitation and O_2 administration. This should be mandatory for dive masters and dive instructors.

Cases such as gas embolism and decompression sickness generally require **100% inspired O_2** from the outset. A system capable of delivering 100% O_2 must be chosen. Even then, an ill fitting mask may allow air to be breathed around the seal, diluting the O_2. Attention to the mask fit and attachment is necessary to prevent this. It is especially likely if the patient sleeps. If a demand valve is used, make sure the patient does not breathe air through the nose at the same time. This can be prevented by using a nose clip (improvise if necessary) or a diver's face mask.

Whenever O_2 is administered there is a serious **fire hazard** since increased concentrations of O_2 accelerate burning and can make ordinarily non-combustible materials burn furiously. The area where the O_2 is administered should be well ventilated and sources of ignition and combustible materials (including cigarettes) should be avoided. The system should be turned on slowly and should be tried and running before it is applied to the patient's face.

Further information may be obtained from the text "Oxygen First Aid for Divers" (1992) — by John Lippmann, J.L. Publications, Australia.

Acknowledgment is made to Jim Corey and John Lippmann for some data used in this Chapter.

Chapter 41

TRAINING & SAFETY CHECKLIST

SAFETY INFORMATION AND BACKUP

- Diving manuals and library (see Appendix A).
- Diving medical and safety manuals and texts (see Appendix A).
- Diving medical organisations (see Appendix B).
- Medical Insurance — DAN has organised this for North Americans and is attempting to extend this world wide.

DIVER TRAINING

- Physical fitness – 200 metres unassisted swim in less than 5 minutes (minimum level).
- Medical examination fitness for diving. Includes audiogram, expiratory spirometry.
- Entry level diving certificate. Qualified by a diving instructor from a reputable training organisation.
- Advanced level training.
- Diving rescue and resuscitation training.
- Specialised courses for the specific diving environment.

DIVE PLAN

- Boat operator's safety and equipment check.
- Dive plan — includes terrain understanding, navigation plan,
  air supply, ascent rate, safety and decompression stops.
- Basic diving equipment check and maintenance.
- Dive responsibility, documentation and buddy system.
- Diving rescue equipment — includes BC, emergency air supplies,
  alarm signals, etc.
- Lost diver strategy.
- Diving rescue plan - includes boat / buoy / diver backups.
- First-Aid kit and resuscitation equipment. (See Chapters 39 and 40).
- Emergency contact numbers (local).

FOR DIVE OPERATORS

- A good lawyer!

Chapter 42

RESUSCITATION REVIEW

It is not possible to learn the techniques of resuscitation from a book. To acquire these skills, the authors recommend that all divers undertake a resuscitation course from one of the many organisations worldwide which teach these techniques. Once learnt, the skills need to be practised regularly, just as do diving emergency procedures.

The protocol used here is meant as a reminder to divers who have already experienced such training. It is based on that recommended by the Australian Resuscitation Council. Organisations in other countries may have slightly different protocols, but if they come from reputable organisations they should be equally effective.

WHAT IS RESUSCITATION?

Resuscitation is the restoration or preservation of life using maintenance of the A–B–C — Airway, Breathing, and Circulation — to preserve oxygenation to vital tissues. The most important tissue to protect from hypoxia is the brain.

Expired Air Resuscitation (EAR) is designated as the best method of initially ventilating the lungs. If the rescuer has the equipment and skill to ventilate the victim with an Oxygen Resuscitator, then that is preferable.

ASSESSMENT OF THE DIVING CASUALTY

In addition to the following measures, it is important to protect the victim from further injury and to control bleeding if present.

Is the Victim Conscious?

Most problems arise in an unconscious victim. Shake the victim and shout at him. If he does do not respond, he is unconscious – or dead!

If the victim is **conscious** he will normally take care of his own airway and breathing. Exceptions to this are the sea snake and blue ringed octopus envenomation, where the victim is conscious but paralysed. In these cases the victim will not respond to shaking and shouting, so the management for an unconscious victim (which is appropriate) will be undertaken.

If the victim is **unconscious** he will be in danger of hypoxic hypoxia from obstruction of the airway or inhibition of breathing, or of stagnant hypoxia from lack of circulation (see Chapter 20).

With an unconscious victim, take care of the following systems :

• AIRWAY
• BREATHING
• CIRCULATION

This is easily remembered by the mnemonic — A B C.

Maintenance of airway, breathing and circulation takes precedence over other forms of care. Without these functions, the victim is certain to die.

A — AIRWAY

An unconscious victim loses muscle control. Loss of control of the muscles of the throat and tongue can cause the airway to become obstructed. This is particularly likely when the victim is lying on his back, mainly due to the tongue falling backwards into the throat, due to gravity.

The airway can be further obstructed by vomit, saliva or foreign material. This would normally be swallowed or spat out by a conscious person, while any material which entered the larynx or trachea would elicit the reflexes of coughing and laryngeal closure. These reflexes may be lost in the unconscious patient.

To prevent airway obstruction :

❑ Turn the victim on the side.

This causes the tongue to fall sideways (not backwards into the throat) and allows liquids in the mouth and throat to drain out of the mouth under gravity (the victim must be positioned with the mouth lower than the larynx to allow this).

❑ Tilt the head backwards.

This further opens the airway.

❑ Clear the mouth.

Sweep the fingers through the mouth to clear out foreign material, or a tongue which has fallen backwards.

❑ Look for signs of airway obstruction.

These include lack of normal respiratory movements of the chest and abdomen, indrawing of the chest as the abdomen moves outwards and inability to feel air movement at the nose and mouth. Airway obstruction can be partial, in which case breathing may be noisy and laboured.

❑ Support the jaw.

Using a chin-lift procedure (such as the 'pistol grip') or jaw thrust manoeuvre, the airway can be further opened if necessary. These techniques are taught in resuscitation courses.

B — BREATHING

Even with a clear airway the victim may not breathe because of respiratory muscle paralysis, cerebral injury, hypoxia or other reasons.

Check for breathing – look, listen and feel.

Look for respiratory movements of the chest and abdomen. Listen and feel for air moving from the nose and mouth.

If the victim is breathing, keep him on his side and keep the airway clear.

If the victim is not breathing :

❑ Turn on back, commence expired air resuscitation (EAR).

The theory and practice of this are covered in a resuscitation course. The steps are :

> – clear the airway
> – tilt the head back
> – blow into the patient
> – look, listen and feel for exhalation

Give five full inflations in ten seconds, then :

❑ Check the carotid pulse.

If this is present continue with expired air resuscitation (EAR).

❑ If no pulse, commence external cardiac comression (ECC).

C — CIRCULATION

If there is no carotid pulse or heart beat, there is no effective circulation. This may be due to cardiac arrest (or cessation of effective heart beat) or excessively low blood pressure from blood loss or other causes.

Recognition of cardiac arrest.

The victim has no circulation to the brain so he is :

– unconscious
– not breathing
– no carotid pulse or heart beat

❑ **External cardiac compression.** Circulation can be restored with this technique. The heart is compressed by pressure on the sternum, forcing blood into the major arteries and producing some circulation to the vital organs. The combination of artificial respiration and external cardiac compression is called CPR.

CARDIOPULMONARY RESUSCITATION (CPR)

When the heart stops, so does the breathing. It is necessary to maintain respiration and cardiac function simultaneously. This is CPR.

❑ **Give five EAR breaths, then**

❑ **Check for circulation (carotid pulse).** If present maintain airway and breathing.

❑ **If no carotid pulse — start external cardiac compression (ECC)**

Practical details of this are covered in a resuscitation course. Remember, compress :

– vertically
– over the lower half of the sternum
– with the heel of the hand
– with no pressure on the ribs
– to a depth of 4–5 centimetres (1.5–2 inches) in adults
– a rate not less than 60 per minute
– time of compression equal to relaxation

CPR with one rescuer

2 respiratory inflations to 15 cardiac compressions in about 15 seconds (this gives the patient at least 60 compressions and 8 breaths per minute).

CPR with two rescuers

1 inflation and 5 compressions in about 5 seconds (giving the patient at least 12 cycles –12 inflations and 60 compressions – per minute). Co-ordinate the inflation with the relaxation phase of the fifth compression so that there is no pause in compressions.

Recovery checks

It is important to check if compression is effective and also for signs of return of normal pulse or heart beat. Check the carotid pulse during compression for effective circulation after one minute, and then at least every two minutes. If there is no pulse with compression of the heart, more effective cardiac compression or medical intervention is needed.

If there is a pulse with compression, then stop compression for five seconds and feel for a pulse from spontaneous heartbeat. If this is present, cease compressions but continue Expired Air Resuscitation (EAR) until breathing returns, repeatedly feeling for the pulse at the wrist or neck. If this stops, check the carotid pulse and respond appropriately.

Duration of CPR

Continue CPR until :

  – the victim recovers
  – expert help arrives
  – a physician pronounces the victim dead
  – it is physically impossible to continue.

SEE RESUSCITATION SUMMARY OVERLEAF

RESUSCITATION SUMMARY

A – Airway
B – Breathing
C – Circulation

Conscious + Breathing present — Pulse Present

Place victim in a comfortable position.
Observe ABC.
Provide O_2 if possible.

Unconscious + Breathing present — Pulse Present

Place victim on side.
Maintain a clear Airway.
Observe B and C.
Provide O_2 if possible.

Unconscious + Not breathing — Pulse Present

Turn victim on back. Ensure Airway.
Commence Expired Air Resuscitation with five full inflations.
Continue at about 15 breaths per minute.
Check pulse after 1 minute, then at least every 2 minutes.
Provide O_2 if possible.

Unconscious + Not breathing — Pulse Not Present

With victim on back, give CPR.
Single rescuer — 2 inflation to 15 compressions / 15 seconds.
Two rescuers — 1 inflation to 5 compressions / 5 seconds.
Check pulse after 1 minute and then at least every 2 minutes.
Provide O_2 if possible.

Appendix A

DIVING MEDICAL LIBRARY

DIVING MANUALS

- US Navy Diving Manual Vol. 1– Air Diving.
- British Subaqua Club (BSAC) Diving Manual.
- National Oceanic and Atmospheric Administration (NOAA) Diving Manual
- Professional Association of Diving Instructors (PADI) – Open Water Diving Manual.
- National Association of Underwater Instructors (NAUI) – Diving Manual.

NEWSLETTERS

• **Undercurrent** – this doubles both as a consumer guide to holiday dive sites, as well as a forum for the presentation of recent technical data, diving accidents, etc. :
Address : PO BOX 1658 Sausalito, California 94965, U.S.A.

• **Triage** – a quarterly newsletter of the National Diving and Hyperbaric Medical Technology, mainly of value to diving medics, with special emphasis on the off shore oil industry :
Address : JESMC Department of Hyperbaric Medicine, Suite 112, 4400 General Meyer Ave, New Orleans LA 70131, U.S.A.

• **Alert Diver** – a quarterly newsletter of the Divers Alert Network. An excellent informative newsletter regarding diving medical safety and accident information, produced by DAN :
Address : BOX 3823 Duke University Medical Centre, Durham, North Carolina 27710, U.S.A.

• **NAUI Sources** – The journal of underwater education, previously referred to as NAUI News. This is a monthly newsletter, and includes an excellent lift-out called "Technical Issues":
Address : PO BOX 14650, Montclair, CA 91763 - 1150, U.S.A.

• **Pressure** – a bi-monthly newsletter of the Undersea and Hyperbaric Medical Society, with information of a social, academic and educational nature, relevant to the Society and its members – mainly physicians and paramedics:
Address : Undersea and Hyperbaric Medical Society 9650 Rockville Pike, Bethesda Marylands 20814, U.S.A.

• **SPUMS Journal** – a bi-monthly journal/newsletter of the South Pacific Underwater Medical Society. This contains both original diving medical articles and reviews, and also summaries of other diving medical research conducted throughout the world:
Address : The Editor, 80 Wellington Parade, East Melbourne, Victoria 3002, Australia.

• **PADI Undersea Journal** – a quarterly magazine essentially for diving instructors but of interest to others.

• **Aqua Corps** including Technical Diver. A recent addition, includes contentious issues and "technical" diving reports. Address : PO BOX 1497 Atos, California 95001, U.S.A.

NB. Many other countries have their own variations of the above newsletters, with local insertions.

DIVING MEDICAL TEXTS

• **Diving Medicine – for Scuba Divers** * — (1992) by Edmonds, McKenzie and Thomas. Available from J.L. Publications, P.O. Box 381, Carnegie, Victoria, Australia, and the Diving Medical Centres, Australia (see Appendix B) and DAN in the U.S.A.

• **The DAN Emergency Handbook** * — by John Lippmann & Stan Bugg. Available from the Divers Alert Network (DAN) in the USA.

• **Dangerous Marine Creatures** * — (1989) by Carl Edmonds, published by Reed, Balgowlah Australia and available from Diving Medical Centres, Australia (see Appendix B) and DAN in the USA.

• **Diving and Subaquatic Medicine,** 3rd edition (1991) — by Edmonds Lowry and Pennefather. For physicians and scientifically sophisticated divers. Published by Butterworths Heinemann, Oxford.

• **The Underwater Handbook,** a Guide to Physiology and Performance for the Engineer (1976) — by C. W. Shilling, M. F. Werts & N. R. Schandolmeier. Published by the Undersea and Hyperbaric Medical Society, Maryland.

• **Diving Medicine** (1976) — by Richard Strauss, published by Grune and Stratton, New York.

• **Diving Medicine** (1990) — by Bove and Davis, published by Saunders, Philadelphia.

• **Field Guide for the Diver Medic** (1983) — by C. G. Dougherty, published by the National Association of Diving Medical Technicians, Texas.

• **The Med Dive Specialist Handbook** (1990) — by Kathy Work, published by Dive Rescue Inc., Colorado.

• **The Physicians Guide to Diving Medicine** (1984) — by Shilling, Carlston and Mathias. Published by Plenum Press, New York.

• **Diving Accident Management** (1990) — the 41st Undersea and Hyperbaric Medical Workshop, edited by Bennett and Moon, and published by the Undersea and Hyperbaric Medical Society, sponsored by the National Oceanic and Atmospheric Administration, and the Divers Alert Network.

• **Oxygen First-Aid for Divers** * (1992) — by John Lippman, J.L. Publications, P.O. Box 381, Carnegie, Victoria, Australia.

* Suitable for recreational divers

Appendix B

EMERGENCY and INFORMATION CONTACTS

SOCIETIES

Apart from the instructor organisations (NAUI, PADI, SSI, NASDS (formerly FAUI), YMCA, BSAC, etc.) there are certain societies which would be very useful for any concerned and knowledgeable diving paramedic to belong to.

These include the following :

• **Divers Alert Network (DAN)** — BOX 3823 Duke University Medical Centre, Durham, NC 27710 (USA and the American continent, offshore and USA islands and trust territories).

• **Undersea and Hyperbaric Medical Society** — Affiliate membership. 9650 Rockville Pike, Bethesda, Maryland, U.S.A.

• **South Pacific Underwater Medicine Society (SPUMS)** — C/- The Australasian College of Occupational Medicine (ACOM), P.O. Box 2090, St. Kilda West, Melbourne, Victoria 3182, Australia (mainly the South Pacific region, centred in Australasia).

• **British Subaqua Club (BSAC)** — (mainly for diving around the United Kingdom).

Diver Alert Network (DAN)

The major international organisation for supply of medical advice to divers, referrals for diving accidents, information about recompression facilities, diving medical insurance and medivac availability, etc.

DAN Address : BOX 3823 Duke University Medical Centre, Durham, NC 27710, U.S.A.
Emergency number   — within USA : (919) 684–8111
Information number   — within USA : (919) 684–2948

A — DAN or DES (Diver Emergency Service) for Australia, New Zealand and surrounding areas.
  • for within Australia : (008) 088–200
  • outside Australia : 618–223–2855
E — DAN for European sector : (Italy) 85–899–0125
J — DAN for the Japanese sector.

Diving Medical Centres (Australia)

For diving medical texts, diving medical courses for physicians and dive instructors, research projects, medical advice, referrals, consultations and treatment of diving accidents.

Diving Medical Centre
66 Pacific Highway
St .Leonards, Sydney,
NSW 2065.
Ph : (02) 437–6681

Diving Medical Centre
132 Yallambee Road
Jindalee, Brisbane,
Q'ld. 4074.
Ph : (07) 376–1414 and
376–1056.

Emergency Telephone Numbers

Other areas to call are as follows :

Australia : Office In Charge **Royal Australian Navy**
School of Underwater Medicine
Balmoral NSW 2091.
From outside Australia   — 612–960–0333
From within Australia   — (02) 960–0333 or (02) 960–0444

The **Diving Emergency Service** (DES) or Divers Alert Network
From within Australia   — (008) 088–200 or
From outside Australia   — 618–223–2855

Canada : Toronto General Hospital
Hyperbaric Unit
(416) 340–4131

New Zealand : Royal New Zealand Naval Hospital
(09) 458–454

United Kingdom : HMS Vernon – Portsmouth
(0705) 818–888. Ask for the Duty Officer or Lieutenant Commander.

USA :   The Divers Alert Network (DAN)
                  919–684–8111 for emergencies or
                  919–684–2948 for non-urgent information

Your Area :   _____
                 _____
                 _____

                 Telephone :

                 _____
                 _____
                 _____

                 Telephone :

                 _____
                 _____
                 _____

                 Telephone :

Others :   _____
                 _____
                 _____

                 Telephone :

Others :   _____
                 _____
                 _____

                 Telephone :

Others :   _____
                 _____
                 _____

                 Telephone :

Others :   _____
                 _____
                 _____

                 Telephone :

Others :   _____
                 _____
                 _____

                 Telephone :

Appendix C

DCIEM
SPORT
DECOMPRESSION
TABLES

DCIEM Sport Diving Tables

A: First Dive No-D Limits

Table A gives you the No-Decompression Limits for First Dives and the Decompression Stop Times needed for dives which exceed the No-Decompression Limits.

A **No-Decompression Limit** (No-D Limit) is the maximum Bottom Time that you may spend on a dive without having to conduct a Decompression Stop before surfacing. *New divers are advised to stay within the No-D Limits.*

To find your No-D Limit for a given depth, enter Table A from the Depth column and follow the row of numbers across to the bold, vertical lines. The largest number to the left of the bold, vertical lines is your No-D Limit (expressed in minutes) for a First Dive.

Beside each number is a **Repetitive Group (RG)** letter. Repetitive Groups are dive exposure guides. To find your Group letter, use the exact or next greater Bottom Time. If no Group letter appears beside your Bottom Time, allow 24 hours to elapse before your next dive.

The proper **Ascent Rate** for using the DCIEM Sport Diving Tables is 60 feet (18 metres) plus or minus 10 feet (3 metres) per minute.

The section to the right of the bold, vertical lines is used only for Decompression Dives. The required **Decompression Stops** are given in minutes at the bottom of each column.

EXAMPLE: First Dive to 70'/21m for 40 minutes

        No-D Limit is 35 minutes
        Decompression Stop is 5 min at 10'/3m
        Repetitive Group for 40 min at 70' is 'F'

B: Surface Intervals

A **Surface Interval** is the time elapsed between surfacing from a dive and beginning the actual descent on the following dive. In Table B, Surface Intervals are expressed in hours and/or minutes.

Enter Table B using the Group letter from your last dive. Match your Group letter with your Surface Interval. The amount of residual nitrogen remaining in your body is indicated in the form of a Repetitive Factor (RF) - the highest Factor being 2.0.

As your Surface Interval increases, your RF decreases. When your RF reaches 1.0, your nitrogen level will be back to normal. Any dive conducted while your RF is greater than 1.0 is a **Repetitive Dive**.

If your RF has diminished to 1.0, use Table A to plan your next dive.

If your RF is greater than 1.0, use the No-D Limits in Table C.

Before conducting a Repetitive Dive, allow enough Surface Interval time to elapse for a Repetitive Factor to appear in Table B.

If you must dive before a Repetitive Factor appears, use the following emergency guidelines for short Surface Intervals:

    i.   For dives to the SAME DEPTH: add the actual Bottom Times together and use the Effective (total) Bottom Time to determine your Repetitive Group in Table A;

    ii.   For dives to DIFFERENT DEPTHS: use the 'Step system' (explained in the Multi-level diving section) to find the equivalent time for your First Dive RG at the second depth. Add the actual Bottom time at the second depth and use the Effective (total) Bottom Time to find your new RG.

Flying After Diving

After a single No-Decompression Dive, allow your Repetitive Factor to drop to **1.0** before flying.

After a Repetitive Dive or a Decompression Dive, allow for a Surface Interval of **at least 24 hours** before flying.

C: Repetitive Dive No-D Limits

The No-D Limits for Repetitive Dives are given in Table C.

On a Repetitive Dive, the No-D Limit is reduced because of residual nitrogen remaining from the preceding dive. To find the No-D Limit for a Repetitive Dive, match the depth with your Repetitive Factor (RF) taken from Table B.

EXAMPLE: Depth of 40'/12m with RF of 1.5
                No-D Limit = 100 minutes

If you stay within the No-D Limits and do not conduct another Repetitive Dive, no calculations are necessary. After 18 hours, you can begin your next dive using the No-D Limits in Table A.

If you plan to conduct another Repetitive Dive (3rd dive), you will need to find your **Effective Bottom Time (EBT)** for dive #2. To find your **EBT**, either multiply the actual Bottom Time by your Repetitive Factor or refer to the 'EBT Table'.

The Repetitive Group for dive #2 is found in Table A according to the depth and Effective Bottom Time.

EXAMPLE: Depth of Repetitive Dive is 40'/12m
                RF is 1.5   *No-D Limit is 100 minutes*

                Actual Bottom Time is 60 minutes
                EBT = 60 min X 1.5 = 90 minutes

                Repetitive Group is 'G'

Whenever the actual Bottom Time on a Repetitive Dive exceeds the No-D Limit given in Table C, a Decompression Stop is required. **Decompression Stops** for Repetitive Dives are found in Table A according to the depth and Effective Bottom Time.*

On a Decompression Repetitive Dive, the EBT may result in a figure that is less than the Table A No-D Limit although the actual Bottom Time exceeds the Table C No-D Limit. If this occurs, conduct a 5 minute Stop at a depth of 10'/3m.

UDT᪣ QWIK EBT TABLE

Minutes ↓ ↓		1.1	1.2	1.3	1.4	1.5	1.6	1.7	1.8	1.9	2.0
10		11	12	13	14	15	16	17	18	19	20
	1	2	2	2	2	2	2	2	2	2	2
20		22	24	26	28	30	32	34	36	38	40
	2	3	3	3	3	3	4	4	4	4	4
30		33	36	39	42	45	48	51	54	57	60
	3	4	4	4	5	5	5	6	6	6	6
40		44	48	52	56	60	64	68	72	76	80
	4	5	5	6	6	6	7	7	8	8	8
50		55	60	65	70	75	80	85	90	95	100
	5	6	6	7	7	8	8	9	9	10	10
60		66	72	78	84	90	96	102	108	114	120
	6	7	8	8	9	9	10	11	11	12	12
70		77	84	91	98	105	112	119	126	133	140
	7	8	9	10	10	11	12	12	13	14	14
80		88	96	104	112	119	128	136	144	152	160
	8	9	10	11	12	12	13	14	15	16	16
90		99	108	117	126	135	144	153	162	171	180
	9	10	11	12	13	14	15	16	17	18	18

Match the actual Bottom Time (given in the left hand column) with your Repetitive Factor.

EXAMPLE: Actual Bottom Time is 65 minutes
Repetitive Factor is 1.5

Effective Bottom Time for 65 minutes
is 60 minutes = 90 minutes
plus 5 minutes = <u>8 minutes</u>
Effective Bottom Time = 98 minutes

Minimum Surface Intervals for No-D Dives

Table C and Table B can be used together to find the minimum Surface Interval needed to conduct a No-Decompression Repetitive Dive. Use Table C to find the Repetitive Factor that corresponds with your actual Bottom Time. Use Table B to match this RF with the Group letter from your last dive. The **Minimum Surface Interval** is given at the top of the matching column in Table B.

EXAMPLE: First Dive - 80'/24m for 25 minutes
Repetitive Group = E
Repetitive Dive - 60'/18m for 31 minutes

in Table C - RF of 1.3 is required at the beginning of the Repetitive Dive

in Table B - Group E diver acquires RF of 1.3 after a Surface Interval of 2 hours.

Adjustments for Multiple Repetitive Dives

Whenever you conduct three or more dives in a series, the Group letter for each Repetitive dive must be higher than that of the preceding dive. *DCIEM recommends a limit of 3 dives in a series.*

If your Group letter is lower than or the same as that of the preceding dive and the Surface Interval before your next dive is less than six (6) hours, make the following adjustment:

Add one letter to the RG from the preceding dive and apply the adjusted Group letter to your current Repetitive Dive.

EXAMPLE: First Dive RG = D   Second Dive RG = B
- less than six hours before 3rd Dive
Raise the Second Dive RG letter to 'E' (First Dive RG 'D' + 1 letter)

No adjustment is needed if the Surface Interval before the next dive is six hours or longer.

If 3 or more dives a day are conducted on 3 consecutive days, allow for a 24 hour Surface Interval after the 3rd day.

MULTI-LEVEL DIVES

A **Multi-level Dive** is a dive during which Bottom Time is spent at two or more depths before surfacing.

During a Multi-level Dive, the decompression that would occur during a normal ascent to the surface is interrupted by the additional ascents in the Multi-level profile.

The following guidelines are designed for No-Decompression Dives with multi-level profiles, and apply only to the DCIEM tables.

GENERAL GUIDELINES

Plan each Multi-level Dive as a NO-DECOMPRESSION Dive;

If a No-D Limit is exceeded, abort the dive and proceed to the Deompression Stop(s) specified in Table A.

Conduct the DEEPEST PART of the dive FIRST. Ascend at least 20'/6m to and between teach additional Step in the dive profile. At depths greater than 100'/30m, ascend at least 30'/9m;

FINISH the dive in SHALLOW water in a depth range between 10'/3m and 20'/6m. Spend at least 5 minutes at this depth and add the time spent to your Bottom Time.

After each dive, allow for a Surface Interval of at least one hour.

FIRST DIVE MULTI-LEVEL PROCEDURES

In Table A, find your Repetitive Group for Step 1 according to the depth and actual Bottom Time.

EXAMPLE: Step 1 is at 90'/27m for 15 minutes,
                (No-D Limit is 20 minutes)
                RG for Step 1 is 'C'

Use Table A to find the equivalent time for RG 'C' at Step 2. Add your actual Bottom Time to the equivalent time for RG 'C'. The total time is your Effective Bottom Time (EBT) at Step 2. Your EBT must not exceed the No-D Limit given for Step 2.

                Step 2 is at 50'/15m for 20 minutes,
                (No-D Limit is 75 minutes)
                Equivalent time for 'C' = 30 minutes
                Actual Bottom Time = 20 minutes
                Effective Bottom Time= 50 minutes
                RG for Step 2 is 'E'

Find the equivalent time for RG 'E' at Step 3. Add your actual Bottom Time to the equivalent time. Your Effective Bottom Time must not exceed the No-D Limit for Step 3.

                Step 3 is at 20'/6m for 20 minutes,
                (No-D Limit at 20' is 'infinity')
                Equivalent time for 'E' = 150 minutes
                Actual Bottom Time = 20 minutes
                Effective Bottom Time = 170 minutes
                RG for Step 3 is 'F'

REPETITIVE DIVE MULTI-LEVEL PROCEDURES

On a Repetitive Dive, your actual Bottom Time at Step 1 must not exceed the No-D Limit given in **Table C**.

EXAMPLE: Repetitive Factor is 1.3

                Step 1 is at 70'/21m,
                (No-D Limit in Table C is 21 minutes)
                Actual Bottom Time = 20 minutes
                EBT = 20 min X 1.3 = 26 minutes
                Repetitive Group for Step 1 is 'E'

The RG for Step 1 is taken from Table A according to the depth and Effective Bottom Time. *Your RG for Step 1*

must be equal to or greater than the RG from your preceding dive.

EXAMPLE: If the RG from the preceding dive was 'F' and the RG for Step 1 is 'E',
                raise 'E' to 'F' before Step 2.

Because you must ascend at least 20'/6m between Steps, Step 2 should be conducted at a depth of 50'/15m or less.

Your Effective Bottom Time (EBT) at Step 2 must not exceed the No-D Limit given in **Table A**.

                Step 2 is at 50'/15m for 10 minutes,
                (No-D Limit is 75 minutes)
                Equivalent time for RG 'F' = 60 minutes
                Actual Bottom Time = 10 minutes
                Effective Bottom Time = 70 minutes
                RG for Step 2 is 'G'

Before surfacing, spend at least 5 minutes at a depth between 10'/3m and 20'/6m. Regardless of whether you conduct this as the final Step in the dive or as a safety stop, the time you spend at this depth must be included in your Effective Bottom Time.

                Step 3 is at 20'/6m for 10 minutes,
                (No-D Limit is 'infinity')

Equivalent time for RG 'G' = 240 minutes
Actual Bottom Time = <u>10 minutes</u>
Effective Bottom Time = 250 minutes
RG for Step 3 is 'H'

SUMMARY

FIRST DIVE: Your actual Bottom Time at Step 1 must not exceed the No-D Limit given in **Table A**. Your EBT (or total bottom time) at each subsequent Step must not exceed the No-D Limit given for that Step.

REPETITIVE DIVE: Your actual Bottom Time at Step 1 must not exceed the No-D Limit given in **Table C**. The Repetitive Group taken from Step 1 must be equal to or greater than the RG from your preceding dive. Your Effective Bottom Time at each subsequent Step must not exceed the No-D Limit given in Table A.

Finish the dive in shallow water (between 10' and 20') and allow for a Surface Interval of at least one hour after each dive.

D: Depth Corrections
(for Altitude Dives)

Table D is used to convert the actual depth at high altitude to an **Effective Depth** that corresponds with the Table A and Table C depth figures intended for use at sea level. Table D provides the Depth Corrections and Actual Decompression Stop Depths needed to conduct dives at altitudes between 1,000 feet (300 metres) and 10,000 feet (3,000 metres) above sea level.

Depth Corrections are necessary when diving at altitude because the reduced atmospheric pressure at the surface of the dive site makes the Altitude Dive equivalent to a much deeper dive at sea level. When you arrive from a lower altitude, your body will already have some residual nitrogen as a result of the decrease in atmospheric pressure.

Use the following procedures only after you have acclimatized at the altitude of the dive site for 12 hours:

1. Establish the altitude of the dive site and the actual depth of the Altitude Dive;

2. Convert the actual depth to EFFECTIVE DEPTH by adding the Depth Correction given in Table D;

3. Apply the Effective Depth and actual Bottom Time to Table A to determine the decompression requirements for the Altitude Dive (for Repetitive Dives, refer to the No-D Limits given in Table C);

4. If the Altitude Dive is a Decompression Dive, conduct the Decompression Stop at the **Actual Stop Depth** specified in Table D;

5. Decompress at the Actual Stop Depth for the Decompression Stop Time given in Table A.

EXAMPLE:
        Altitude = 6,000'/1,800m
        Actual Depth = 60'/18m
        Bottom Time = 35 minutes
        Depth Correction = +20'/6m

        EFFECTIVE DEPTH = 80'/24m
        Dec. Stop = 10 min at 10'/3m (from Table A)

        Actual Decompression Stop Depth is 8'/2.5m[*]

At altitudes above 5,000'/1,500m, reduce your **Ascent Rate** to 50'/15m per minute.

If you must dive before 12 hours have elapsed, begin by using the NEXT GREATER Depth than the actual depth. Using the example given above, you would begin the depth correction procedure as if the actual depth were 70 feet/21 metres. The Effective Depth would be 90'/27m (70'/21m + 20'/6m).

The decompression required at Actual Stop Depths would be 5 minutes at 16'/5m, and 10 minutes at 8'/2.5m[*]

The imperial and metric figures given for Actual Stop Depths are not direct conversions. Because of the effect of rounding the numbers on the imperial table, the imperial equivalents may differ slightly from the metric figures.

The DCIEM Sport Diving Tables and Procedures are copyrighted, and produced under government license by Universal Dive Techtronics, Inc., (UDT). The procedures for using the Sport Diving Tables were prepared by Ron Nishi of DCIEM and Gain Wong of UDT.

The final revisions to the DCIEM sport diving procedures were approved on December 23, 1991. Divers should follow the revised guidelines. The DCIEM diving tables may not be reproduced without the written authorization of Universal Dive Techtronics, Inc. All Rights Reserved.

The Defence and Civil Institute of Environmental Medicine (DCIEM), Universal Dive Techtronics, Inc., and the Department of National Defence (Canada) disclaim any and all responsibilities for the use of the DCIEM Sport Diving Tables and Procedures.

DCIEM
SPORT DIVING TABLES

A: AIR DECOMPRESSION

Depth	No-Decompression Bottom Times (minutes)				Decompression Required Bottom Times			
20' 6m	30 A 60 B 90 C 120 D	150 E 180 F 240 G 300 H	360 I 420 J 480 K 600 L	720 M ∞				
30' 9m	30 A 45 B 60 C 90 D	100 E 120 F 150 G 180 H	190 I 210 J 240 K 270 L	300 M	360	400		
40' 12m	22 A 30 B 40 C	60 D 70 E 80 F	90 G 120 H 130 I	150 J	160 K 170 L	180 M 190	200	215
50' 15m	18 A 25 B	30 C 40 D	50 E 60 F	75 G	85 H 95 I	105 J 115 K	124 L	132 M
60' 18m	14 A 20 B	25 C 30 D	40 E	50 F	60 G	70 H 80 I	85 J	92 K
Decompression Stops in minutes		**at 10' 3m**			**5**	**10**	**15**	**20**
70' 21m	12 A 15 B	20 C	25 D	35 E	40 F	50 G	60 H 63 I	66 J
80' 24m	10 A 13 B	15 C	20 D	25 E	29 F	35 G	48 H	52 I
90' 27m	9 A	12 B	15 C	20 D	23 E	27 F	35 G	40 H 43 I
100' 30m	7 A	10 B	12 C	15 D	18 D	21 E	25 F 29 G	36 H
110' 33m		6 A	10 B	12 C	15 D	18 E	22 F	26 G 30 H
120' 36m		6 A	8 B	10 C	12 D	15 E	19 F	25 G
130' 39m			5 A	8 B	10 C	13 D	16 F	21 G
140' 42m			5 A	7 B	9 C	11 D	14 F	18 G
150' 45m			4 A	6 B	8 C	10 D	12 E	15 F
Decompression Stops in minutes		**at 20' 6m**			-	-	5	10
		at 10' 3m			5	10	10	10

- **ASCENT RATE** is 60' (18m) plus or minus 10' (3m) per minute
  NO-DECOMPRESSION LIMITS are given for first dives
- **DECOMPRESSION STOPS** are taken at mid-chest level for the times indicated at the specified stop depths

→ Table B for **Minimum Surface Intervals** and Repetitive Factors
→ Table C for **Repetitive Dive No-Decompression Limits**
→ Table D for **Depth Corrections** required at Altitudes above 1000' (300m)

Note: From time to time changes may occur to the rules governing the use of these tables or to the tables themselves. For diving, refer to the most recent edition of the tables available commercially.

B: SURFACE INTERVALS

Rep. Group	0:15 ⟶ 0:29	0:30 ⟶ 0:59	1:00 ⟶ 1:29	1:30 ⟶ 1:59	2:00 ⟶ 2:59	3:00 ⟶ 3:59	4:00 ⟶ 5:59	6:00 ⟶ 8:59	9:00 ⟶ 11:59	12:00 ⟶ 14:59	15:00 ⟶ 18:00
A	1.4	1.2	1.1	1.1	1.1	1.1	1.1	1.1	1.0	1.0	1.0
B	1.5	1.3	1.2	1.2	1.2	1.1	1.1	1.1	1.1	1.0	1.0
C	1.6	1.4	1.3	1.2	1.2	1.2	1.1	1.1	1.1	1.0	1.0
D	1.8	1.5	1.4	1.3	1.3	1.2	1.2	1.1	1.1	1.0	1.0
E	1.9	1.6	1.5	1.4	1.3	1.3	1.2	1.2	1.1	1.1	1.0
F	2.0	1.7	1.6	1.5	1.4	1.3	1.3	1.2	1.1	1.1	1.0
G	-	1.9	1.7	1.6	1.5	1.4	1.3	1.2	1.1	1.1	1.0
H	-	-	1.9	1.7	1.6	1.5	1.4	1.3	1.1	1.1	1.1
I	-	-	2.0	1.8	1.7	1.5	1.4	1.3	1.1	1.1	1.1
J	-	-	-	1.9	1.8	1.6	1.5	1.3	1.2	1.1	1.1
K	-	-	-	2.0	1.9	1.7	1.5	1.3	1.2	1.1	1.1
L	-	-	-	-	2.0	1.7	1.6	1.4	1.2	1.1	1.1
M	-	-	-	-	-	1.8	1.6	1.4	1.2	1.1	1.1

Repetitive Factors (RF) given for Surface Intervals (hr:min)

C: REPETITIVE DIVING

Depth		1.1	1.2	1.3	1.4	1.5	1.6	1.7	1.8	1.9	2.0
30'	9m	272	250	230	214	200	187	176	166	157	150
40'	12m	136	125	115	107	100	93	88	83	78	75
50'	15m	60	55	50	45	41	38	36	34	32	31
60'	18m	40	35	31	29	27	26	24	23	22	21
70'	21m	30	25	21	19	18	17	16	15	14	13
80'	24m	20	18	16	15	14	13	12	12	11	11
90'	27m	16	14	12	11	11	10	9	9	8	8
100'	30m	13	11	10	9	9	8	8	7	7	7
110'	33m	10	9	8	8	7	7	6	6	6	6
120'	36m	8	7	7	6	6	6	5	5	5	5
130'	39m	7	6	6	5	5	5	4	4	4	4
140'	42m	6	5	5	5	4	4	4	3	3	3
150'	45m	5	5	4	4	4	3	3	3	3	3

Repetitive Dive No-D Limits given in minutes according to Depth and RF

D: DEPTH CORRECTIONS

Actual Depth		1000' ⟶ 1999 / 300m ⟶ 599		2000' ⟶ 2999 / 600m ⟶ 899		3000' ⟶ 3999 / 900m ⟶ 1199		4000' ⟶ 4999 / 1200m ⟶ 1499		5000' ⟶ 5999 / 1500m ⟶ 1799		6000' ⟶ 6999 / 1800m ⟶ 2099		7000' ⟶ 7999 / 2100m ⟶ 2399		8000' ⟶ 10000 / 2400m ⟶ 3000	
30'	9m	10	3	10	3	10	3	10	3	10	3	10	3	20	6	20	6
40'	12m	10	3	10	3	10	3	10	3	10	3	20	6	20	6	20	6
50'	15m	10	3	10	3	10	3	10	3	20	6	20	6	20	6	20	6
60'	18m	10	3	10	3	10	3	20	6	20	6	20	6	20	6	30	9
70'	21m	10	3	10	3	10	3	20	6	20	6	20	6	30	9	30	9
80'	24m	10	3	10	3	20	6	20	6	20	6	30	9	30	9	40	12
90'	27m	10	3	10	3	20	6	20	6	20	6	30	9	30	9	40	12
100'	30m	10	3	10	3	20	6	20	6	30	9	30	9	30	9	40	12
110'	33m	10	3	20	6	20	6	20	6	30	9	30	9	40	12		
120'	36m	10	3	20	6	20	6	30	9	30	9	30	9				
130'	39m	10	3	20	6	20	6										
140'	42m	10	3														

Add Depth Correction to Actual Depth of Altitude Dive

| 10' | 3m | 10 | 3.0 | 10 | 3.0 | 9 | 3.0 | 9 | 3.0 | 9 | 3.0 | 8 | 2.5 | 8 | 2.5 | 8 | 2.5 |
| 20' | 6m | 20 | 6.0 | 19 | 6.0 | 18 | 5.5 | 18 | 5.5 | 17 | 5.0 | 16 | 5.0 | 16 | 5.0 | 15 | 4.5 |

Actual Decompression Stop Depths (feet/metres) at Altitude

Published under government licence by Universal Dive Techtronics, Inc. Ste 203 2651 Viscount Way Richmond B.C. CANADA V6V 1M6

Appendix D

U.S. NAVY DECOMPRESSION TABLES

DECOMPRESSION PROCEDURES AND TABLES FROM U.S. NAVY DIVING MANUAL

Repetitive Dive Procedure

A dive performed within 12 hours of surfacing from a previous dive is a repetitive dive. The period between dives is the surface interval. Excess nitrogen requires 12 hours to be effectively lost from the body. These tables are designed to protect the diver from the effects of this residual nitrogen. Allow a minimum surface interval of 10 minutes between all dives. For any interval under 10 minutes, add the bottom time of the previous dives to that of the repetitive dive and choose the decompression schedule for the total bottom time and the deepest dive. Specific instructions are given for the use of each table in the following order:

(1) The *No-Decompression Table* or the *Navy Standard Air Decompression Table* gives the repetitive group designation for all schedules which may precede a repetitive dive.

(2) The *Surface Interval Credit Table* gives credit for the desaturation occurring during the surface interval.

(3) The *Repetitive Dive Timetable* gives the number of minutes of residual nitrogen time to add to the actual bottom time of the repetitive dive to obtain decompression for the residual nitrogen.

(4) The *No-Decompression Table* or the *Navy Standard Air Decompression Table* gives the decompression required for the repetitive dive.

U.S. NAVY STANDARD AIR DECOMPRESSION TABLE

Instructions for Use

Time of decompression stops in the table is in minutes.

Enter the table at the exact or the next greater depth than the maximum depth attained during the dive. Select the listed bottom time that is exactly equal to or is next greater than the bottom time of the dive. Maintain the diver's chest as close as possible to each decompression depth for the number of minutes listed. The rate of ascent *between* stops is not critical for stops of 50 feet or less. Commence timing each stop on arrival at the decompression depth and resume ascent when the specified time has lapsed.

For example — a dive to 82 feet for 36 minutes. To determine the proper decompression procedure: The next greater depth listed in this table is 90 feet. The next greater bottom time listed opposite 90 feet is 40. Stop 7 minutes at 10 feet in accordance with the 90/40 schedule.

For example — a dive to 110 feet for 30 minutes. It is known that the depth did not exceed 110 feet. To determine the proper decompression schedule: The exact depth of 110 feet is listed. The exact bottom time of 30 minutes is listed opposite 110 feet. Decompress according to the 110/30 schedule unless the dive was particularly cold or arduous. In that case, go to the schedule for the next deeper and longer dive, i.e., 120/40.

Depth (feet)	Bottom time (min)	Time to first stop (min : sec)	Decompression stops (feet)					Total ascent (min : sec)	Repetitive group
			50	40	30	20	10		
40	200	—	—	—	—	—	0	0:40	(*)
	210	0:30	—	—	—	—	2	2:40	N
	230	0:30	—	—	—	—	7	7:40	N
	250	0:30	—	—	—	—	11	11:40	O
	270	0:30	—	—	—	—	15	15:40	O
	300	0:30	—	—	—	—	19	19:40	Z
50	100	—	—	—	—	—	0	0:50	(*)
	110	0:40	—	—	—	—	3	3:50	L
	120	0:40	—	—	—	—	5	5:50	M
	140	0:40	—	—	—	—	10	10:50	M
	160	0:40	—	—	—	—	21	21:50	N
	180	0:40	—	—	—	—	29	29:50	O
	200	0:40	—	—	—	—	35	35:50	O
	220	0:40	—	—	—	—	40	40:50	Z
	240	0:40	—	—	—	—	47	47:50	Z
60	60	—	—	—	—	—	0	1:00	(*)
	70	0:50	—	—	—	—	2	3:00	K
	80	0:50	—	—	—	—	7	8:00	L
	100	0:50	—	—	—	—	14	15:00	M
	120	0:50	—	—	—	—	26	27:00	N
	140	0:50	—	—	—	—	39	40:00	O
	160	0:50	—	—	—	—	48	49:00	Z
	180	0:50	—	—	—	—	56	57:00	Z
	200	0:40	—	—	—	1	69	71:00	Z
70	50	—	—	—	—	—	0	1:10	(*)
	60	1:00	—	—	—	—	8	9:10	K
	70	1:00	—	—	—	—	14	15:10	L
	80	1:00	—	—	—	—	18	19:10	M
	90	1:00	—	—	—	—	23	24:10	N
	100	1:00	—	—	—	—	33	34:10	N
	110	0:50	—	—	—	2	41	44:10	O
	120	0:50	—	—	—	4	47	52:10	O
	130	0:50	—	—	—	6	52	59:10	O
	140	0:50	—	—	—	8	56	65:10	Z
	150	0:50	—	—	—	9	61	71:10	Z
	160	0:50	—	—	—	13	72	86:10	Z
	170	0:50	—	—	—	19	79	99:10	Z
80	40	—	—	—	—	—	0	1:20	(*)
	50	1:10	—	—	—	—	10	11:20	K
	60	1:10	—	—	—	—	17	18:20	L
	70	1:10	—	—	—	—	23	24:20	M
	80	1:00	—	—	—	2	31	34:20	N
	90	1:00	—	—	—	7	39	47:20	N
	100	1:00	—	—	—	11	46	58:20	O
	110	1:00	—	—	—	13	53	67:20	O
	120	1:00	—	—	—	17	56	74:20	Z
	130	1:00	—	—	—	19	63	83:20	Z
	140	1:00	—	—	—	26	69	96:20	Z
	150	1:00	—	—	—	32	77	110:20	Z
90	30	—	—	—	—	—	0	1:30	(*)
	40	1:20	—	—	—	—	7	8:30	J
	50	1:20	—	—	—	—	18	19:30	L
	60	1:20	—	—	—	—	25	26:30	M
	70	1:10	—	—	—	7	30	38:30	N
	80	1:10	—	—	—	13	40	54:30	N
	90	1:10	—	—	—	18	48	67:30	O
	100	1:10	—	—	—	21	54	76:30	Z
	110	1:10	—	—	—	24	61	86:30	Z
	120	1:10	—	—	—	32	68	101:30	Z
	130	1:00	—	—	5	36	74	116:30	Z
100	25	—	—	—	—	—	0	1:40	(*)
	30	1:30	—	—	—	—	3	4:40	I
	40	1:30	—	—	—	—	15	16:40	K
	50	1:20	—	—	—	2	24	27:40	L
	60	1:20	—	—	—	9	28	38:40	N
	70	1:20	—	—	—	17	39	57:40	O
	80	1:20	—	—	—	23	48	72:40	O
	90	1:10	—	—	3	23	57	84:40	Z
	100	1:10	—	—	7	23	66	97:40	Z
	110	1:10	—	—	10	34	72	117:40	Z
	120	1:10	—	—	12	41	78	132:40	Z

Depth (feet)	Bottom time (min)	Time to first stop (min : sec)	Decompression stops (feet)					Total ascent (min : sec)	Repetitive group
			50	40	30	20	10		
110	20	—	—	—	—	—	0	1:50	(*)
	25	1:40	—	—	—	—	3	4:50	H
	30	1:40	—	—	—	—	7	8:50	J
	40	1:30	—	—	—	2	21	24:50	L
	50	1:30	—	—	—	8	26	35:50	M
	60	1:30	—	—	—	18	36	55:50	N
	70	1:20	—	—	1	23	48	73:50	O
	80	1:20	—	—	7	23	57	88:50	Z
	90	1:20	—	—	12	30	64	107:50	Z
	100	1:20	—	—	15	37	72	125:50	Z
120	15	—	—	—	—	—	0	2:00	(*)
	20	1:50	—	—	—	—	2	4:00	H
	25	1:50	—	—	—	—	6	8:00	I
	30	1:50	—	—	—	—	14	16:00	I
	40	1:40	—	—	—	5	25	32:00	L
	50	1:40	—	—	—	15	31	48:00	N
	60	1:30	—	—	2	22	45	71:00	O
	70	1:30	—	—	9	23	55	89:00	O
	80	1:30	—	—	15	27	63	107:00	Z
	90	1:30	—	—	19	37	74	132:00	Z
	100	1:30	—	—	23	45	80	150:00	Z
130	10	—	—	—	—	—	0	2:10	(*)
	15	2:00	—	—	—	—	1	3:10	F
	20	2:00	—	—	—	—	4	6:10	H
	25	2:00	—	—	—	—	10	12:10	J
	30	1:50	—	—	—	3	18	23:10	M
	40	1:50	—	—	—	10	25	37:10	N
	50	1:40	—	—	3	21	37	63:10	O
	60	1:40	—	—	9	23	52	86:10	Z
	70	1:40	—	—	16	24	61	103:10	Z
	80	1:30	—	3	19	35	72	131:10	Z
	90	1:30	—	8	19	45	80	154:10	Z
140	10	—	—	—	—	—	0	2:20	(*)
	15	2:10	—	—	—	—	2	4:20	G
	20	2:10	—	—	—	—	6	8:20	I
	25	2:00	—	—	—	2	14	18:20	J
	30	2:00	—	—	—	5	21	28:20	K
	40	1:50	—	—	2	16	26	46:20	N
	50	1:50	—	—	6	24	44	76:20	O
	60	1:50	—	—	16	23	56	97:20	Z
	70	1:40	—	4	19	32	68	125:20	Z
	80	1:40	—	10	23	41	79	155:20	Z
150	5	—	—	—	—	—	0	2:30	C
	10	2:20	—	—	—	—	1	3:30	E
	15	2:20	—	—	—	—	3	5:30	G
	20	2:10	—	—	—	2	7	11:30	H
	25	2:10	—	—	—	4	17	23:30	K
	30	2:10	—	—	—	8	24	34:30	L
	40	2:00	—	—	5	19	33	59:30	N
	50	2:00	—	—	12	23	51	88:30	O
	60	1:50	—	3	19	26	62	112:30	Z
	70	1:50	—	11	19	39	75	146:30	Z
	80	1:40	1	17	19	50	84	173:30	Z
160	5	—	—	—	—	—	0	2:40	D
	10	2:30	—	—	—	—	1	3:40	F
	15	2:20	—	—	—	1	4	7:40	H
	20	2:20	—	—	—	3	11	16:40	J
	25	2:20	—	—	—	7	20	29:40	K
	30	2:10	—	—	2	11	25	40:40	M
	40	2:10	—	—	7	23	39	71:40	N
	50	2:00	—	2	16	23	55	98:40	Z
	60	2:00	—	9	19	33	69	132:40	Z
	70	1:50	1	17	22	44	80	166:40	Z
170	5	—	—	—	—	—	0	2:50	D
	10	2:40	—	—	—	—	2	4:50	F
	15	2:30	—	—	—	2	5	9:50	H
	20	2:30	—	—	—	4	15	21:50	J
	25	2:20	—	—	2	7	23	34:50	L
	30	2:20	—	—	4	13	26	45:50	M
	40	2:10	—	1	10	23	45	81:50	O
	50	2:10	—	5	18	23	61	109:50	Z
	60	2:00	2	15	22	37	74	152:50	Z
	70	2:00	8	17	19	51	86	183:50	Z

Depth (feet)	Bottom time (min)	Time to first stop (min : sec)	Decompression stops (feet)					Total ascent (min : sec)	Repetitive group
			50	40	30	20	10		
180	5	—	—	—	—	—	0	3:00	D
	10	2:50	—	—	—	—	3	6:00	F
	15	2:40	—	—	—	3	6	12:00	I
	20	2:30	—	—	1	5	17	26:00	K
	25	2:30	—	—	3	10	24	40:00	L
	30	2:30	—	—	6	17	27	53:00	N
	40	2:20	—	3	14	23	50	93:00	O
	50	2:10	2	9	19	30	65	128:00	Z
	60	2:10	5	16	19	44	81	168:00	Z
190	5	—	—	—	—	—	0	3:10	D
	10	2:50	—	—	—	1	3	7:10	G
	15	2:50	—	—	—	4	7	14:10	I
	20	2:40	—	—	2	6	20	31:10	K
	25	2:40	—	—	5	11	25	44:10	M
	30	2:30	—	1	8	19	32	63:10	N
	40	2:30	—	8	14	23	55	103:10	O
	50	2:20	4	13	22	33	72	147:10	Z
	60	2:20	10	17	19	50	84	183:10	Z

* See table 1-11 for repetitive groups in no-decompression dives

TABLE 1-11 — *NO-DECOMPRESSION LIMITS AND REPETITIVE GROUP DESIGNATION TABLE FOR NO-DECOMPRESSION AIR DIVES*

Depth (feet)	No-decompression limits (min)	Repetitive groups (air dives)														
		A	B	C	D	E	F	G	H	I	J	K	L	M	N	O
10	—	60	120	210	300	—	—	—	—	—	—	—	—	—	—	—
15	—	35	70	110	160	225	350	—	—	—	—	—	—	—	—	—
20	—	25	50	75	100	135	180	240	325	—	—	—	—	—	—	—
25	—	20	35	55	75	100	125	160	195	245	315	—	—	—	—	—
30	—	15	30	45	60	75	95	120	145	170	205	250	310	—	—	—
35	310	5	15	25	40	50	60	80	100	120	140	160	190	220	270	310
40	200	5	15	25	30	40	50	70	80	100	110	130	150	170	200	—
50	100	—	10	15	25	30	40	50	60	70	80	90	100	—	—	—
60	60	—	10	15	20	25	30	40	50	55	60	—	—	—	—	—
70	50	—	5	10	15	20	30	35	40	45	50	—	—	—	—	—
80	40	—	5	10	15	20	25	30	35	40	—	—	—	—	—	—
90	30	—	5	10	12	15	20	25	30	—	—	—	—	—	—	—
100	25	—	5	7	10	15	20	22	25	—	—	—	—	—	—	—
110	20	—	—	5	10	13	15	20	—	—	—	—	—	—	—	—
120	15	—	—	5	10	12	15	—	—	—	—	—	—	—	—	—
130	10	—	—	5	8	10	—	—	—	—	—	—	—	—	—	—
140	10	—	—	5	7	10	—	—	—	—	—	—	—	—	—	—
150	5	—	—	5	—	—	—	—	—	—	—	—	—	—	—	—
160	5	—	—	—	5	—	—	—	—	—	—	—	—	—	—	—
170	5	—	—	—	5	—	—	—	—	—	—	—	—	—	—	—
180	5	—	—	—	5	—	—	—	—	—	—	—	—	—	—	—
190	5	—	—	—	5	—	—	—	—	—	—	—	—	—	—	—

Instructions for Use

I. No-decompression limits:

This column shows at various depths greater than 30 feet the allowable diving times (in minutes) which permit surfacing directly at 60 feet a minute with no decompression stops. Longer exposure times require the use of the Standard Air Decompression Table (table 1-10).

II. Repetitive group designation table:

The tabulated exposure times (or bottom times) are in minutes. The times at the various depths in each vertical column are the maximum exposures during which a diver will remain within the group listed at the head of the column.

To find the repetitive group designation at surfacing for dives involving exposures up to and including the no-decompression limits: Enter the table on the *exact or next greater depth* than that to which exposed and select the listed exposure time *exact or next greater* than the actual exposure time. The repetitive group designation is indicated by the letter at the head of the vertical column where the selected exposure time is listed.

For example: A dive was to 32 feet for 45 minutes. Enter the table along the 35-foot-depth line since it is next greater than 32 feet. The table shows that since group D is left after 40 minutes' exposure and group E after 50 minutes, group E (at the head of the column where the 50-minute exposure is listed) is the proper selection.

Exposure times for depths less than 40 feet are listed only up to approximately 5 hours since this is considered to be beyond field requirements for this table.

TABLE 1-12 — *SURFACE INTERVAL CREDIT TABLE FOR AIR DECOMPRESSION DIVES*
(REPETITIVE GROUP AT THE END OF THE SURFACE INTERVAL (AIR dive))

NEW GROUP DESIGNATION

Begin	Z	O	N	M	L	K	J	I	H	G	F	E	D	C	B	A
Z	0:10 / 0:22	0:23 / 0:34	0:35 / 0:48	0:49 / 1:02	1:03 / 1:18	1:19 / 1:36	1:37 / 1:55	1:56 / 2:17	2:18 / 2:42	2:43 / 3:10	3:11 / 3:45	3:46 / 4:29	4:30 / 5:27	5:28 / 6:56	6:57 / 10:05	10:06 / 12:00
O		0:10 / 0:23	0:24 / 0:36	0:37 / 0:51	0:52 / 1:07	1:08 / 1:24	1:25 / 1:43	1:44 / 2:04	2:05 / 2:29	2:30 / 2:59	3:00 / 3:33	3:34 / 4:17	4:18 / 5:16	5:17 / 6:44	6:45 / 9:54	9:55 / 12:00
N			0:10 / 0:24	0:25 / 0:39	0:40 / 0:54	0:55 / 1:11	1:12 / 1:30	1:31 / 1:53	1:54 / 2:18	2:19 / 2:47	2:48 / 3:22	3:23 / 4:04	4:05 / 5:03	5:04 / 6:32	6:33 / 9:43	9:44 / 12:00
M				0:10 / 0:25	0:26 / 0:42	0:43 / 0:59	1:00 / 1:18	1:19 / 1:39	1:40 / 2:05	2:06 / 2:34	2:35 / 3:08	3:09 / 3:52	3:53 / 4:49	4:50 / 6:18	6:19 / 9:28	9:29 / 12:00
L					0:10 / 0:26	0:27 / 0:45	0:46 / 1:04	1:05 / 1:25	1:26 / 1:49	1:50 / 2:19	2:20 / 2:53	2:54 / 3:36	3:37 / 4:35	4:36 / 6:02	6:03 / 9:12	9:13 / 12:00
K						0:10 / 0:28	0:29 / 0:49	0:50 / 1:11	1:12 / 1:35	1:36 / 2:03	2:04 / 2:38	2:39 / 3:21	3:22 / 4:19	4:20 / 5:48	5:49 / 8:58	8:59 / 12:00
J							0:10 / 0:31	0:32 / 0:54	0:55 / 1:19	1:20 / 1:47	1:48 / 2:20	2:21 / 3:04	3:05 / 4:02	4:03 / 5:40	5:41 / 8:40	8:41 / 12:00
I								0:10 / 0:33	0:34 / 0:59	1:00 / 1:29	1:30 / 2:02	2:03 / 2:44	2:45 / 3:43	3:44 / 5:12	5:13 / 8:21	8:22 / 12:00
H									0:10 / 0:36	0:37 / 1:06	1:07 / 1:41	1:42 / 2:23	2:24 / 3:20	3:21 / 4:49	4:50 / 7:59	8:00 / 12:00
G										0:10 / 0:40	0:41 / 1:15	1:16 / 1:59	2:00 / 2:58	2:59 / 4:25	4:26 / 7:35	7:36 / 12:00
F											0:10 / 0:45	0:46 / 1:29	1:30 / 2:28	2:29 / 3:57	3:58 / 7:05	7:06 / 12:00
E												0:10 / 0:54	0:55 / 1:57	1:58 / 3:22	3:23 / 6:32	6:33 / 12:00
D													0:10 / 1:09	1:10 / 2:38	2:39 / 5:48	5:49 / 12:00
C														0:10 / 1:39	1:40 / 2:49	2:50 / 12:00
B															0:10 / 2:10	2:11 / 12:00
A																0:10 / 12:00

Repetitive group at the beginning of the surface interval from previous dive

ENTER HERE

Instructions for Use

Surface interval time in the table is in *hours* and *minutes* (7 : 59) means 7 hours and 59 minutes). The surface interval must be at least 10 minutes.

Find the *repetitive group designation letter* (from the previous dive schedule) on the diagonal slope. Enter the table horizontally to select the surface interval time that is exactly between the actual surface interval times shown. The repetitive group designation for the *end* of the surface interval is at the head of the vertical column where the selected surface interval time is listed. For example, a previous dive was to 110 feet for 30 minutes. The diver remains on the surface 1 hour and 30 minutes and wishes to find the new repetitive group designation: The repetitive group from the last column of the 110/30 schedule in the Standard Air Decompression Tables is "J." Enter the surface interval credit table along the horizontal line labeled "J." The 1-hour-and-30-minute surface interval lies between the times 1 : 20 and 1 : 47. Therefore, the diver has lost sufficient inert gas to place him in group "G" (at the head of the vertical column selected).

*NOTE. — Dives following surface intervals of more than 12 hours are not considered repetitive dives. *Actual* bottom times in the Standard Air Decompression Tables may be used in computing decompression for such dives.

TABLE 1-13. — *REPETITIVE DIVE TIMETABLE FOR AIR DIVES*

RESIDUAL NITROGEN TIMES (MINUTES)

Repetitive groups	Repetitive			dive				depth			(ft)			(air		dives)
	40	50	60	70	80	90	100	110	120	130	140	150	160	170	180	190
A	7	6	5	4	4	3	3	3	3	3	2	2	2	2	2	2
B	17	13	11	9	8	7	7	6	6	6	5	5	4	4	4	4
C	25	21	17	15	13	11	10	10	9	8	7	7	6	6	6	6
D	37	29	24	20	18	16	14	13	12	11	10	9	8	8	8	8
E	49	38	30	26	23	20	18	16	15	13	12	12	11	10	10	10
F	61	47	36	31	28	24	22	20	18	16	15	14	13	13	12	11
G	73	56	44	37	32	29	26	24	21	19	18	17	16	15	14	13
H	87	66	52	43	38	33	30	27	25	22	20	19	18	17	16	15
I	101	76	61	50	43	38	34	31	28	25	23	22	20	19	18	17
J	116	87	70	57	48	43	38	34	32	28	26	24	23	22	20	19
K	138	99	79	64	54	47	43	38	35	31	29	27	26	24	22	21
L	161	111	88	72	61	53	48	42	39	35	32	30	28	26	25	24
M	187	124	97	80	68	58	52	47	43	38	35	32	31	29	27	26
N	213	142	107	87	73	64	57	51	46	40	38	35	33	31	29	28
O	241	160	117	96	80	70	62	55	50	44	40	38	36	34	31	30
Z	257	169	122	100	84	73	64	57	52	46	42	40	37	35	32	31

Instructions for use

The bottom times listed in this table are called "residual nitrogen times" and are the times a diver is to consider he has *already* spent on bottom when he *starts* a repetitive dive to a specific depth. They are in minutes.

Enter the table horizontally with the repetitive group designation from the Surface Interval Credit Table. The time in each vertical column is the number of minutes that would be required (at the depth listed at the head of the column) to saturate to the particular group.

For example: The final group designation from the Surface Interval Credit Table, on the basis of a previous dive and surface interval, is "H." To plan a dive to 110 feet, determine the residual nitrogen time for this depth required by the repetitive group designation: Enter this table along the horizontal line labeled "H." The table shows that one must *start* a dive to 110 feet as though he had already been on the bottom for 27 minutes. This information can then be applied to the Standard Air Decompression Table or No-Decompression Table in a number of ways:

(1) Assuming a diver is going to finish a job and take whatever decompression is required, he must add 27 minutes to his actual bottom time and be prepared to take decompression according to the 110-foot schedules for the sum or equivalent single dive time.

(2) Assuming one wishes to make a quick inspection dive for the minimum decompression, he will decompress according to the 110/30 schedule for a dive of 3 minutes or less (27 + 3 = 30). For a dive of over 3 minutes but less than 13, he will decompress according to the 110/40 schedule (27 + 13 = 40).

(3) Assuming that one does not want to exceed the 110/50 schedule and the amount of decompression it requires, he will have to start ascent before 23 minutes of actual bottom time (50 - 27 = 23).

(4) Assuming that a diver has air for approximately 45 minutes bottom time and decompression stops, the possible dives can be computed: A dive of 13 minutes will require 23 minutes of decompression (110/40 schedule), for a total submerged time of 36 minutes. A dive of 13 to 23 minutes will require 34 minutes of decompression (110/50 schedule), for a total submerged time of 47 to 57 minutes. Therefore, to be safe, the diver will have to start ascent before 13 minutes or a standby air source will have to be provided.

Appendix E

IN–WATER O$_2$ RECOMPRESSION THERAPY

AUSTRALIAN UNDERWATER OXYGEN TABLE

Notes :

1. It is recommended that the application of this therapy technique be restricted to trained and experienced diving medical practitioners and paramedics.

2. This technique may be useful in treating cases of decompression sickness in localities remote from recompression facilities. It may also be of use while suitable transport to such a centre is being arranged.

3. In planning, it should be realised that the therapy may take up to 3 hours. The risks of cold, immersion and other environmental factors should be balanced against the beneficial effects.

4. The diver must be accompanied by an attendant at all times.

❑ Equipment.

The following equipment is essential before attempting this form of treatment :

1. Full face mask with demand valve and surface supply *or* helmet with free flow.
2. Adequate supply of 100% oxygen for patient, and air for attendant.
3. Wet suit for thermal protection.
4. Shot with at least 10 metres of rope (a seat or harness may be rigged to the shot).
5. Some form of communication system between patient, attendant and surface.

❏ Method.

1. The patient is lowered on the shot rope to 9 metres, breathing 100% oxygen.
2. Ascent is commenced after 30 minutes in mild cases, or 60 minutes in severe cases, if improvement has occurred. These times may be extended to 60 minutes and 90 minutes respectively if there is no improvement.
3. Ascent is at the rate of 1 metre every 12 minutes.
4. If symptoms recur, remain at depth a further 30 minutes before continuing ascent.
5. If oxygen supply is exhausted, return to the surface, rather than breathe air underwater.
6. After surfacing, the patient should breathe 1 hour on 100% oxygen, one hour off, for a further 12 hours.

Table Aust 9 (RAN 82), *short oxygen table*

DEPTH (metres)	ELAPSED TIME Mild	ELAPSED TIME Serious	RATE OF ASCENT
9	0030-0100	0100-0130	
8	0042-0112	0112-0142	
7	0054-0124	0124-0154	12 minutes
6	0106-0136	0136-0206	per metre
5	0118-0148	0148-0218	(4 min/ft)
4	0130-0200	0200-0230	
3	0142-0212	0212-0242	
2	0154-0224	0224-0254	
1	0206-0236	0236-0306	

Total table time 2 hours 6 min — 2 hours 36 min for mild cases
2 hours 36 min — 3 hours 6 min for serious cases

INDEX.

ACKNOWLEDGEMENTS

To my diving buddy and wife, Cindy, for her invaluable criticisms, suggestions and proof-reading. To my son, Mark, who inspired the predecessor of this text, "A Diving Manual for Mark", which I prepared for him. The motivation was to ensure that he had more factual information than that available from his open water scuba diving course. He is now a competent and perceptive diver, partly from his understanding of this text. Thanks also to Patracia Larke and Enid Page for their secretarial services.

Carl Edmonds.

I would like to thank my wife, Ann, for tolerating my on and off affair with a word processor, and also my daughter Deborah, Des Lund, Tammy Lye, Shirley Warner, and Joanne Wright who helped me in the gestation of this book.

Bart McKenzie

I wish to thank my daughter, Natalia, for her assistance in producing some of the diagrams used within this book. I also wish to thank my wife, Denise, for her tireless support and patience regarding my often frustrating use of a computer and its noisy printer late at night — its completion represents something she believed would never really eventuate!

Bob Thomas

Finally, the authors wish to thank the U.S. Navy and the Canadian Defence and Civil Institute of Environmental Medicine (DCIEM) for permission to include their diving decompression tables in this book.

Other books available from J.L. Publications

The DAN Emergency Handbook by John Lippmann and Stan Bugg. Melbourne: J.L. Publications, 1990.

A guide to the identification of and first aid for SCUBA diving injuries. An essential reference for all divers.

Deeper Into Diving by John Lippmann. Melbourne: J.L. Publications, 1990.

A very detailed technical review of most of the available decompression systems and of the physical and physiological aspects of deeper diving. An essential reference for divemasters, instructors and other diving professionals.

The Essentials of Deeper (Sport) Diving by John Lippmann. New York: Aqua Quest Publications Inc., 1992.

An overview of the theory and requirements of deeper diving. Interesting and useful reading for all divers.

Oxygen First Aid for Divers by John Lippmann. Melbourne: J.L. Publications, 1992.

A detailed review of the equipment and procedures for pre-hospital oxygen administration to injured divers. *Interesting reading for all divers. Essential for divemasters and instructors.*

J.L. Publications

P.O. Box 381, Carnegie, Victoria, 3163, Australia.

Tel/Fax: 61-3-569 4803